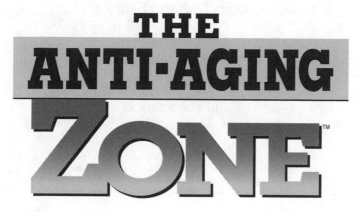

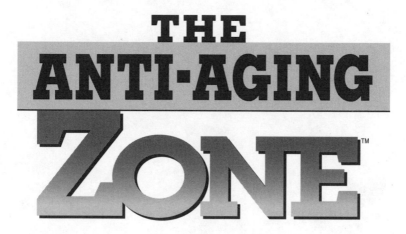

THE ANTI-AGING ZONE™

BARRY SEARS, Ph.D.

ReganBooks
An Imprint of HarperCollins*Publishers*

HARPERCOLLINS books may be purchased for educational, business, or sales promotional use. For information please write: Special Markets Department, HarperCollins Publishers, Inc., 10 East 53rd Street, New York, NY 10022.

Text graphics by Elaine Wilkens

FIRST EDITION

Library of Congress Cataloging-in-Publication Data on file at the Library of Congress.
ISBN 0-06-039243-6

98 99 00 01 02 10 9 8 7 6 5 4 3 2 1

To Mike Palm,
a good friend and early supporter
of the Zone.

CONTENTS

PART V
WHAT ELSE SHOULD YOU KNOW?

ACKNOWLEDGMENTS

I am truly fortunate to have a very talented support team associated with me as I continue to write books on the Zone. The first and foremost member of this team is my wife, Lynn, who has edited some very complex concepts into a clear and hopefully concise format for the lay reader. Next is my brother, Doug, who has been my business partner and best friend for the past 17 years and has likewise made valuable editing comments based on his many years of experience in this field.

I would be highly remiss if I didn't profusely thank both my administrative assistant, Beth Twiss, who organized my otherwise chaotic schedule so that this book could be completed, and Scott C. Lane for his excellence in developing the Zone recipes found in this book and others he has designed for my previous books.

I also wish to thank Todd Silverstein and Jill Sullivan for their overall editing comments that contributed greatly to this book. A special thanks goes to Dr. Michael Norden, the author of *Beyond Prozac,* and Pat Puglio of the Barnes Research Foundation for their comments on selected chapters.

Of course my final thanks always goes to the staff of Regan Books, especially Amye Dyer, who did the final editing on this manuscript. But as always without the continuing support of Judith Regan, none of the Zone books would have ever been published.

INTRODUCTION

With the exception of Stephen Hawking's *A Brief History of Time*, I can think of no other best-selling book that has been less understood than *The Zone*. Written to educate cardiovascular physicians about a group of mysterious hormones known as eicosanoids, *The Zone* has not been easy reading for the general public. Needless to say, I was totally surprised by its success in the popular marketplace. Unfortunately, amid this public acclaim, I felt that two important concepts from the book got along the way. First, *The Zone* was perceived as a diet book, which it is not. It was written to put forward new treatments for diabetes and heart disease by lowering insulin levels and altering eicosanoid balance when you treat food as if it were a "drug." Second, the most important implication of *The Zone* is almost completely overlooked: the idea that the Zone Diet is also an anti-aging program too. In this book, I begin to explore this anti-aging concept in greater detail.

The secret of the Zone Diet's anti-aging potential is more fully understood by closely examining the hormones either generated or influenced by the food we eat and how these hormones communicate with one another so that our bodies can function at high levels of efficiency.

With as many theories on aging as there are researchers in the field, there is only one consensus in the world of anti-aging: the only proven way to reverse aging is to restrict calories. No one disagrees about this. It has been demonstrated over and over for the past 60 years. Yet, this fact has been given only passing notice since everyone assumes that calorie restriction in humans is equivalent to constant starvation and deprivation. But what if it's possible to enjoy the benefits of calorie restriction without deprivation or hunger? If the answer is yes, this means that you have a proven anti-aging "drug" that everyone could be using tomorrow. That "drug" exists today, and it's the Zone Diet. My goal is to show you how and why the Zone Diet works to reverse the aging process.

This book actually began several years ago. Soon after I wrote *The Zone*, I was invited to give a talk at an endocrinology conference sponsored by the Broda Barnes Foundation. I delivered my lecture on insulin and eicosanoids and thought I was pretty hot stuff. That is until I heard the other lecturers and realized the hormonal landscape was far more complex and interrelated than I had ever imagined. While I could make cogent arguments about food controlling insulin and eicosanoids, I knew that I had to go back to square one to master the interactions of these complex hormonal systems that are mediated by food if I was to fully understand the aging process. This book represents the fruit of that journey.

We will never know everything about aging, any more than it is likely we will eliminate heart disease and cancer in our lifetime, but there is already enough data for developing an effective anti-aging program that can start today without any fear of side effects and with proven benefits. That program is the Anti-Aging Zone Lifestyle Pyramid, and the base of that pyramid is the Zone Diet.

Fortunately, in the last few years hormones have become the focus of virtually everyone's vocabulary. Melatonin, serotonin, DHEA, growth hormone, estrogen, and testosterone are new cocktail party conversation topics. This makes talking of hormones easier and less formidable. The growing awareness by baby boomers about their own approaching mortality coupled with their extraordinary desire to forestall life's inevitable outcome forms the basis of my hope that the concept of Zone Diet as the foundation for successful anti-aging will be accepted and acted upon.

In my first book, *The Zone*, I described a little-known group of hormones known as eicosanoids and how food ultimately controls their production. But since very few people could even spell eicosanoids, let alone understand what they did, I focused my subsequent books on insulin control since people were familiar with that hormone and because it has such a significant impact on eicosanoid formation. But in this book I must return to discussing eicosanoids in greater detail because it's only through the dietary control of these hormones that you can reverse the aging process.

This book is not meant to be a technical encyclopedia of hormonal action nor is it a watered-down version on the complexities of the aging process peppered with testimonials. This book is meant to give you a practical insight into understanding how hormones control the aging process, and what you can do with easy-to-implement lifestyle choices to alter that process. It is a book that you may have to read several times, like a textbook, because of the intricate relationships between hormones. This is why I recommend that you use the chapter index to find those topics that are of immediate interest to you, read them, and then come back to explore other chapters. However, I suggest that many readers, after reading the first chapter, go directly to Part II of this book, "Beginning Your Anti-Aging Zone Lifestyle Today," that starts with Chapter 6. Then come back to the other chapters as a reference. In addition, because many of the terms used in this book may initially seem foreign, I recommend that you use the Glossary in the Appendix to help you learn some of the basic terminology that will be fundamental to understanding how to reverse aging.

My goal is to unravel some of the mystery and hype surrounding hormones and the aging process. To control this process, the one "drug" you have to take is food. How to use that "drug" to alter the aging process is the premise of this book. The technology is there. The research has been done. All that remains is your desire to use that "drug" correctly.

PART I

HORMONES AND AGING

CHAPTER 1

THE QUEST:
LONGER LIFE OR BETTER LIFE?

From the beginning of written history, man's quest for a longer life, if not immortality, has been a constant theme. In fact a longer life might have seemed like immortality for early man since the average life span through Roman times was about 22 years of age.

Some of the earliest recorded anti-aging literature came from the Egyptian papyrus, "Book for Transforming an Old Man into a Youth of Twenty." Written nearly 2,600 years ago, it promised to reverse the aging process, not to achieve longer life. Throughout Greek and Roman literature there are continued references to magic elixirs for living longer and, often equally important, improved sexual potency. The idea of immortality was something only to be found among the pantheon of the Greek and Roman gods.

While ancient Western thought viewed death as an inevitable process to make way for the next generation, ancient Eastern philosophy embraced the balance of opposing forces as the road to immortality. Yet both ancient Western and Eastern literature suggest that if one could only eat the food of the gods, immortality might be ensured. As we approach the new millennium, we now realize that the ancients had the essence of truth in their quest. While no one can ever become immortal, we can use food to balance powerful forces within our bodies to slow, if not reverse, the process we call aging. This food is not the property of the gods. It is in your own kitchen.

Anti-aging is not just a matter of simply living longer, but also living better. I personally don't want to reach the age of 120 if I am enfeebled and need constant assistance to take care of myself. I'd much rather live to a more modest age and enjoy a better quality of life. In essence, you want to maintain functionality (being able to take care of yourself) as long as possible before death. Although life expectancy was much shorter in the past, functionality was usually maintained until death. Today we have a greater life expectancy than at any time in history, but much of our extended time on earth includes a greater number of years of declining function before death. The concept of a slow death in a nursing home surrounded by nonfunctional people is a frightening picture. The baby boomers have seen this new face of aging and, frankly, they are scared. It is not a fear of death but a fear of declining physical and mental function.

A good way of describing anti-aging is that it is the process of dissociating biological age from chronological age. Chronological age is easy. Just count your birthdays. Biological age is a little more complex. Determining the biological changes (and therefore your functionality) that take place during aging has been one of the primary research areas of gerontology (the study of aging) over the past 30 years. During this time period, a number of biological markers of aging have been identified for humans. A true biological marker of aging must be universal. You can't call cancer a marker of aging since not everyone who ages gets cancer. On the other hand, loss of muscle mass in both males and females seems to be a universal marker. Reversing the biological markers of aging is the true goal of any successful anti-aging program.

By reversing these biological markers, your body can once more appear years younger even though it's not. Furthermore, you will maintain physical and mental performance at levels that you were accustomed to at an earlier stage in life. These biological markers provide you with a scientific starting point that can indicate whether or not your anti-aging program is actually working. After all, anti-aging is a science, not an art form. These biological markers of aging are ultimately governed by hormonal changes that take place as you age. Therefore the key to reversing aging is our ability to alter our hormones.

The first scientific evidence that the aging process could be reversed by hormonal modulation appeared in the latter part of the nineteenth century. The beginning of this new age began when Charles-Edouard Brown-Séquard, a member of the French Academy, reported that self-injections of ground-up animal testicles reversed the aging process with a corresponding increase in his sexual potency. Needless to say, his discovery was greeted with great enthusiasm. Nor could he be accused of being a snake-oil salesman because he gave his new youth elixir to other physicians at no charge with the provision that they not charge their patients. Unfortunately, Brown-Séquard's research was also met with great derision throughout Europe because his results couldn't be replicated by others. Yet a century later we now understand that he had indeed crossed the barrier and discovered that anti-aging was possible through hormonal modulation. In fact, aging revolves around hormones. The right balance of hormones will slow the aging process; the wrong balance will accelerate it. It's not necessarily the lack of certain hormones that is the fundamental cause of aging, but really how hormones lose their ability to communicate with each other to maintain equilibrium. The goal of this book is to present a new anti-aging manifesto: how to use your diet to improve hormonal communication and therefore reverse aging.

And more importantly for you is the fact that many of these biological markers can be reversed by the most powerful anti-aging drug readily available to everyone. What's the name of this drug? It's food, assuming you are willing to treat food with the same respect that you would treat any prescription drug. Food is a powerful "drug" because it alters hormonal responses. Used properly, food can improve hormonal communication. If you can achieve that goal, you will begin to reverse the aging process. On the other hand, the improper use of food can speed the aging process. Essentially, after each meal you want to ask yourself the question: "Did I reverse the aging process or did I accelerate it?"

In my first book, *The Zone*, I began to outline the hormonal consequences of the diet and its implications for treatment of chronic diseases. In my following books, *Mastering the Zone, Zone Perfect Meals in Minutes*, and *Zone Food Blocks*, I tried to show how easy it is to prepare the foods you already like to eat into a powerful drug simply by making a few adjustments with the balance of the protein, carbohydrate, and fat content of your meals. In this book, I go back to the biological foundation (i.e., hormones) that defines our existence and demonstrate how to alter that foundation, starting with your next meal.

Many readers may want to simply begin the lifestyle modifications that are the essence of anti-aging. If so, I suggest that you go directly to Part II of this book that begins with Chapter 6 so that you can begin your anti-aging program with your very next meal. Then return to the other chapters of the book to understand the science behind anti-aging. Others may wish to understand the science of aging first. Those readers should go to the next chapter. Regardless of where you start, if you are interested in reaching the Anti-Aging Zone, then read on.

CHAPTER 2

WHY ARE WE LIVING LONGER?

That's a good question. Genetically, man hasn't changed much in the last 100,000 years, so it can't be better genes. So what else may explain our increased longevity? Before I turn to that question, it helps to define some basic terms about aging. The first is average life span. An average life span (or life expectancy) is simply the average age at which 50 percent of a given population have died. Obviously, if you have a lot of childhood mortality, then the average life span will be short. Second is maximum life span. This is the upper limit of age that is unlikely to be surpassed. The third is longevity. Longevity is how close you get to the maximum life span before you die. And finally there is aging, which is defined as the general deterioration of the body with increasing age. With these definitions, let's go back to our basic question: Why are we living longer?

Our best estimates are that the average life span of neo-Paleolithic man some 10,000 to 15,000 years ago was approximately 18 years. However, this is a very misleading figure since there was an incredibly high level of childhood mortality, primarily at birth, that skews this average life span to an early age. Obviously, you have to have a long enough life span to give birth to the next generation and raise the young in order for a continuation of the species. Since we are still here, this means that neo-Paleolithic man (not to mention his ancestors) had a long enough life span to continue populating the earth.

The maximum life span for humans appears to be 120 years, which probably hasn't changed in the past 100,000 years. It is also unlikely that it will change very soon. It turns out that the maximum life span of any species can be predicted by the relative size of the brain compared to body weight. The brain size of man has been constant for the last 100,000 years. Furthermore, the number of people with legitimate, verifiable birth records who have reached the age of 120 in the past century can be counted on the fingers of one hand. As I will point out later, it is unlikely that the number of people reaching an age of 120 will increase greatly in the the next century.

It's important to keep in mind that while maximum life span hasn't changed, life expectancy has increased because of its heavy dependence on the death rates of young children. The less rapidly the young die, the greater the average life expectancy of the population. But what about aging? Although aging is defined as the general deterioration of the body with increasing age, a more quantitative definition of aging is the amount of time required to double the likelihood of death after you reach adulthood. This is a far better definition of aging than average life span because childhood mortality is no longer a factor. This definition of aging is also known as the mortality doubling time. Currently in the United States and other industrialized countries, the mortality doubling time is between 7 and 10 years after you reach the age of 40. If the mean doubling time is 10 years, then if you are 50 you will be twice as likely to die at this age than at age 40. It also means that at age 60 you will be two times more likely to die than at age 50 and four times more likely to die than at age 40. You can quickly see that as you age your chances of dying are exponentially greater. Why is this definition of aging important? Because it allows you to define anti-aging in terms of increased mortality doubling time without having to exceed the maximum life span.

In addition to the quantity of life (as measured by longevity), the quality of life (maintaining functionality for as long as possible) is an equally important consideration for any successful anti-aging program. If you are living longer but have not slowed the aging process (i.e., the general deterioration of the body), then you have achieved little. You may have a longer life, but with far less quality (i.e., decreased functionality). Not a very inviting trade off.

Before I explore why we are living longer, let me address the question of why we should die in the first place. Three possible explanations have been put forward and can be summarized as follows: (1) we die for the good of the species; (2) we live fast and die young; and (3) we die because we live in an increasingly less hostile environment. Thus genes that have nothing to do with procreation of the species but are associated with the development of chronic diseases and resulting death.

Let's evaluate them one by one. Dying for the good of the species has an altruistic tone to it, but it doesn't make sense. Most animals (including humans until the development of writing about 5,000 years ago) have no way of communicating knowledge from one generation to the next other than by example. The older the animal, the more experience it accumulates and the more wisdom can be passed to its offspring. The smarter the next generation is, the more likely they can successfully procreate and pass their genes onto still another generation. This is why the elderly were especially venerated (at least until recently). Their personal experience contained practical knowledge about what to expect in the world. So why would Nature choose to discard the advantage of accumulated knowledge when it could be retained and communicated by older animals for the good of the species. Therefore, this explanation of dying doesn't seem very likely.

The "live fast, die young" theory, especially popular in the 1920s, was developed by Raymond Pearl, an early gerontologist. This theory surmised that you had a limited number of swings at the plate of life; once those were used up, it was curtain time. This theory was based on the fact that it appeared that the higher the metabolism of the animal, the shorter its life span. Unfortunately, when it was found that some animals (especially birds) have very high metabolisms, but also very long lifetimes, this theory became untenable.

Finally, we are left with the evolutionary theory of dying. After our genes are passed to the next generation, evolution doesn't really care what happens to the parents. Death, according to this theory, is caused by an accumulation of genetic defects that only manifest themselves well after the next generation has reached maturity. As our environment has become less hostile, people have a decreased probability of random death. The result is an increasing life span, which allows for the accumulation of inherent genetic defects that manifest themselves as chronic disease in an aging population. There are three good examples of this phenomenon.

The first is Huntington's disease, which strikes in middle age with devastating consequences—the complete loss of mental powers. Huntington's was the disease that killed the famous folksinger Woody Guthrie. Lending credence to this evolutionary theory of aging is the fact that Huntington's manifests itself only well after another generation has been produced. From an evolutionary perspective it doesn't matter whether or not that particular gene is present since it would not affect your ability to pass on your other genes. Of course, while it might not matter to Nature, it does matter to you if you happen to carry that gene.

Two other examples that give credence to this evolutionary theory are Alzheimer's and heart disease. There appears to be an increased likelihood of being stricken with Alzheimer's disease if you have the ∈-4 form of the gene that codes for ApoE (a constituent of lipoproteins). This same form of the ApoE gene is associated with higher levels of cholesterol and heart disease. On the other hand, the ∈-2 form of the same ApoE gene seems to confer decreased likelihood for both heart disease and Alzheimer's disease with a corresponding increase in longevity. Because the occurrence of heart disease and Alzheimer's only appear a long time after procreation of the next generation, Nature has never bothered to "choose" between the good or bad forms of the ApoE gene. Either way, you've got plenty of time to reproduce. This is why diseases associated with aging—such as heart disease, cancer, Type 2 diabetes, and arthritis—rarely strikes young adults.

It appears that why we die is most likely due to the appearance of genetic defects that have nothing to do with successful procreation. And because evolution is a cruel master, it doesn't matter what happens to you after you have successfully reared the next generation of your species. For the first time in history, we are trying to wage war against a seemingly immutable law of Nature.

Why we die remains a continuing philosophical and biological debate. How to live a longer and more functional life, on the other hand, is a more practical question. Since longevity is defined as your success in reaching the maximum life span, there are many factors besides your genes that can affect longevity. Infectious disease, accidents, and predators are some of the factors that can decrease the likelihood of reaching your maximum life span.

In fact, the concept of increasing life span may be simply an artifact of civilization. In the wild, there is no such thing as aging. Death in that arena appears to be a random event because it is difficult to predict when it will occur. This is similar to radioactive decay rates, as it is impossible to predict when a particular atom will decay (see Figure 2-1 on page 11).

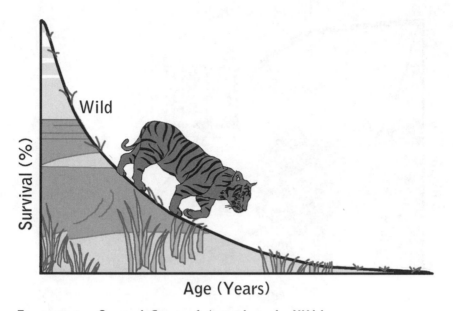

Figure 2-1   Survival Curve of Animals in the Wild

This is why when wild animals are tracked from birth, the decay in their population follows a decay rate like any radioactive isotope. Whatever this decay rate, however, there must be enough of the species left to create the next generation and rear it before random death strikes. This random decay in the wild can be altered by civilization. Put a wild animal in a zoo and its life expectancy follows a different course. The survival rate becomes more rectangular (see Figure 2-2 on page 12).

Why the differences? Animals in zoos get medical care. They don't have to worry about predators. And the most important reason is that they get fed on time. It's a pretty civilized life. The same is true for humans. Our life-expectancy curves have become more rectangular with increasing levels of civilization (see Figure 2-3 on page 13).

It is estimated that it took nearly 3,000 years (from 1000 B.C. to 1900) for the life expectancy of man to increase by 25 years (from the low 20s to 46). In the next 50 years (from 1900 to 1950), life span increased approximately another 25 years (from 46 to 72). That's a 50 percent increase in life expectancy in only 50 years. What happened in that 50-year period that dramatically increased life expectancy? Before 1900, 75 percent of all people died before the age of 65. Now more

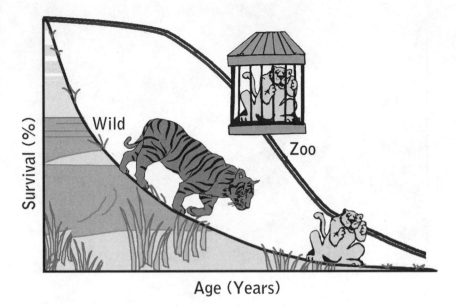

Figure 2-2   Life Expectancy of Animals in the Wild vs. Captivity

than 70 percent will die after age 70. That would suggest that the mortality doubling time has increased, and we have begun to reverse aging. But this is less of a gain than you might initially think. As impressive as these gains may sound, at the turn of the century if you were a male and lived to age 70, it was likely that you would live for another 9 years. Today if you are a male and reach the age of 70, it is likely that you will live another 12 years, only three more years and often with far less functionality. Although life expectancy has increased, there is little indication that the mortality doubling rate has not changed dramatically since detailed birth records were kept beginning some 200 years ago. So if the intrinsic rate of aging has not changed in some 200 years, what changed at the turn of the century to dramatically increase life expectancy?

The average life expectancy in America in 1900 was only 46 years. The leading causes of death in America at that time were infectious diseases spread through respiratory exposure (like tuberculosis and pneumonia), and were unlikely to be greatly affected by improved sanitation (which would affect diseases, like cholera, spread through fecal contamination). Could the dramatic increase in life expectancy in the

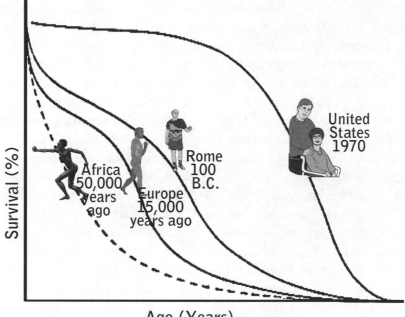

Figure 2-3   Changing Life Expectancy of Humans

first half of this century be a consequence of better control of infectious disease?

Estimates have been made on the increase in life expectancy if certain causes of death, including infectious disease, could be completely eliminated. Not surprisingly, the effect on life span depends upon what the current leading cause of death is and on what potential causes of mortality might theoretically be eliminated. These results are shown in Table 2-1.

TABLE 2-1

Effects on Life Expectancy with Mortality Eradication Depending on the Stage of Development

	SEMIDEVELOPED COUNTRY	DEVELOPED COUNTRY
Infectious disease	19 years	1.7 years
Cancer	9 months	2.5 years
Violence/Accidents	6 months	8 months

If you live in a less-developed society with an average life expectancy of only 40 years of age (and this would have included many industrialized Western countries at the turn of the century), the total elimination of violence and accidents and even cancer have a very limited impact on life expectancy. However, elimination of infectious diseases has a dramatic impact on life expectancy, increasing it by 19 years or nearly 50 percent. This is approximately the same percentage increase in life span that occurred in the first half of this century.

On the other hand, in developed industrialized countries with an average life expectancy of 72 years (like present-day America), if one could eliminate all violence and accidents, only another 8-month increase in average life expectancy would be achieved. You would enjoy a totally crime-free and accident-free society (which is desirable), but not necessarily a longer-living one. And the increase in life expectancy from the elimination of cancer in an industrialized country has a much greater impact on increased life expectancy compared to the elimination of all infectious disease.

Why does the potential elimination of cancer have a far greater impact on life expectancy than elimination of infectious disease in developed countries? First, infectious disease is no longer a great killer in developed countries. Second, the vast majority of cancers strike adults. If you are not dying at an earlier age due to infectious disease, then eliminating cancer is going to make a bigger difference in life expectancy.

However, the number-one killer in industrialized countries is not cancer, but heart disease. It is estimated that if all heart disease could be eliminated, the increase in life expectancy would only be another 4 to 6 years. So even if you could magically eradicate cancer and heart disease overnight in America, the maximum increase in life expectancy would only be an additional 6 to 9 years. This is why it is unlikely that we will ever exceed our maximum life span of 120 years.

So it appears that our control of infectious disease in the first half of this century has been the primary cause of our dramatic improvement in life expectancy. But is the control of infectious disease due to better nutrition or better drugs?

The body's primary defense against infectious disease is a strong functioning immune system. The efficiency of this defense system is controlled to a great extent by the diet, in particular, the protein content of the diet. The first casualty of protein malnutrition is the immune system. In fact, combatting malnutrition in general has been one of man's major challenges since the beginning of recorded history. It is only in this century that adequate supplies of protein became more abundant and more accessible to the general population. Therefore better nutrition is a very likely candidate in explaining the dramatic increase in life expectancy during the first half of this century.

Medical experts, however, are usually quick to take credit for their role in halting the advance of disease (especially infectious disease). But is that credit justified? Before the 1930s the typical physician could best be characterized by Norman Rockwell-like paintings of the family doctor sitting at the patient's bedside hoping the fever would break. All he could really offer was encouragement and prayer, plus some simple remedies and herbs that would be laughed at by his colleagues today. And drug companies 50 years ago were a pale imitation of what they are today. Their major products were patent medicines, which were not exactly herculean in the fight against disease. In fact, many of the over-the-counter (OTC) drugs found in every pharmacy and supermarket today are far more powerful than the state-of-the-art drugs used 50 years ago.

The waning of infectious disease in the first half of this century is commonly thought to be the result of new drug discovery. Yet the conquest of those diseases that were the captains of death at the turn of the century had very little to do with the drugs themselves. For example, almost 70 percent of the decline in pneumonia mortality occurred before the invention of sulfa drugs in 1935 (and frankly those drugs weren't very good anyway). Likewise more than 80 percent of the decline in tuberculosis mortality occurred before any good drug therapy was developed in the 1950s. There are other examples, such as the 90 percent decrease in the mortality of whooping cough and the more than 70 percent decrease in the mortality of scarlet fever and diphtheria before effective vaccines were developed. Polio is the only disease in twentieth-century America that shows a correlation between a drug or vaccine introduced to treat it and the slowing of its infection rate.

However, one feat that the pharmaceutical industry is slow to accept credit for is a new cause of death in this country that never existed at the turn of the century. It is now estimated that the fourth leading cause of death in the United States is adverse drug reactions (ADR). Deaths from ADR are not due to administrative mistakes or patient overdoses but represent deaths in which a drug was used correctly. It is as if we have suddenly invented a new cause of death that never existed before. Bear in mind that the deaths from ADR are far greater than the mortality caused by AIDS, which only ranks tenth as a cause of death in the United States.

The pharmaceutical industry shouldn't take credit for the dramatic increase in life expectancy in the first half of this century, since it appears the primary reason that we are living longer is simply better nutrition. Your best defense against disease is not some new medical treatment, but an active and fully functioning immune system. And your immune system, as you might imagine, is largely controlled by what you eat and the quality of the food you consume. This is why malnutrition (not only in terms of calories but also in terms of protein content) is the greatest contributing factor for reduced longevity. Your immune system is primarily composed of protein and therefore any deficiency in protein intake will dramatically compromise its efficiency. On the other hand, with adequate protein intake, the immune system is able to overcome any infectious disease with greater efficiency.

Obtaining adequate levels of protein has been a very difficult task since the advent of agriculture, because crops are by definition carbohydrate rich and protein poor. This was why hunter-gatherer populations (assuming adequate supplies of wild game) had a better nutritional status and were more healthy than their counterparts who were agrarian based. Surprisingly, Americans have been consuming adequate protein only since the turn of the century. This is why the average size of an American soldier during the Civil War was only 5 feet 5 inches. Now the average height of American males (5 feet 10 inches) and females (5 feet 6 inches) is just about what it was 10,000 years ago for neo-Paleolithic hunter-gatherers who had adequate levels of protein in their diets. Without adequate protein, not only is it impossible to attain your maximum genetically programmed height, but it's also impossible to maintain a highly efficient immune system. (Remember that the lower life expectancy of neo-Paleolithic man was due to living in a much more hostile environment.) With the development of cattle as a readily available source of protein coupled with refrigeration and the development of an efficient transportation system, protein has become a much more common dietary staple for Americans since the turn of the century. The subsequent increase in protein consumption correlates much better with the control of infectious diseases than does the development of new drugs to treat infectious diseases.

Therefore the most important factor as to why we are living longer since the turn of the century may simply be that we are eating better. However, what Americans have been eating in the past 15 years is very different from what they ate in the first 50 years of this century. In this same 15-year time period, we have become increasingly fatter and less healthy as a nation. This indicates that something very wrong is happening to our dietary habits. If eating better is the primary reason why we were living longer in the first half of the century, then it also becomes the key to reverse aging in order to achieve increased longevity in the next century. But the diet to reverse aging has to be very different than the one we have been eating in the last 15 years. In essence, if you want to reverse the aging process, then food is your "drug" of choice. But the door can swing both ways because the improper use of food can also decrease longevity.

Although my definition of an effective anti-aging program is one that increases the mortality doubling-time, it may take one or two generations to truly know the success of any such intervention in humans. Fortunately, there are biological markers of aging which allow us to test anti-aging interventions today. If these biological markers can be reversed, then you will know you're on the right track toward anti-aging. Those biological markers of aging are detailed in the next chapter.

CHAPTER 3

THE BIOLOGICAL MARKERS
OF AGING

Defining the biological markers of aging is essential in the search for a successful anti-aging program. Only by reversing some, if not all, of these markers can you truly state that your anti-aging strategy is successful. Much of our current human data on the biological markers that change with age come from longitudinal aging studies starting with the Baltimore Longitudinal Study of Aging (BLSA) in 1958. Longitudinal studies are truly ambitious because they begin with the largest possible group of young adults and then follow them as they age. So with 40 years of data collection completed with the BLSA and other on-going studies as well, we are beginning to know a few things about aging. First, not all biological markers change universally with age. As an example, systolic blood pressure (the upper number of your blood pressure) universally increases with aging, whereas diastolic blood pressure (the lower number of your blood pressure) does not. Second, and not surprisingly, there is a great range of variability in aging. Some people age quickly, others age more slowly.

To qualify as a biological marker of aging, a marker is defined as a biological process that cannot only be measured and quantified, but is also universal. As I pointed out earlier, cancer is a disease associated with aging, but not everyone gets cancer. It is a possible consequence of aging, not a marker of aging. For humans the primary biological markers of aging appear to be those listed in Table 3-1 on page 19.

Although this is a fairly broad list of physiological changes, they all can be all related to one single factor—excess levels of the hormone insulin. Although this hormone will be discussed in greater detail in a later chapter, it is important to note that excess levels of insulin is probably the greatest single factor that accelerates the aging process because it affects all of the biological markers of aging.

TABLE 3-1

Some Biological Markers of Human Aging

MARKERS THAT INCREASE WITH AGE	MARKERS THAT DECREASE WITH AGE
Insulin resistance	Glucose tolerance
Systolic blood pressure	Aerobic capacity
Percent body fat	Muscle mass
Lipid ratios	Strength
	Temperature regulation
	Immune function

To explore the role of excess insulin on the biological markers of aging, let's first look at the biological markers that increase with age. The increase in insulin resistance (and the resulting increase of insulin in the bloodstream) may have the most far-reaching impact on the aging process because of its effect on other hormonal systems, in particular eicosanoids (which ultimately control the immune system). In simple terms, the job of insulin is to store incoming nutrients (especially carbohydrates) in its appropriate target cells. Without sufficient insulin, your cells would essentially starve, so you have to have a certain level of insulin to ensure appropriate delivery of nutrients. Insulin resistance makes it difficult for insulin to do its primary job. With increased insulin resistance, insulin is still being produced, however, its ability to communicate and relay its message to store nutrients, (in particular blood glucose) is highly compromised. The biological response to increasing insulin resistance is to secrete even more insulin into the bloodstream to drive down blood glucose levels by brute force. This leads to an overproduction of insulin in the bloodstream, which is known as hyperinsulinemia. One of the first indicators of hyperinsulinemia is an increase in stored body fat. Many of the markers of aging are a direct or indirect consequence of hyperinsulinemia.

Hyperinsulinemia is like a loose cannon on the deck of a ship because it can adversely affect other hormonal systems. One key hormonal system is eicosanoids. Eicosanoids are an exceptionally complex group of hormones that represent the molecular foundation of aging, as I will discuss in greater detail in a later chapter. For now, let's just say that eicosanoids are in many ways "master" hormones that control a wide range of physiological systems. This is achieved by balancing opposing actions of "good" and "bad" eicosanoids. The role insulin plays in eicosanoid production is that it causes the production of more "bad" and fewer "good" eicosanoids. For example, the higher the insulin level, the more vasoconstrictive ("bad") eicosanoids are made that increase blood pressure. The less insulin in the bloodstream, the more vasodilating ("good") eicosanoids are made. It is the balance of these opposing eicosanoids that determines blood pressure. Therefore as insulin levels increase so does blood pressure.

With age-associated hyperinsulinemia the percentage of body fat will also increase. Higher levels of insulin promote the storage of any excess calorie intake into the adipose tissue, at the same time preventing the release of stored fat for energy by inhibiting the gate keeper of the fat cell, the hormone-sensitive lipase.

Hyperinsulinemia will also reduce HDL cholesterol levels. Thus it is not surprising that any lipid ratio that uses HDL cholesterol as one of its components will also increase. In addition, excess insulin stimulates the liver to produce more cholesterol thereby increasing the risk of heart disease.

Now let's turn to the biological markers that decrease with age. Here a similar pattern emerges as many of these biological markers are also strongly influenced by excess insulin. A decrease in glucose tolerance is another way of stating that insulin resistance is increased. The body cannot take up glucose from the blood effectively and therefore must increase insulin output. One of the best clinical ways to determine your tolerance to glucose is a blood test that measures the extent of the cross-linking of glucose to proteins in the plasma, in particular the cross-linking of glucose to hemoglobin in the red blood cells. The higher the amount of glycosylated hemoglobin (the end product of the cross-linking of glucose with hemoglobin in red blood cells), the higher the long-term levels of glucose in the bloodstream due to increased glucose intolerance. Simply put, the higher the levels of glycosylated hemoglobin in the bloodstream, the more glucose intolerant you are and the faster you are aging.

Decreased aerobic capacity is another marker of aging, and it appears to decrease by about 1 percent per year after age 20. Aerobic capacity is the ability to deliver adequate levels of oxygen to the muscles, so that lactic acid doesn't build up (causing the muscle to stop working). In athletics, this buildup is called the burn because the actively exercising muscle group is building up lactic acid levels very rapidly, which causes pain. In cardiac patients, the same process is called angina, but occurs at much lower levels of exercise intensity. In cardiovascular patients with angina, their actively exercising muscle (the heart) is not getting enough oxygen and lactic acid builds up.

Obviously, the factors that affect the transfer of oxygen from the air you breath to its final delivery to the muscles are complex. But from a hormonal standpoint there are three distinct areas that contribute to this marker of aging, and all are related to hyperinsulinemia.

The first step that determines overall aerobic capacity is your lung capacity, which is ultimately controlled by eicosanoids that are either bronchodilators ("good" eicosanoids) or bronchoconstrictors ("bad" eicosanoids). Elevated levels of insulin promote the overproduction of broncoconstrictors. If you have ever had an asthma attack, you have been exposed to an overproduction of bronchoconstrictors (i.e., leukotrienes) with a resulting decrease in oxygen transfer. Of course, if you have destroyed lung tissue by smoking, disease, or environmental insults, your lung capacity will be compromised even more as you age.

A second factor that affects oxygen delivery to muscles (and other cells for that matter) is the diameter of the capillaries that surround the lung tissue. The greater the capillary diameter, the greater the rate at which oxygen will be transferred to red blood cells in the bloodstream. Not surprisingly, this process also falls under hormonal control by eicosanoids. Eicosanoids that are vasodilating ("good" eicosanoids) will increase the diameter of the vessels surrounding the lung tissue, whereas eicosanoids that are vasoconstrictors ("bad" eicosanoids) will decrease the diameter of the same blood vessels, thus reducing oxygen transfer. Elevated insulin promotes the overproduction of vasoconstrictors.

The final determinant of oxygen transfer is the delivery of oxygen to the target cells based on the flexibility of your red blood cells. The ability of red blood cells to contort or deform themselves as they squeeze through the capillaries is enhanced by "good" eicosanoids. The more flexible the red blood cells, the greater the amount of oxygen they can deliver to the cell. The production of "good" eicosanoids is decreased as insulin levels increase. Therefore, if any one of the three phases of oxygen transfer is compromised, then an overall decrease in aerobic capacity is the result. Less oxygen is delivered to the cell, and if that cell is an actively exercising cell, then lactic acid builds up and fatigue sets in. This is why physical endurance decreases with age. As you can see, aerobic capacity is largely determined by the balance of "good" and "bad" eicosanoids, which is strongly influenced by insulin levels.

Another important biological marker of aging is the loss of muscle mass and the loss of strength. The best estimate is that you lose about 6 pounds of muscle mass with each decade of aging so that by age 65 you have lost 25 to 30 percent of your muscle mass and strength. Furthermore, it is the loss of muscle mass and strength that has the greatest impact on the lack of functionality as you age. The muscles you are born with are the ones you die with minus any of those that have died during the aging process. Unlike skin cells, muscle cells don't divide. The amount of your muscle mass therefore has less to do with the number of muscle cells you have, but much more to do with their size. The two hormones that control maintenance of muscle size and strength are growth hormone and testosterone. As I will show in later chapters, the levels of both these hormones can be reduced by elevated insulin. Therefore the decrease in muscle mass and strength will be greatly affected by elevated insulin. Viewed in this light, the drop in the levels of growth hormone and testosterone that occur with aging may simply be secondary consequences of this age-related increase in insulin.

Another marker of aging that appears to be universal is lack of temperature regulation. As you age, your ability to tolerate extremes in temperature decreases. You feel more uncomfortable in the summer as your body is less likely to sweat to cool down your core temperature, and you feel more uncomfortable in the winter because less blood circulates to the periphery (fingers and toes). To a great extent, this lack of temperature regulation is controlled by the diameter of your vascular system in your skin, which is ultimately controlled by eicosanoids. Elevated levels of insulin influence the production of those eicosanoids that decrease the diameter of the vascular system causing to impaired circulation and decreased temperature regulation, just as it leads to reduced oxygen transfer.

The final biological marker that decreases with age is your immune system, especially the ability of the white cells to fight disease. Your immune system is controlled by eicosanoids and can be severely depressed by high levels of insulin, which promote the synthesis of "bad" eicosanoids that are immunodepressing.

These biological markers of aging affect everyone regardless of sex or race. What is important to note is the common theme: each biological marker of aging is profoundly influenced by excess insulin and its effect on other hormonal systems. Therefore reducing excess insulin becomes a critical factor in any anti-aging program.

You may be asking why other hormone levels are not considered biological markers of aging. After all, isn't menopause caused by decreased estrogen? And doesn't decreased growth hormone cause loss of muscle mass? Well, yes and no. Many hormones do decrease with age, but others do not. Some, such as insulin and cortisol, can increase; others remain relatively constant. Therefore hormone changes per se may be secondary markers of aging. As an example, the levels of growth hormone decrease dramatically with age. However, if the pituitary gland (the source of growth hormone) is properly stimulated, then growth hormone secretion quickly rises to the same levels produced in your youth. So it's not a decrease in growth hormone levels as much as a decreased response to hormonal signals that accounts for the drop. Thus, the lowered levels of growth hormone when we age (as well as many other hormones) are simply a secondary consequence of a primary mediator of aging: hormonal miscommunication. In fact, all of the measured biological markers of aging may be thought of as a growing degree of hormone miscommunication (facilitated by excess insulin) as we age.

Understanding how hormones communicate biological information and improving that communication becomes the foundation for developing a practical anti-aging program.

CHAPTER 4

HORMONES:
THE SHORT COURSE

Hormones—everyone has heard about them, but very few know much about what they do. As it turns out, understanding hormones (and really the communication between hormones) is essential to understanding the aging process. Fortunately, many of the hormones that are key to successful anti-aging are under your direct control.

So the first question is: What is a hormone? The word hormone is derived from the Greek word *hormao* which means "I arouse to activity." A hormone is a biochemical messenger that is basically a molecular call to action that can work with incredible speed, complexity, and specificity to communicate information. If anything goes wrong with that complex hormonal communication system, you begin to age far faster than you should. Alex Comfort, one of the early pioneers of the study of aging, stated that aging is "an increased liability to die." Therefore any breakdown in your hormonal communication systems will have negative consequences on your longevity by increasing the likelihood of death.

The study of hormones is called endocrinology. However, a better definition of endocrinology is the study of biological communication systems. From that perspective, endocrinology has a lot in common with any communication system that you access when sending information at a distance.

Hormones are the core of your internal communication system. Their evolution was caused by many of the same factors that have made your local telephone company become much more high-tech over time to meet the demands of today's advanced communication needs. Take for example, the car phone. Imagine that your car phone had to have a telephone cord stretching from the car to your home's phone jack. Obviously, this would have to be a very long cord to enable your car to drive any significant distance from the house. That might be OK if you are the first on your block with a car phone, but what if your neighbor wants one too. And then what if everyone on your block wants one, then everyone in the city. You can quickly visualize the mass of phone wires entangling, if not choking the system, and most likely they will be pulled out of their jacks. What you need is a new type of communication system that allows you to use the phone in your car with the same ease as the phone in your home. This is exactly what the telephone companies developed; a wireless system that can send telephone signals effortlessly to your car and enable you to maintain contact with distant points very easily. Five hundred million years ago, Nature faced a very similar problem. That problem was how to better improve cellular communication at a distance.

As long as life consisted of single-celled organisms, communication from one part of the cell to another wasn't too difficult. A chemical signal could be made in one area of the cell and then simply diffuse to another part of the cell to report what was happening on the other side. Now it becomes more complex when you have two cells trying to communicate with each other. A new communication system was required for greater sophistication to ensure that a number of the same type of cells could work together in harmony if the biochemical message leaving the cell could hopefully be picked up by another cell. These processes are called exocytosis (leaving the cell), and endocytosis (entering the cell). If all the cells are the same, this system works reasonably well (depending on how many cells have to be informed of new events). And the biochemicals that are moving from cell to cell are called biological response modifiers. Simply stated, this means they are messengers that tell neighboring cells that something is happening nearby; they also have the ability to modify the biological response of the cell with which they are interacting. But this is like being on an island and sending messages in bottles to other nearby islands hoping they all arrive at the same time.

As an organism becomes even more complex, this form of communication is just too haphazard. Different cells evolve with specific, specialized functions. They need a secure information pipeline so that the right information gets to the right location at the right time. Nature's solution? Nerves that, like telephone lines, can hard-wire different parts of your body together for better, quicker, and more efficient communication.

But what happens when this nervous system becomes too unwieldy, like our analogy of car phones connected by telephone lines. To solve this problem, Nature developed an even more sophisticated system of communication known as hormones. For the sake of this example, let's just say that hormones appear to be the biological equivalent of wireless communications. In reality they are far more complex.

Hormones require complexity to work because they filter information. The biological message they carry is not for every cell in the body, but only for specialized cells. How a hormone finds a particular cell is solved by having receptors in different parts of the cell that only recognize that hormone. These discrete receptors on or in the cell act as a lock-and-key system. If a cell doesn't have a receptor for a hormone, no matter what message that hormone might carry, it can't make the cell alter its biological response.

Sometimes one hormone will have multiple actions. Likewise, one biological function may be affected by many different hormones. For example, at least four different hormonal systems can be utilized to maintain blood glucose levels to ensure adequate brain function. Often adding to this complexity is a very complex feedback relationship between the hormones in the bloodstream and the hypothalamus that governs their levels.

Now that you have some basic ideas on how hormones communicate, let me explain how they operate in a little more detail. Most hormones convey their information by using the superhighway of the body; the bloodstream. Known as endocrine hormones, these hormones move very quickly from their site of synthesis to their point of action using the bloodstream as their transportation highway. Familiar endocrine hormones include insulin, cortisol, growth hormone, thyroid hormones, estrogen, and testosterone. All are made in a very distinct gland or organ and then released into the bloodstream to locate their target tissues—interacting with a discrete receptor on a specialized target cell and then delivering a very powerful message to the target cell to take action.

All endocrine hormones are ultimately controlled by the body's own "Wizard of Oz," also known as the hypothalamus. Located deep within the brain, the hypothalamus is continually receiving signals from the body (i.e., temperature, blood pressure, blood glucose levels, hormone levels, etc.) through connections to the central nervous system. Depending on these continued dynamic inputs, the hypothalamus then secretes what are known as hormone-releasing hormones, which travel a very short distance through a direct connection to the pituitary gland. Although the pituitary gland is in the brain, it is one of the few of its parts that is in direct contact with the bloodstream. This tiny gland makes ten different hormones that can be released directly into the bloodstream depending on the amount of releasing factor secreted from the hypothalamus. Some of these pituitary hormones (like growth hormone) directly enter the bloodstream. Other hormones that leave the pituitary seek out target tissues in the adrenals, thyroid, ovary, and testes, releasing still more hormones that affect the final hormonal action on cells.

As these secondary hormone levels from the distant glands rise in the bloodstream, they signal back to the hypothalamus via sensors in the central nervous system. Finally, to complete the cycle, the hypothalamus through its sensing mechanisms registers the rising hormone levels (which it dispatched in the first place) in the bloodstream. The hypothalamus can also sense the final biological action, which the released hormones were intended to initiate when they first began their journey. In either case, once the hypothalamus gets wind of what's happening, it shuts down the production of the specific releasing hormones temporarily stopping the pituitary from secreting any more of that particular hormone. This complex feedback communication system is your hormonal lifeline. The better it functions, the slower you age. The less efficiently it functions, the more rapidly you age. The central role of the hypothalamus is shown in Figure 4-1 on page 28.

It should be obvious from this figure that to make this communication system work flawlessly, all the parts must work in tight harmony. Any miscommunication in this system is like a weak link in a chain that leads to hormonal chaos and accelerated aging.

But the hypothalamus, pituitary, and the glands in the adrenals, thyroid, ovary, and testes are not the only places where hormones are made. They are also produced in the pancreas, the pineal gland, and in the glands located in the throat. In fact there are nine known groupings of endocrine hormone glands. Three are in the brain (pineal, pituitary, and hypothalamus), three more are in the throat (thyroid, parathyroids, and thymus), two are in the abdominal region (adrenal

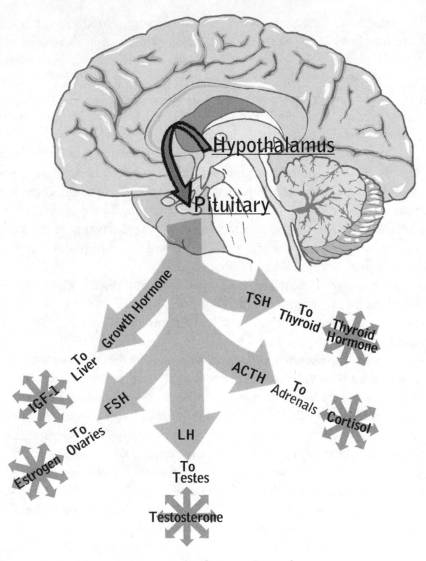

Figure 4-1   Hypothalamus is the Starting Point for
            Most Endocrine Hormones

and pancreas), and one is in the gonads (testes for males, ovaries for females). And they vary in size from the pancreas (which weighs about three ounces) to the pineal (which is about the size of a grape seed). How these sites process incoming information and send out the corresponding hormonal messengers is an extremely sophisticated and precise communication system (see Figure 4-2 on page 29).

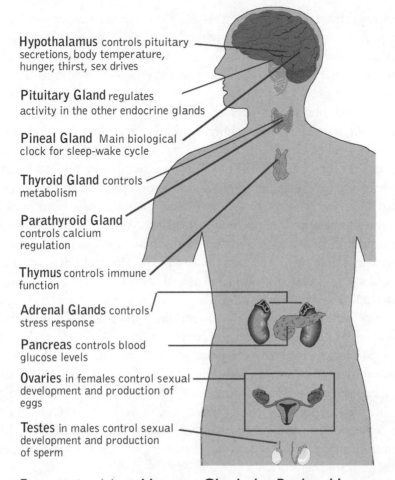

Hypothalamus controls pituitary secretions, body temperature, hunger, thirst, sex drives

Pituitary Gland regulates activity in the other endocrine glands

Pineal Gland Main biological clock for sleep-wake cycle

Thyroid Gland controls metabolism

Parathyroid Gland controls calcium regulation

Thymus controls immune function

Adrenal Glands controls stress response

Pancreas controls blood glucose levels

Ovaries in females control sexual development and production of eggs

Testes in males control sexual development and production of sperm

Figure 4-2   Major Hormone Glands that Produce Hormones

Now let's add to the complexity of this communication system by talking about hormonal axes. Hormones are like a thermostat in your house. They maintain biological functions within tight zones. To do this effectively, sets of hormones often have opposite physiological functions, so that their constant battling will keep a particular biological function within a zone. When sets of hormones act like this, they are called an axis. To make this concept clearer, visualize the axis that goes through the earth. At the extremes of the axis are different seasons. When it's winter in the Northern Hemisphere, it's summer in the Southern Hemisphere. Between these two extremes lie the Tropics, where the temperature is fairly uniform year round. The farther

you move from the center of this axis, the greater the seasonal variations in the weather. This is what hormonal axes do. They keep a
particular biological function within a zone, and the farther you move
from the center of that axis, the more variations you find in that biological function.

For example, the control of blood glucose is critical for optimal
brain function. The primary hormonal axis that controls blood glucose
is the insulin-glucagon axis. Insulin drives down blood glucose, glucagon raises blood glucose. As long as these two hormones are balanced
in their opposing physiological actions, blood glucose is stabilized and
brain function is optimal. On the other hand, if this hormonal axis
becomes unbalanced, brain function suffers. An everyday example of a
disruption in this axis occurs after eating a big bowl of pasta for lunch,
then almost falling asleep three hours later. The carbohydrates in the
pasta have stimulated a rapid release of insulin into the bloodstream
and that drives down blood glucose levels. Unfortunately, the pasta
contains very little protein that is required to stimulate the hormone
glucagon which, in turn, raises blood glucose. The end result is that
your pasta-rich meal has temporarily disrupted the insulin-glucagon
axis, which makes you sleepy due to a significant drop in brain function because its primary fuel (blood glucose) is no longer available
in optimal amounts. Even more complex axis systems include
the hypothalamus-pituitary-gonad and hypothalamus-pituitary-adrenal
communication loops because they have more numerous control
points within them.

Hormonal axis systems are a relatively recent evolutionary development because only very complex biological systems require such
tight controls. The less developed an organism, the less likely these
hormonal axis systems are necessary. This is why endocrine hormones
also represent a much more recent evolutionary development than the
first hormones developed by living organisms, which are known as
autocrine hormones.

Autocrine hormones are released from a cell and then come back
to act upon the same cell or its immediate neighbor as long as the
appropriate receptor is in the membrane of the target cell. They don't
need to travel through the bloodstream to find their target tissues since
the target is right next door. Although these were the earliest hormones developed by Nature, they remained the most resistant to study
until very recently because they can't be sampled in the bloodstream

(since they don't use it), they work at vanishingly low concentrations (because they are so powerful), and they self-destruct in seconds (their call to action is too intense to persist). Eicosanoids derived from dietary fat are among the most powerful of these autocrine hormones.

Between the extremes of endocrine and autocrine hormones in both complexity and evolutionary development are the paracrine hormones. These hormones are usually controlled by discrete channels or physical structures to ensure that they are not circulating over a wide area. Typical paracrine hormones include the releasing hormones that travel from the hypothalamaus to the pituitary via a stalk (really a defined duct known as the hypophyseal portal vessel) or neurotransmitters (like serotonin) that are released by a nerve, then cross a small space (known as the synaptic junction) to interact with another nerve in order to generate a biological message.

These three types of hormonal systems (endocrine, autocrine, and paracrine) constitute your biological communication system; all three components must work in concert if you plan to reverse aging.

Because hormones filter information, have elegant feedback control systems, and relay discrete information that is encrypted for only specialized cells, it's best to visualize hormones as the biological equivalent of the Internet, only more complex. We think of the Internet as a very complex monument of information transfer. And in many ways it is. More than 40 million people are currently using the Internet, trying to communicate a wide variety of information in real time. Now try visualizing 60 trillion cells trying to communicate much more complex information with each other. This is what happens every second within your body. Just like the Internet, all this biological information has to go through a central server that relays the information with fidelity to other parts of the body via hormones. If anything happens to that central server, the information on the Internet becomes a cacophony of meaningless information. Similarly in your biological Internet, there is a central server (the hypothalamus) that is the key to maintaining the fidelity of hormonal communication flow (see Figure 4-3 on page 32).

However, the communication fidelity of hormonal messengers to and from this central server is maintained by a backup system that is controlled by autocrine hormones. The more efficiently these autocrine hormones work, the better the communication between cells and the hypothalamus becomes. The end result of this improved commu-

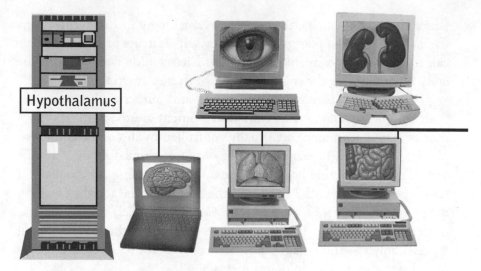

Figure 4-3   Your Biological Internet

nication is a slowdown, if not reversal, of the aging process. Fortunately, the key autocrine hormones of your biological Internet, are eicosanoids, which can be controlled by diet. Knowing how to use your diet to maintain the fidelity of information transfer to and from the central server (i.e., hypothalamus) throughout your biological Internet becomes the molecular basis for creating a successful anti-aging program.

The fact that diet plays such a critical role in hormonal communication doesn't seem to be very high tech. Likewise, the role of food in evolution is also overlooked. There is a growing body of knowledge that looks at food as an important evolutionary driving force. How to obtain food more efficiently, how to digest food with greater ease, and how to make better use of the energy contained in food become primary factors in determining evolutionary pathways. Obviously, the more well-nourished an organism, the more likely it will pass its genes to the next generation. From this viewpoint, organisms that developed more sophisticated hormonal systems based on the food they ate had a better chance of survival and were more likely to pass on their genes. Therefore, not surprisingly, those hormones directly regulated by the diet will have the greatest effect on survival and therefore the greatest potential for anti-aging if you can optimize their performance.

How food controls the communication between hormonal systems is the foundation of your anti-aging strategy. While it may be impossible to extend your maximum life span, you can improve longevity and maintain your functionality by increasing the mortality doubling time. How that can be achieved requires some understanding of the actual mechanisms that cause aging.

CHAPTER 5

MECHANISMS OF AGING:
THE FOUR PILLARS OF AGING

Aging is pretty simple to define. It's the general deterioration of the body over time. This rate of deterioration can be quantified by the mortality doubling time. In addition, 40 years of research has given us an insight into the biological markers of aging. But what are the molecular mechanisms behind aging? What happens in our bodies at the cellular level that causes the changes in these biological markers? Once unifying factors for various mechanisms of aging are identified, then you can devise an anti-aging battle plan that allows you to attack the aging process at its molecular core.

It has often been said that there are almost as many proposed mechanisms of aging as there are researchers in the field. This is because what is termed as aging is really a multifactorial process with no one single control mechanism. This means that several processes are probably occurring on simultaneously that result in aging. However, I believe that if you carefully distill all the mechanisms of aging, you find consistent themes that lead to what I describe as the four pillars of aging, So what are the pillars of aging? They are as shown in Table 5-1.

TABLE 5-1

Four Pillars of Aging

- Excess insulin
- Excess blood glucose
- Excess free radicals
- Excess cortisol

The reduction and eventual control of the pillars of aging are the keys to successful anti-aging. More important to you, each can be lowered through diet and lifestyle within a very short period of time.

Most of this chapter is devoted to detailing various mechanisms of aging and how they are related to one or more of the four pillars. If you want to know how to reduce the four pillars of aging with your next meal, you might want to jump forward to the next chapter. On the other hand, if you are interested in the details of how various aging mechanisms define the four pillars, then read on.

How do you measure the success of any anti-aging program? By reversing the biological markers of aging, but ultimately by increasing the mortality doubling time. Although mortality doubling time was discussed briefly in an earlier chapter, it is worth reviewing since it is my definition of anti-aging. Mortality doubling time for a given age after reaching adulthood (let's call it x), is how many years (let's call that y) that have to go by until the mortality rate is doubled. Today in America that number is about 8 years. This means if you are 40, then your likelihood of death will be twice as great at age 48. It also means that your likelihood of death will be four times as great at 56, and 16 times as great at age 64. The older you get, the greater the increase in the likelihood of dying. This is how insurance companies establish their premiums. It turns out that the doubling time for human mortality has been fairly constant after age 40, averaging between 7 and 10 years (after subtracting out mortality due to accidents and death) in a wide variety of societies since historic records have been kept. Although we are living longer due to improvements in civilization (environment, sanitation, medicine, etc.), the rate of aging (by the criteria of mortality doubling time) does not appear to have changed significantly over the past 200 years (and maybe not even in the last 20,000 years), even though life expectancy has dramatically increased during the same time period.

So how can we test whether or not mortality doubling time can be increased? As usual, with experimental animals. As any animal ages, the probability of death increases. As discussed earlier, death can be random—depending on the hostility of the environment. Long life is seldom observed in Nature; the survival curve of animals in the wild reflects that fact—death is almost by pure random chance. However, remove much of the hostility in the environment, and the longevity curve will become more rectangular. When this happens, death now comes from the diseases associated with aging. Remove all risks, as you can under laboratory conditions, and you can then test various interventions to assess whether or not they have reversed the aging process. Under these conditions to be a true anti-aging intervention there must be some indication that it can actually increase the maximum life span in test animals while simultaneously increasing their life expectancy. The end result is an increase in mortality doubling time. This is shown in Figure 5-1.

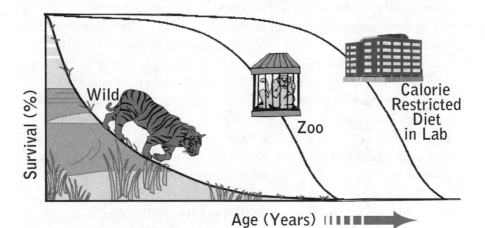

Figure 5-1   Rectangularization of the Survival Curve Under Laboratory Conditions

This curve illustrates why you have to be careful in the interpretation of longevity curves. Increased longevity may simply be the slowing of chronic diseases associated with aging and not due to any fundamental change in the aging process itself. This would indicate that the intervention is a secondary, not a primary, factor in aging. Therefore what you are looking for when testing different anti-aging interventions is to both rectangularize the longevity curve while also increasing maximum life span. The methodology just described is how anti-aging interventions are tested today to determine whether or not a proposed mechanism of aging is valid.

There are two schools of thought on various mechanisms of aging. The first school holds that aging is programmed. The other school contends that aging is simply a combination of random events that accumulate with time. Even today, any proposed mechanism about human aging should be considered a working hypothesis whose truth or falsehood will be difficult to prove within our lifetimes. However, since animals under highly controlled laboratory conditions die of many of the same diseases that characterize death in aging humans, it is reasonable to assume that many of the same factors that can be modified to increase mortality doubling time in test animals are applicable to humans.

About a decade ago, Bernard Strehler proposed the parameters that any reasonable mechanism of aging should meet. First, an aging mechanism must explain why there are losses in physiological function. Second, it must explain why these losses in physiological function are gradual. Third, it must postulate that the physiological losses that occur in aging are intrinsic. This means they cannot be corrected (otherwise we would achieve immortality), but they can be modified (which would increase the maximum life span in experimental animals). Finally, the physiological losses associated with aging must be universal (i.e., a biological marker of aging).

Using these postulates of aging, we can then investigate many of the most likely mechanisms to see which is the most likely to produce optimal results with the least amount of effort (after all, we are still human). But as you will see, when it comes to mechanisms of aging, there is a tremendous overlap suggesting that there may be some underlying factors that are probably working at the same time.

Let's take programmed aging first. The most remarkable example of this type of aging occurs in Pacific salmon. At some point in the Pacific salmon's life span, it develops the overwhelming desire to return to its birth site to spawn. Like world-class athletes, Pacific salmon overcome formidable physical barriers (including fishermen) to return to the site of their birth. After spawning, the Pacific salmon then begin aging with incredible speed, often dying within days. The cause of this rapid aging? It's due to a massive increase in the hormones called corticosteroids secreted from the adrenal glands. The surge in these hormones shuts down many of the essential physiological functions of the salmon (including its immune system), thus making it very vulnerable to infection. This same type of programmed death after mating is also found in certain mammals, such as marsupial mice. Although Pacific salmon and marsupial mice are genetically different from humans, many of the corticosteroids that lead to their rapid aging are the same as those found in our own bodies. However, this sudden surge of corticosteroids violates one of Strehler's postulates of aging (gradual loss of function). Nonetheless, the role of increasing corticosteroid levels offers a tantalizing clue about aging.

A more sophisticated approach to programmed aging in humans is known as the neuroendocrine mechanism of aging. This theory, first proposed by Valdimar Dilman, a Russian pioneer in aging research, is based upon some type of preset mechanism (almost acting like a clock) within the brain that sets in motion hormonal changes that begin to accelerate the aging process. A likely candidate for the location of this "clock" is the hypothalamus. The hypothalamus is hormone control central. It integrates incoming biochemical signals and sends out hormonal responses to maintain biological equilibrium. Since virtually all physiological systems in the human body (including the immune system) are affected by hormones, this theory has an attractive quality to it. The neuroendocrine theory suggests that something can be done to modify the clock and therefore the hormonal changes influenced by it.

Another interesting variation on this line of thinking is known as the glucocorticoid cascade mechanism, which links increased cortisol levels with the aging process. (Cortisol is the most abundant corticosteroid synthesized by the body.) Put forward by Robert Sapolsky, a researcher at Stanford University, this mechanism describes cortisol-induced toxicity. There are neurons in the brain that are very sensitive to excess cortisol. As some of these cortisol-sensitive neurons die, the feedback mechanism that controls the release of cortisol becomes damaged, and increasing amounts of cortisol are released from the adrenal glands. As damage to the cortisol-sensitive neurons increases, the cycle continues and cortisol begins to flood the system just as with Pacific salmon, but at a slower rate. Could a programmed release of cortisol be the "clock" of Dilman's mechanism? Why would excess cortisol be important to aging? Because the primary mode of cortisol's action, and other corticosteroids like it, is the inhibition of eicosanoid formation. Eicosanoids not only control the immune system, but also control the cardiovascular, digestive, central nervous, and a myriad of other biological systems in your body. Obviously, an overproduction of cortisol can have potentially devastating effects systemwide. Of course, anyone who has ever taken synthetic corticosteroids, such as prednisone (the most widely prescribed corticosteroid drug), knows this all too well. Within a month everything in the body begins to go haywire. This systemic damage is due to the nondiscriminate inhibition of all eicosanoid synthesis. This is why excess cortisol is one of the pillars of aging.

Another mechanism of aging suggests the possibility that there is a programmed cessation of DNA replication that leads to aging. Based on the early pioneering work of Leonard Hayflick, who studied replication in fibroblasts (skin cells), this mechanism suggests that cells may only be able to divide so many times before they stop. Fibroblast cells can be isolated and easily replicated under laboratory conditions. He noticed that after about 50 generations the cells would simply stop dividing and die. He could stop the process by freezing the cells in liquid nitrogen. Once unfrozen, they would continue to divide until they reached 50 generations and then would die. It was as if there were an internal clock telling the cell when to stop dividing. The unfortunate part of this attractive theory is that skin cells are known to rapidly divide, but nerve and muscle cells (the ones you really care about) don't. The nerve and muscle cells you are born with are the cells you die with (minus those that have expired before you do).

However, the original Hayflick mechanism of cell aging has now been modified to take into account the concept of telomeres. Telomeres are small fragments at the ends of DNA that are shortened every time a new cell division takes place. After a certain amount of telomere shortening, cell division stops. So the length of the telomere might be a molecular clock within the DNA telling the cell when it's time to stop dividing. In the lab, the length of the telomere can be increased by a telomerease enzyme. The theory goes that if you could find a telomerease stimulator, then cells would continue to divide as they did in their youth because a longer telomere length signals continued division. Of course, there might be a slight problem with this approach. Cells that don't stop dividing when they are supposed to are called cancer cells. How to increase the telomerease activity in human cells and control it so it doesn't turn a normal cell into a cancer cell is a perplexing question.

This on/off process of DNA replication is controlled by the body's production of growth factors, and insulin is one of the most powerful. The more insulin you make, the more cells are encouraged to grow, and growing cells need more proteins, which only come from turning on the DNA more often. One way to control telomere length is simply not to have the cell continually turned on to make more proteins, and that is done by reducing excess insulin. So excess insulin appears to be another clue in the aging process.

While programmed damage to the hypothalamus through a "clock" or the cessation of DNA replication after a defined number of replications represents one school of thought on aging mechanisms; the other school of thought can be lumped together under the phrase that life is a crapshoot. This school of thought suggests that aging is a consequence of the random accumulation of mistakes acquired during the course of living that ultimately take their toll.

The first of these random-chance theories was the "wear-and-tear" theory in the late nineteenth century. The basis of this theory was simple enough. Cells were assumed to be like other pieces of machinery that cannot work forever and eventually give out. However, the difference between a machine and a human is that our cells are constantly renewing themselves. In fact, it is estimated that within a two-year period every molecule in our body has been replaced. So asking why our bodies wear down despite constantly repairing themselves was postponed for a more detailed understanding of cellular biochemistry.

In the 1950s, Denham Harman (the founding father of the free radical theory of aging) proposed that aging is a consequence of an overproduction of free radicals. You've probably heard of these dreaded free radicals. But what are they and why are they so bad? A free radical is simply the name for a molecule that has an unpaired electron. Without the body's normal production of free radicals, you would die because they are integral in producing cellular energy from food, defending you against opportunistic infections, and making the hormones needed to maintain communications in your body. It's that unpaired electron that makes free radicals reactive so that they can do their assigned jobs. That's not so bad until you learn that Nature hates unpaired electrons and that any excess free radicals not immediately used in chemical reactions will go to excessive lengths to steal another electron from some other molecule to make itself whole again. Unfortunately, during this robbing from-Peter-to-pay-Paul process, another free radical is formed, and this newly formed free radical may possess some very undesirable consequences, including the oxidation of fats, proteins, and DNA. When one of these important biochemicals becomes a free radical, significant molecular damage can be inflicted and aging is accelerated.

This is why the body has developed so many sophisticated defense systems (both antioxidant enzymes and molecules) to keep these newly formed free radicals under close control. Any breakdown of your free radical control systems will lead to an overproduction of excess free radicals that can accelerate the aging process. These defense systems act as a biological control rod, not unlike the control rods in nuclear reactors. In fact, the best example of a rapid overproduction of free radicals occurs in victims exposed to atomic radiation. Fortunately, we have had only two examples in World War II (unless you count the Chernobyl reactor catastrophe) on the effect that massive exposure to radiation has on free radical production in humans. The elevated production of free radicals overwhelmed the victims' internal defense systems, and long-term irreversible damage to their DNA was the result. For example, X-ray therapy for cancer patients is essentially a controlled atomic bomb blast that tries to restrict excess free radical generation to a very defined area. Anyone who has been through radiation treatments for cancer knows it has significant biological side effects. These side effects are due to excess free radical production.

The free radical mechanism of aging focuses on the overproduction of free radicals and the potential accumulated damage they can cause when not properly controlled. So, it's not the free radical mechanism of aging, but really the *excess* free radical mechanism of aging.

Let's see how and why free radicals are formed. The oxygen we breathe is a relatively inactive molecule. Unless you extract an electron from oxygen to form a free radical, it can't react with other molecules to maintain the dynamic processes that control our bodies. Once you make an oxygen free radical (also known as a reactive oxygen species), aerobic life begins. Keep in mind that for 3 billion years, there was only anaerobic life on earth, since these early single-cell organisms did not require oxygen for survival. With the advent of photosynthetic organisms about a billion years ago, oxygen began to accumulate in the atmosphere. Anaerobic organisms had to evolve to exist in this new oxygen-rich (and therefore toxic) environment. They did so by developing new ways to reduce oxygen to water and extract the energy of that conversion for themselves (see Figure 5-2 on page 42).

Energy generation during aerobic metabolism drives your cells. That energy is stored in a molecule known as adenosine triphosphate (ATP). But to make ATP you need to make oxygen free radicals. Although ATP is essential to human life, the body has a limited ability

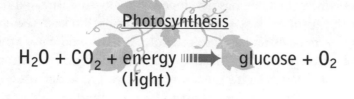

Photosynthesis

$$H_2O + CO_2 + energy \Longrightarrow glucose + O_2$$
(light)

Aerobic

$$glucose + O_2 \Longrightarrow energy + CO_2 + H_2O$$
(ATP)

Figure 5-2

to store it, so limited in fact that you can only go all out physically for about 10 seconds before your internal stores of ATP are exhausted. Once the internal supplies of ATP are used up, you have to replace this small amount of stored ATP by making more ATP, which requires the production of more free radicals.

What exactly do these life-giving oxygen free radicals look like? The most prominent ones are shown in Table 5-2

Superoxide anion is the most common oxygen-free radical since it consists of an oxygen molecule where one electron has been stripped away (usually by some enzymatic reaction involving iron-containing enzymes). This is the first step in a very complex process that leads to the formation of ATP. This same superoxide free radical can help kill invading bacteria or facilitate the synthesis of hormones like estrogen, testosterone, corticosteroids, and eicosanoids. All of these biological

TABLE 5-2

Examples of Oxygen Free Radicals

	$O_2{\cdot}^-$ or
Superoxide anion	$O_2{\cdot}^-$
Hydroxyl radical	$OH{\cdot}$
Hydrogen peroxide	H_2O_2
Peralkoxy radical	$ROO{\cdot}$

activities require superoxide formation. Unfortunately, in each of these important biological functions, some oxygen free radicals will escape, resulting in potential free radical damage. The free radical that escaped will try to steal some other neighboring molecule's electron to make itself whole. If this neighbor happens to be a fat, protein, or DNA, then one of these molecules becomes a new free radical. This is called free radical propagation that continues until the free radical is either destroyed (i.e., quenched by some antioxidant reaction) or it forms a cross-link with another free radical to form polymerized products. Polymerized products pose serious problems because they can accelerate aging.

Due to the high degree of polyunsaturation in essential fatty acids, their electrons can easily be removed by an oxygen free radical, leaving behind a new free radical that can readily interact with oxygen to form a peralkoxy free radical (see Table 5-2 on page 42). The same polyunsaturation that made the peralkoxy free radical easy to form also stabilizes this new free radical so that it can inflict even greater damage as it seeks out other cellular components from which it can strip electrons. Because of the high proclivity of essential fatty acids to oxidation, they become the primary targets of free radical-induced damage in the cell. In addition, once an essential fatty acid is oxidized, it can no longer be a substrate to make eicosanoids, the primary hormones critical for maintaining information fidelity on your biological Internet.

When a protein free radical is formed (and these are more difficult to make), it can now react with glucose molecules to produce advanced glycosylated endproducts (AGEs) that do nothing but stick to things and cause more biological damage.

If a free radical attacks part of a DNA molecule, it makes a genetic mutation that unless corrected will be the cause of continued defective protein production in the next replication cycle. It is estimated that for every 100,000 free radicals formed only one DNA residue becomes oxidized. That doesn't seem like a lot of damage until you realize that you have 60 trillion cells making free radicals 24 hours a day. It is estimated that some 6 percent of all free radicals escape and become "rogue" free radicals. The end result of these free radicals attacking other biological components (like essential fatty acids, proteins, and DNA) is called oxidative damage (i.e., damage caused by reactive oxygen free radicals) and a growing accumulation of cellular damage. This adds up to accelerated aging at the molecular level. This is why excess free radicals are another pillar of aging.

Considering all the potential damage that excess free radicals can cause to a cell, it is not surprising that we have developed unique cellular defense systems whose sole purpose is to quench excess free radicals before they create any lasting cellular damage. The enzyme superoxide dimutase is one such example. It will seek out superoxide free radicals and convert them to hydrogen peroxide. Other enzymes, such as catalase and gluathione peroxide, reduce hydrogen peroxide to water before it can combine with another superoxide free radical to form the hydroxyl free radical, the most destructive of all free radicals.

However, these enzyme systems alone are not sufficient to keep free radicals under control. This is why having adequate levels of antioxidation enzymes, along with adequate levels of diet-derived antioxidant molecules, such as vitamin E and vitamin C, is the core of your free radical defense system. Vitamin E and vitamin C sacrifice themselves to break up (i.e., quench) the free radical chain reaction and thus must be replaced in the diet on a continuing basis since your body cannot make either one.

Since vitamin E and vitamin C are such important antioxidants, these questions should be asked: Why doesn't our body make these important biochemicals? Why are we forced to get them from our diet? A partial answer may be the physical limits of your DNA. DNA is like a disk drive in a personal computer. It can carry a lot of information but eventually it becomes full. It may be that during the course of evolution loss of the genes responsible for the synthesis of vitamin E and vitamin C freed up extra genetic space for coding other important proteins. Whatever the answer, our inability to make these important antioxidants means that we are genetically designed to eat lots of fruits and vegetables (a rich source of vitamin C) and adequate level of fats (the best source of vitamin E) to help control free radical formation. As we age, our internal anti-oxidant enzymes become less active. Couple that with a decrease in the consumption of diet-derived antioxidants, the end result will be even more excess free radical production, which leads to accelerated aging.

The original free radical mechanism of aging promoted by Harman stated that excess free radicals attack nuclear DNA causing errors to be made, which would promote defective protein synthesis in the future. This theory had to be modified when it was found that the nucleus of the cell contains certain repair mechanisms that excise damaged parts of nuclear DNA and replace them on a regular basis to maintain the fidelity of the DNA's genetic information.

This mechanism of aging was later modified based on a better understanding of where free radicals are primarily produced. We usually assume that the majority of free radicals come from the environment or self-induced free radical generation by smoking. Actually, most of the free radicals in the body come from two distinct functions you need to survive.

The first is eating food. The calories in food must be converted to a form of energy the body can use. That energy molecule is ATP, which is the molecular fuel required to run our cells. To form ATP from food requires the breakdown of oxygen to form free radicals in the cells (and primarily in the mitochondria, which is the cellular factory where ATP is constantly generated). The process of energy generation from the food you eat creates massive amounts (more than 90 percent) of free radicals in the body. And the more food you eat, the more free radicals are generated. Herein lies the problem: you have to eat, but how much? Is there some zone of calories, not too little (or not enough ATP will be generated), but not too much (or overproduction of free radicals will be generated) that exists for optimal control of aging? The answer is yes, and as I will explain later, it becomes the key to anti-aging.

The other generator of free radicals is your immune system. One of the best ways to kill invading organisms is to bombard them with a burst of free radicals. And this is exactly how your lymphocytes (i.e., white cells) work. This is your front line of defense against germs, and obviously you want your free radical weaponry primed for action. Food and a strong immune system are two things you must have to maintain life, yet together they generate most of the free radicals in your system.

This isn't to say that external sources of free radicals (such as pollution or smoking) are not important, but they have a smaller impact on total free radical production than excess food consumption does. Obviously, it makes perfect sense to live in pollution-free environments and not smoke in order to cut down further on excess free radical formation. But keep in mind, the greatest source of excess free radicals remains the over-consumption of calories.

The refinement of the free radical mechanism of aging made it reasonable to assume that if the cell's power plant (i.e., mitochondria) gives out, the cell will soon follow. The mitochondria of the cell are unique because they have their own DNA for controlling the replication of the critical proteins required for the generation of cellular energy. This mitochondrial DNA is separate from the DNA located in the nucleus of the cell, and it controls the synthesis of the vast majority of the proteins required for ATP generation.

Unlike nuclear DNA, mitochondrial DNA doesn't have the internal repair system that replaces damaged parts of this genetic material. The mitochondrial DNA codes for 13 separate proteins that are critical in ATP production. This is why as you age, the mitochondria tends to become less efficient in making ATP (this is called uncoupling). This means that more and more of the free radicals produced in the mitochondria escape and continue to do damage in other parts of the cell, while at the same time you are making less ATP for cellular energy. This is a double whammy for aging: less energy production coupled with increased oxidative damage.

Basically, mitochondrial DNA is at ground zero for free radical damage and is much more likely to become damaged with increasing age than nuclear DNA. This is confirmed by studies that demonstrate that mitochondrial DNA has more mutations than nuclear DNA and becomes less efficient in producing ATP over time. Thus the stability of mitochondrial DNA may indicate your eventual longevity. Why is this important? Unlike nuclear DNA, which is composed of equal genetic contributions from your mother and father, mitochondrial DNA is derived solely from your mother. As a consequence, your ultimate longevity may not lie in choosing your parents more carefully, but in choosing your mother with greater care—especially if she comes from a family with a good history of longevity.

As I will explain in more detail later, it is possible to slow down the rate of free radical generation in the mitochondria without decreasing the production of ATP through calorie restriction. This is pretty close to the Holy Grail regarding the free radical mechanism of aging. Let it suffice for now to know that the more food you consume, the more free radicals you make. Excess free radical production is primarily a consequence of excess calorie consumption.

A newer mechanism of aging focuses on the role of advanced glycosylated end products (AGEs). AGEs are cross-linked products of carbohydrates and protein, and this cross-linking can be accelerated in the presence of free radicals. Unlike age spots on the skin which contain lipofuscin (cross-linked protein and fat), and have no impact on aging (although they are an external indicator of the aging process), AGEs have a profound impact on accelerating the chronic diseases that are associated with aging. Any time you have sustained levels of elevated blood glucose, you will generate a buildup of AGE modified proteins. Glucose is a very reactive molecule. The higher the concentration of blood glucose, the more likely it will irreversibly bind to equally reactive amino acids in proteins to ultimately form an AGE modified protein.

The first step in this complex series of reactions is the formation of a Schiff's base which occurs when glucose forms a weak bond to an animo group (usually a lysine or arginine residue) in the protein. This can then go through a chemical rearrangement to generate an Amadori adduct that begins the complex process of AGE formation, which is called a Maillard reaction. (See Figure 5-3.)

Actually, the Maillard reaction was discovered through food technology in 1912. You see it every time you add a glaze to protein. The carbohydrate-rich glaze you put on the ham (which is protein) gives rise to AGEs which polymerize to give that golden crust that everyone loves so much. The same polymerization takes place within your body if you have too much glucose floating in the bloodstream. The more AGEs you make in your body, the faster you age because glucose-modified proteins are much "stickier." As a result, they tend to adhere

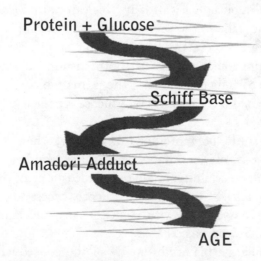

Protein + Glucose

Schiff Base

Amadori Adduct

AGE

Figure 5-3   AGE Product Generation

to the surface of arteries and capillaries, leading to increased athero-sclerosis, blindness, impotence, and kidney disease. High levels of AGEs are found in diabetics (because of their high blood glucose levels). Perhaps not surprisingly, these individuals have higher rates of atherosclerosis, stroke, blindness, impotence, and kidney failure than age-matched individuals.

Some researchers have combined the two mechanisms into a free radical-induced AGE formation. With this combined approach, the normally slow progression of AGE formation is dramatically enhanced in the presence of excess free radicals. Nonetheless, unless blood glucose is elevated, it becomes very difficult to make AGE products even in the presence of excess free radicals.

Another consequence of excess blood glucose on aging has gained even greater credence with our improved understanding of the neurobiology of the hypothalamus. There are three regions of the hypothalamus known as the ventromedial nucleus (VMN), the dorsomedial nucleus (DMN), and the lateral hypothalmic area (LHA). These regions appear to work together as an integrated network controlling neuroendocrine and neuroautonomic function. One of the functions of this integrated network is to maintain adequate levels of blood glucose to the brain. The VMN neurons that are part of this glucose regulatory network are very prone to damage by elevated levels of glucose. The result of this accumulated damage to the glucose-sensitive neurons in the VMN is an increase in pancreatic activity, including an increase in insulin output. Eventually, this can cause insulin resistance which forces the pancreas to secrete even more insulin in an effort to reduce blood glucose levels. The end result is a decrease in glucose tolerance. As previously discussed, both insulin resistance and decreased glucose tolerance are among the primary biological markers of the aging process. Thus excess blood glucose represents the final pillar of aging.

As I stated in the beginning of this chapter, when you stand back from all of these diverse mechanisms of aging, you begin to see constant themes emerge as unifying factors. At least one of the four pillars of aging (excess insulin, excess blood glucose, excess free radicals, and excess cortisol) is associated with virtually every mechanism of aging as seen in Table 5-3 on page 49.

The four pillars explain why many of the consequences of aging are highly interrelated. Excess calorie consumption causes excess free

TABLE 5-3

PILLAR OF AGING	MECHANISM
Excess Insulin	Increased calorie consumption
	Increased DNA turnover
Excess Blood Glucose	Increased AGE formation
	Neural death in VMN
Excess Free Radicals	Increased calorie consumption
	Increased AGE formation
Excess Cortisol	Neural death in the hippocampus
	Decreased eicosanoid synthesis

radical formation. Eating too many calories (especially too many carbohydrates) will also cause an increase in both insulin and blood glucose levels. Elevated insulin is a growth factor that causes cells to turn over more quickly and shorten the telomeres on the DNA. Increased blood glucose levels increase the production of AGEs. Increased insulin also inhibits the restoration of blood glucose by glucagon, thus forcing the body to secrete more cortisol as a backup system to try and increase blood glucose levels for the brain. Increased cortisol decreases eicosanoid formation, which is the underlying basis for maintaining the fidelity of hormonal communication. Although each pillar of aging speeds the aging process, combined they represent a powerful synergistic force when working in concert to accelerate aging more rapidly.

What about hormones that decrease with age? As we age, certain hormone levels do decrease. Obvious examples are estrogen in females, testosterone in males, and growth hormone, DHEA, and melatonin in everyone. Simple thinking would predict that by restoring these hormones to a more youthful level, we should be able to reverse aging. In many cases this approach has some credence, as hormonal replacement can impact the appearance of aging (and often functionality). But are changes in hormone levels a primary mechanism of aging or simply a consequence of decreased hormonal communication with the hypothalamus? The answer appears to be the latter. As an example, growth hormone secretion in the elderly can be reestablished to youthful levels by the appropriate stimulation of the pituitary gland. Growth hormone is still there in the pituitary, it just has more trouble being secreted. Thus, aging may not be as much about hormonal depletion as it is

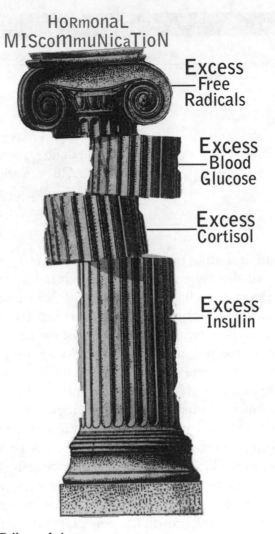

Figure 5-4   Pillars of Aging

about maintaining hormonal equilibrium, and this will be reflected in various ratios of hormones. So even if hormone levels drop, and if the ratios of key hormones are maintained, communication is not compromised. Also, notice that two of the four pillars of aging deal with excess levels of certain hormones (insulin and cortisol), not their deficiency.

The hormonal miscommunication connection is a much more comprehensive anti-aging mechanism than the others because it is impacted by each of the four pillars of aging, which are unifying factors derived from the various aging mechanisms. Hormones must talk to one another to maintain the body at peak efficiency. The hormonal miscommunication mechanism views aging as increasing hormonal static that interferes with communication within your biological Internet. Aging from this perspective suggests that increasing hormonal miscommunication occurs with increasing chronological age. Anti-aging, therefore, is best described as decreasing hormonal miscommunication as you age. I personally favor this approach as it gives hope for the possibility of reestablishing hormonal communication by nondrug, lifestyle interventions.

Therefore, what the four pillars of aging support is the real foundation of aging: increased hormonal miscommunication. Notice also that all the pillars of aging are not equal. The most important is excess insulin. This is shown in Figure 5-4 on page 50.

Any practical strategy to reverse aging must be able to reduce each of these four pillars, and ideally all at the same time. The more successfully you reduce each pillar of aging (especially excess insulin), the more you reduce hormonal miscommunication which is the foundation of aging. The most powerful tool you have to accomplish that goal is your diet.

PART II

BEGINNING YOUR ANTI-AGING ZONE LIFESTYLE TODAY

CHAPTER 6

GUARANTEED ANTI-AGING:
CALORIE RESTRICTION

Fortunately there is one magic elixir that can turn back the hands of time to improve the quality of life as we age. And there is no controversy about the use of this "drug" to reverse aging. The answer to successful anti-aging has been with us for millennia, but we never realized it. It turns out that the food we eat can provide the pathway to a longer life with better functionality, but only if we are willing to treat food with the same respect as we treat a drug.

Despite the plethora of fad diets that come and go, it is not by eating any special type of magical food that one reverses aging, but simply by eating less of it. Known as calorie restriction, it has been demonstrated for the past 60 years to be the only proven technique to reverse the aging process. In fact, in every animal species ever tested, restricting calorie intake has always produced a longer and a more functional life with less chronic disease under controlled laboratory conditions. In addition you will approximately double mortality doubling times. If that isn't a prescription for age reversal, I don't know what is.

The first recorded anti-aging experiments based on calorie restriction were not conducted on animals, but on humans in the sixteenth century. Luigi Cornaro, an Italian nobleman, was about 50 years old, when, disgusted with his deteriorating health (caused by gluttony and overindulgence), he turned to a more Spartan lifestyle. One that emphasized abstinence, moderation, and a diet consisting of coarse grain bread, meat broth with eggs, and new wine. Almost immediately his health turned around, and he lived another 48 years. Before he died (at the age of 98), he wrote one of the most popular diet books ever (at least before the twentieth century) entitled *Discourses on the Tem-*

perate Life. The premise was simple: eat enough food to maintain yourself, but never eat too many calories. Today we call that calorie restriction.

Calorie restriction is not the same as malnutrition, extended fasting, or starvation. These dietary practices accelerate the aging process because key macronutrients (essential amino acids and essential fatty acids) are deficient. Furthermore extended fasting or starvation also generate deficiencies in micronutrients (vitamins and minerals). Calorie restriction, on the other hand, should provide adequate levels of both protein (thereby preserving lean body mass) and essential fat (necessary for the production of eicosanoids), as well as enough carbohydrates to maintain adequate brain function. At the same time, it should provide adequate levels of micronutrients. Finally, calorie restriction means eating smaller meals throughout the day, to control nutrient intake just like taking an intravenous drug.

While there is total consensus that calorie restriction works to reverse aging, the tricky part of calorie restriction is its practical application to humans. The benefits of calorie restriction in rodents appear to be based only on the total number of calories consumed, but not all calories are the same if you consider the long-term functioning of an organism. You need adequate amounts of protein (but not too much) to meet your daily requirement of essential amino acids. You need adequate amounts of fat (but not too much) to meet your daily requirement of essential fatty acids. The key to practical calorie restriction is to determine the minimum level of carbohydrate you need to function efficiently. The intake of carbohydrate will increase insulin levels, but you will always need some insulin to drive nutrients into cells because without adequate levels of insulin, your cells will essentially starve to death. But having the appropriate amount of carbohydrate allows the body to perform its daily functions, but without the overproduction of free radicals, glucose, or insulin. However, too low an intake of carbohydrates will place the body into an abnormal state known as ketosis. In essence you need a zone of carbohydrates (not too much, not too little) plus similar zones of protein and fat to achieve calorie restriction with the desired anti-aging benefits.

How powerful is calorie restriction if it meets all of these requirements? If you reduce your usual total calorie intake by 40 percent, you get some pretty impressive results. Just how impressive is shown in Table 6-1 on page 57.

TABLE 6-1

Physiological Benefits of Calorie Restriction

Increased maximum life span
Increased neurotransmitter receptors
Increased learning ability
Increased immune system function
Increased kidney function
Increased length of female fertility

Decreased fat accumulation
Decreased loss of bone mass
Decreased blood glucose levels
Decreased insulin levels
Decreased cancer
Decreased autoimmune disease
Decreased blood lipid levels
Decreased heart disease
Decreased diabetes

If there is a Holy Grail of anti-aging, calorie restriction is pretty close to it. On the other hand, maybe it's not that calorie restriction actually provides these benefits, but that gluttony promotes the decrease in longevity. That is why gluttony remains one of the seven deadly sins as well as the most widely practiced one in America, where you can eat all you want at any time of day. Just like control animals in calorie restriction experiments, it appears that unrestricted eating is the best way to accelerate aging and reduce longevity.

So why does calorie restriction produce such magical results? Actually it works on three different levels. The first level involves the free radical mechanism of aging. As discussed earlier, the more free radicals you are exposed to, the faster you age. And one of the best ways to be bombarded by excess free radicals is to consume too many calories.

Your body is an extremely efficient piece of machinery that can absorb virtually all the food you consume. The trouble is that it has to do something with all that incoming food. The only choices for your body are to (a) turn these incoming calories into something that can be either used immediately for energy or (b) process these calories into some form that can be stored and eventually used for energy in the future. In either case, your body has to use oxygen to initate these biochemical processes. At the molecular level, the processing of incoming calories requires ATP. Since your body stores very little ATP in the cells, you have to make more ATP, which requires the production of more free radicals. The fewer calories you consume, the less energy is required to process the incoming food and the fewer free radicals you make. The fewer free radicals you make, the longer you live. Actually, it's pretty simple.

Calorie restriction reduces oxidative damage not only because less oxygen is consumed, but also because there is a greater efficiency in making ATP with fewer escaping free radicals. When calorie restriction begins, there is a transient drop in metabolism—but within a few weeks, the metabolism of calorie-restricted animals (based on their lean body mass) is equal to, if not higher than, those animals fed to their hearts' content. As a result of calorie restriction, metabolism actually becomes more efficient with reduced free radical formation. This is the molecular equivalent of having your cake and eating it too.

Calorie restriction also causes an increase in protective enzymes, such as superoxide dimutase (that reduces the superoxide free radicals into hydrogen peroxide), and both glutathione peroxidase and catalase (that reduce hydrogen peroxide into water). In addition, the synthesis of melatonin also increases with calorie restriction. This is important since melatonin is a very efficient scavenger of hydroxyl free radicals. The increased production of antioxidative defense systems through calorie restriction further decreases the likelihood of forming the destructive hydroxyl free radicals, which are the true villains that promote cellular damage.

The second important way that calorie restriction works to reverse aging is by reducing excess blood glucose levels. Glucose can combine with protein to make advanced glycosylated end products (AGEs). As discussed earlier, these AGEs represent a real problem for the body. They are sticky and tend to adhere to places they shouldn't. They accelerate the occlusion of blood vessels and capillaries that serve the eyes, heart, brain, and kidneys. The clinical consequences of increased AGEs are a corresponding increase in blindness, heart attack, stroke, and kidney failure.

Another complicating factor for elevated blood glucose levels is glucose induced toxicity in the hypothalamus. As discussed earlier, the hypothalamus is the central control point for integrating and orchestrating incoming information and sending out the correct hormones in response to this information. The ventriomedial nucleus (VMN) in the hypothalamus is primarily responsible for sensing the amount of glucose in the bloodstream and controlling the activity of the pancreas, whose job it is to stabilize blood sugar. In the presence of continually high glucose levels, the glucoreceptors in the VMN become damaged, leading to pancreatic hyperactivity. Blood glucose levels are not as well regulated, and larger swings in blood glucose peaks and valleys are experienced. The higher the blood glucose (due to excess carbohydrate consumption), the more damage the VMN incurs, and this promotes additional increases in insulin secretion. This increased insulin promotes insulin resistance which in turn decreases your tolerance to glucose, both of which are primary markers of aging.

The third and perhaps the most important way calorie restriction retards aging is by reducing excess insulin levels. Since insulin is secreted in response to incoming calories (and primarily carbohydrates), fewer calories consumed mean less insulin is secreted. By making less insulin you favorably increase the production of the "good" eicosanoids that ultimately control the communication fidelity of your biological Internet. Thus, lower insulin means better hormonal communication throughout the body. On the other hand, eating too many calories containing an abundance of carbohydrates is the best way to accelerate aging. This is exactly what Americans have been doing for the past 15 years.

Another important benefit of reduced insulin secretion is the stabilization of blood glucose levels. If you are producing excess cortisol in an attempt to restore blood glucose levels (due to lack of protein to stimulate glucagon), then simply following a calorie-restricted diet that contains adequate protein will eliminate that need, since excess cortisol is no longer required to maintain an adequate supply of glucose to the brain. Excess cortisol not only inhibits the formation of eicosanoids, but also kills cortisol-sensitive cells in the brain and the thymus. The result is decreased brain and immune function. Two very good reasons to lower excess cortisol levels.

As I will describe in a later chapter, much of the information flow in your biological Internet is controlled by eicosanoids acting as a backup system to maintain the transmission of hormonal signals. By controlling insulin, you reestablish a more appropriate eicosanoid balance, or zone, thus restoring better hormonal communication. Since essential fatty acids (the precursors of eicosanoids) are the most likely targets for free radical attacks, any reduction of excess free radical formation will only benefit eicosanoid formation and improve hormonal communication will be maintained.

It is through these three different but related molecular mechanisms (decreased free radical production, decreased blood glucose levels, and decreased insulin levels) that calorie restriction appears to increase not only longevity (less death from diseases associated with aging) in animals, but also to increase the maximum life span (slowing of the general deterioration of the body with time). But remember that the true criteria for any anti-aging intervention is the increase in the mortality doubling time. Calorie restriction in rats (the most studied species) nearly doubles the mortality doubling time from an average of 101 days to 197 days.

Much of our knowledge on calorie restriction comes from small animal studies (in particular mice and rats). From an evolutionary standpoint, rats and mice may have very different metabolic mechanisms than man. Fortunately, they are not the only species upon which such studies have been conducted. One of the animals most genetically similar to man is the rhesus monkey, which makes it useful to ask what are the benefits of calorie restriction in these animals before jumping to humans. Such experiments are ongoing, and they appear to confirm all the previous small animal data. Rhesus monkeys on a calorie-restricted diet have less obesity, lower blood pressure, lower cholesterol, lower blood glucose, and lower fasting insulin than the same animals fed a higher level of calories. Also levels of several hormones (melatonin and DHEA) that normally decrease during aging, begin to rise with calorie restriction. If we are to believe 60 years of animal research coupled with some very compelling primate trials, then it is not too great a leap of faith to believe that calorie restriction (but not malnutrition) is the single easiest way to improve longevity, because it reduces all four pillars of aging simultaneously.

But does it really work in humans? Let's take as one example the society with the largest percentage of legitimate centenarians: the Okinawans. The Okinawans have more than four times the number of centenarians per 100,000 population as the Japanese do, and their death rate of people between the ages of 60 and 64 is 60 percent lower than the Japanese. In fact, their death rate from stroke, cancer, and heart disease is approximately 60 percent less than the Japanese. The diet of Okinawans is also slightly different from the Japanese. Okinawans eat a higher amount of pork and less rice than the Japanese, and they also consume three times as many vegetables and double the amount of fish. However, the Okinawan diet typically contains between 20 to 40 percent fewer calories than the standard Japanese diet. Therein lies a major clue to their longevity: calorie restriction. But it is calorie restriction that includes adequate protein, adequate essential fat (from the fish), and moderate amounts of carbohydrates (primarily from low glycemic vegetables which have a very low carbohydrate density) that is the key.

Do we have other examples that demonstrate the effect of calorie restriction in humans? Yes. During World War II, Norwegians were subjected to a high degree of calorie restriction because much of the indigenous food supply was shipped to Germany. It is estimated that the typical Norwegian's calorie consumption dropped by nearly 40 percent in comparison to prewar levels, and their primary source of protein was fish. Perhaps, not surprisingly, their mortality from heart attacks dropped by 50 percent in a four-year period. After the war, when their consumption of calories increased again, the heart attack rate quickly jumped back to the pre-World War II levels.

An even more recent experiment in calorie restriction was the Biosphere experiment in which seven volunteers locked themselves in isolation and were limited to their own resources to grow food. Calorie restriction was nearly 30 percent less than before they entered the Biosphere, but every cardiovascular risk parameter was significantly lower after six months.

But each of the above human examples would be considered by many to be deprivation diets. Can the benefits of calorie restriction be achieved without continuous hunger and deprivation (which would be especially difficult in the land of plenty)?

Does such a diet exist that real people can adhere to without being constantly hungry? Yes, it's called the Zone Diet.

CHAPTER 7

THE ZONE DIET:
CALORIE RESTRICTION WITHOUT HUNGER OR DEPRIVATION

In the next to last chapter in my first book, *The Zone*, I pointed out that one of the many long-term benefits of the Zone Diet is its impact on aging. Why? Because the Zone Diet is a calorie-restricted diet, but surprisingly one without deprivation or hunger. The Zone Diet is based on maintaining key hormonal systems in zones (not too high, not too low). It is rich in vitamins and minerals since the Zone Diet uses primarily low-density carbohydrates (like fruits and vegetables) rich in these micronutrients and provides adequate protein and essential fat. The Zone Diet is based upon treating food with the same respect as any prescription drug by understanding food from a hormonal perspective. The core of the Zone Diet is the realization that this is the way we were genetically designed to eat. In the final analysis, the Zone Diet is about hormonal thinking, which is very different than caloric thinking. The food doesn't change, it is only how you perceive food that changes. And food provides the hormonal control and restoration of hormonal communication that are the keys to any successful anti-aging program.

Our genes have not changed in the last 100,000 years. During much of that evolutionary time, high-density carbohydrates like starches and grains were never part of man's diet. In fact, grains were only introduced 10,000 years ago with the dawn of agriculture. This doesn't mean we have to eat the same diet as neo-Paleolithic man (even though our genes are the same). After all, we are about to enter the twenty-first century. But it does mean that we can use our new knowledge about the hormonal effects of food to construct diets that generate the optimal hormonal responses at every meal (and with a far greater variety of foods than at any time in the history of man) based on our genetic makeup. This makes the Zone Diet infinitely flexible and adaptable for any culture and every culinary taste or philosophy.

The Zone Diet may be the most misunderstood nutritional program in history. First, it is not a diet in the typical sense. The word diet usually implies short-term deprivation, and then reverting back to old dietary habits. The Zone Diet is a lifelong program. Second, the Zone Diet is not about losing weight. It is a program designed to use food as a drug to control insulin and by doing so, it improves the production of "good" eicosanoids that help maintain information flow in your biological Internet. Fat loss is simply a pleasant side effect of improved insulin control. Third, the Zone Diet is not a high-protein diet because it provides adequate (not excessive) protein in controlled amounts throughout the day to maintain your lean body mass.

There is little need to go into the how-tos of the Zone Diet since I have done that in great detail in *The Zone, Mastering the Zone, Zone Perfect Meals in Minutes,* and *Zone Food Blocks.* These books show you how to prepare your anti-aging "drug" at every meal with ease. The important thing is to be consistent at every meal. Hormonally you are only as good as your last meal, and hormonally you are only as good as your next meal. Anti-aging is a lot like pregnancy, either you are or you aren't. If your last meal did not reverse the aging process, then it accelerated it. All you have to do is be consistent. But that's true of taking any drug.

If you're not familiar with basic Zone concepts, let me give you a thumbnail sketch. The first key is to have some low-fat protein at every meal and snack. The maximum amount of protein you would consume at any meal is no larger or thicker than the palm of your hand. Then divide your plate at each meal into three equal-sized sections. Whatever the volume of protein you plan to eat, put it in one of these sections. The other two sections you will fill primarily with low glycemic vegetables, and then always have a piece of fruit for dessert. Add a dash of monounsaturated fat like olive oil, slivered almonds, or gucamole, and there you have a Zone meal. Just make every meal like that. Snacks are the same but only about one-third the size of a Zone meal. A typical day in the Zone consists of three Zone meals and two Zone snacks with never more than five hours passing between a Zone meal or two to three hours after having a Zone snack. Notice at no point have you counted calories or grams, you are simply using your eyeball to balance your plate to make a hormonally correct meal.

So, with this quick summary on the Zone Diet, let's go back and list the key factors essential for successful calorie restriction. These are listed in Table 7-1.

TABLE 7-1

Key Factors for an Anti-aging Calorie Restriction Diet

- Adequate protein
- Adequate essential fats
- Adequate levels of carbohydrate for optimal brain function
- Adequate vitamins and minerals

Once you achieve these goals, any excess calories will increase free radical formation. However, anything less than the above will lead to malnutrition. Both possibilities (too few calories or too many calories) will increase the rate of aging.

Let's start with protein first. Of the 20 amino acids used in building protein, 8 of them can't be made by the human body. These are called the essential amino acids. The reason they are essential is that without them in the diet you would die.

The body is constantly making new protein to replace enzymes, synthesize antibodies, renew cell membranes, make new structural proteins, etc. It's as if you have a very complex assembly line using a very precise blueprint (consisting of messenger RNA) to make exceptionally complex products (proteins) which require a minimum supply of parts (amino acids). If one of these key parts (an essential amino acid) is missing, the production of new protein stops. You have 60 trillion factories (cells) in your body where these production lines are working 24 hours per day. If enough essential amino acids aren't present in the parts bin of each cell, local production stops. It's basically an amino acid strike. The body will sense this manufacturing discord and immediately start tearing down existing muscle to obtain the missing parts. New protein production goes on, but to the detriment of existing muscle mass. That's not a very good way of slowing the aging process: tearing down muscle to obtain spare parts (essential amino acids) that could easily be supplied by the diet. This is why you want to have adequate dietary protein in order to preserve existing muscle mass. Furthermore, you want to spread this protein intake throughout the day so that the body is never exposed to too much protein at one time. When that occurs, any excess protein (including essential amino acids) that cannot be immediately utilized in the part bins are converted to stored fat. The first step in this process of fat storage of excess protein intake is the breakdown of the amino group of the constituent amino acids, which will put a significant load on the kidneys. So not only do you want adequate protein (with sufficient amounts of essential amino acids), but you want that protein entering the system in small amounts throughout the day like the intravenous drip of a drug.

The second requirement for successful calorie restriction is the intake of adequate amounts of essential fatty acids. These include both omega-3 and omega-6 essential fatty acids. Like essential amino acids, the human body cannot make these essential fatty acids, therefore they must also be part of the diet. They are important because they are the building blocks of eicosanoids, the hormones that maintain the fidelity of information transfer to your biological Internet.

The designations omega-3 and omega-6 describe the positions in the fatty acids that contain double bonds. The positions of the double bonds determine their three-dimensional structure, and thus what type of eicosanoids are formed. If you are eating adequate levels of low-fat protein, then you are getting enough omega-6 essential fatty acids. However, omega-3 essential fatty acids, especially the longer-chained ones—such as eicosapentaenoic acid (EPA)—are not so easy to come by. These are found in cold-water fish. There is nothing magical about fish other than they simply happen to be at the end of the food chain that starts with plankton. If plankton live in cold-water locations, they have to make EPA, which acts as a biological anti-freeze. The fish at the top of the food chain simply accumulate these fatty acids either as fish body oils or in the liver. Cod-liver oil, a rich source of long-chain omega-3 essential fatty acids, such as EPA, has been used for hundreds of years in spite of its disgusting taste. However, a more civilized way to ensure adequate amounts of EPA is to eat cold-water fish like salmon.

Then there is the third macronutrient component—carbohydrates. Unlike essential amino acids and essential fatty acids, there is no such thing as essential carbohydrates because the body can manufacture glucose from either protein or fat. There is, however, a need for sufficient carbohydrates to maintain adequate brain function and to stimulate enough insulin release to drive all of the macronutrients into their respective cells for utilization. However, any excess carbohydrate above this minimum threshold will increase insulin levels, which accelerates the rate of aging as discussed earlier.

Finally, there are vitamins and minerals found in both protein and carbohydrate sources. Since animal protein sources tend to be at the top of the food chain, they also accumulate vitamins and minerals. Carbohydrates, on the other hand, present a greater challenge as the concentration of vitamins and minerals can vary greatly. Usually the higher the carbohydrate density (i.e., starches and grains), the fewer vitamins and minerals per calorie of carbohydrate. On the other hand, the lower-density carbohydrates (like most vegetables) will have a much higher level of vitamins and minerals per calorie of carbohydrate. Fruits are intermediate in both carbohydrate density and amounts of vitamins and minerals per calorie of carbohydrate. Therefore, the solution to this dilemma of how to limit carbohydrate intake but maximize vitamin and mineral intake is to make sure that most of your carbohydrates come from vegetables, consume moderate amounts of fruits, and really ease off eating the starches and grains. By doing so, you maximize your vitamin and mineral intake without consuming excess carbohydrate calories.

The final key to a successful anti-aging diet is to maintain tight control of insulin. Excess carbohydrates have a powerful stimulatory effect on insulin. Excess protein has a very slight stimulatory effect on insulin, but a strong stimulatory effect on the counterregulatory hormone glucagon that moderates insulin levels. Therefore the balance of protein to carbohydrate at *each* meal is important for insulin stabilization.

What about fat? Fat has no effect on insulin or glucagon. However, fat does slow the entry rate of any carbohydrate into the bloodstream and also sends hormonal signals to the brain registering satiety. Therefore, if extra fat is added to the diet, it should be in the form of monounsaturated fat since it cannot be made into eicosanoids, and thus preserves the critical balance of omega-3 to omega-6 essential fatty acids needed for eicosanoid synthesis.

Taking all of this into account would seem like a formidable task to ensure that all these conditions are met. Yet this was my goal in developing the Zone Diet. It was designed to control insulin levels with the least amount of calories consistent with maximum physical and mental performance throughout the day. As you can see, the Zone

Diet operates under more complex constraints than a typical calorie-restricted diet used in experimental test animals. But the important thing for you is to realize that all of this intricate hormonal control technology is incredibly easy to access with the Zone Diet.

But just to convince you that you won't starve on the Zone Diet, let's go back to understand how Zone meals can achieve the benefits of calorie restriction without hunger or deprivation. In fact, for many people, eating all the food required on the Zone Diet may be difficult.

The suggested calorie intake for the typical American female is 2,000 calories per day, and 2,500 calories per day for the typical American male. So to achieve the anti-aging benefits of calorie restriction (a 40 percent reduction in usual calorie consumption), the typical American female should consume about 1,200 calories per day, and the average American male about 1,500 calories per day. Obviously, you would realize all the benefits of calorie restriction, but who could exist by eating so few calories? Perhaps a far better question to ask is who could eat all of this food if they followed the Zone Diet.

To reinforce the fact that Zone meals provide more than adequate amounts of food, on the following pages I have included three days of anti-aging Zone meals and snacks for the typical American male and female. Each day would provide approproximately 1,200 calories for a female and 1,500 calories for a male. These meals were constructed by Master Chef Scott C. Lane, who also designed the meals in *Mastering the Zone* and *Zone Perfect Meals in Minutes*.

TABLE 7-2

Three Days in the Zone for Typical Women and Men

DAY 1 FOR THE TYPICAL FEMALE

BREAKFAST

SMOTHERED VEGETABLE CHEESE OMELETTE

½ cup egg substitute
1 ounce low-fat shredded Cheddar cheese
¼ cup canned mushrooms, chopped

½ cup frozen bell peppers, chopped
¼ cup frozen pearl onions
¾ cup tomatoes, seeded and diced
¼ cup salsa*
¾ teaspoon cornstarch
½ orange, quartered
1 teaspoon olive oil, divided
¼ teaspoon garlic, minced
⅛ teaspoon celery salt
¼ teaspoon Worcestershire Sauce
1 teaspoon cider vinegar
Salt and pepper to taste

In a medium nonstick sauté pan heat ⅔ teaspoon oil. Add mushrooms and saute for 3 minutes. Stir in peppers and cook an additional 3 minutes. Add onions, tomatoes salsa, and cornstarch to form a sauce. (Mix cornstarch with a little water to dissolve it before adding to pan.) Heat remaining oil in a second sauté pan. In a small bowl combine egg substitute, garlic, celery salt, Worcestershire Sauce, cider vinegar, salt and pepper. Pour into second sauté pan. Cook until almost set. Spoon vegetable mixture onto half of omelette. Fold over and cook for an additional 3 to 5 minutes. Lift with spatula onto serving dish. Top with shredded cheese and serve. Garnish with quartered orange.

*NOTE: Salsa comes with different levels of heat. Choose one that best fits your taste.

LUNCH

SAUTÉED STEAK WITH VEGETABLE MEDLEY

3 ounces sirloin steak, ¾" thick
1½ cups tomatoes, chopped
¼ cup frozen pearl onions
¾ cup frozen green beans
1½ cups frozen chopped spinach
¼ cup cooked kidney beans
½ kiwi, sliced

1 teaspoon olive oil, divided
1 teaspoon garlic, minced
$\frac{1}{4}$ teaspoon Worcestershire Sauce
$\frac{1}{8}$ teaspoon celery salt
2 teaspoons cider vinegar
$\frac{1}{2}$ teaspoon parsley, chopped
Salt and pepper to taste

In a medium nonstick sauté pan, heat $\frac{1}{3}$ teaspoon oil. Combine all vegetables and seasonings and sauté 5 to 7 minutes until crisp-tender. In a second sauté pan heat remaining oil and sauté steak until cooked to the desired degree. Place steak on one side of serving dish, vegetables on the other side of serving dish; garnish with kiwi slices.

LATE AFTERNOON SNACK

GRANNY SMITH APPLE WRAPPED IN HAM

$1\frac{1}{2}$ ounces, deli-style ham, diced
$\frac{1}{2}$ Granny Smith apple, cored and diced*
1 macadamia nut, finely diced

Wrap ham around diced apple pieces and secure with a toothpick. Arrange on serving dish and garnish with diced macadamia nut.

*NOTE: Dip diced apple pieces in lemon juice to prevent browning (oxidation) from occurring.

DINNER

NEW ORLEANS CREOLE-STYLE CHICKEN

3 ounces chicken tenderloins, $\frac{1}{2}$" cubes
$\frac{1}{4}$ cup frozen chopped onion
$\frac{1}{2}$ cup Zoned Barbecue Sauce (*see page 84*)
$\frac{1}{2}$ cup canned mushrooms, sliced
$\frac{3}{4}$ cup celery, sliced
$1\frac{1}{2}$ cups frozen red and green pepper strips
1 teaspoon olive oil

1 teaspoon chili powder
½ teaspoon dry red wine
2 teaspoons garlic, minced

Heat oil in medium nonstick sauté pan, add chicken, onion, mushrooms, celery, pepper strips, chili powder, wine and garlic. Stir-fry until chicken is cooked and vegetables are tender. Stir in Zoned Barbecue Sauce and cook an additional 3 minutes. Spoon onto heated plate and serve.

LATE EVENING SNACK

WINE AND CHEESE

4 ounces of wine
1 ounce of cheese

DAY 2 FOR THE TYPICAL FEMALE

BREAKFAST

OMELETTE FLORENTINE

½ cup egg substitute
½ ounce Cheddar cheese, fat-free shredded
¾ ounce deli-style ham, diced
¼ cup, frozen onion, diced
1½ cups frozen chopped spinach
¾ cup tomatoes, chopped
¼ cup, salsa*
¼ cup cooked kidney beans, rinsed
2 teaspoons cornstarch
1 teaspoon olive oil, divided
¼ teaspoon garlic, minced
⅛ teaspoon chili powder
1 teaspoon apple cider vinegar
¼ teaspoon cilantro, chopped

⅛ teaspoon celery salt
Salt and pepper to taste

In a medium nonstick sauté pan, heat ⅓ teaspoon of oil. Combine onion, spinach, tomato, salsa, kidney beans, and seasonings. (Mix cornstarch with a little water to dissolve it before adding to pan.) Cook for 5 to 8 minutes, stirring occasionally. In a second sauté pan, heat remaining oil. Using a medium bowl blend egg substitute, ham, salt, and pepper. Pour egg mixture into pan and stir to distribute ham evenly. Cook until set. Flip omelette over with spatula and cook another 2 minutes. Place omelette on serving plate and spoon spinach mixture onto half of omelette. Fold omelette over and sprinkle with cheese and serve.

*NOTE: Salsa comes with different levels of heat. Choose one that best fits your taste.

LUNCH

MEDITERRANEAN BEEF SALAD

3 ounces beef eye of round, ⅛″ slices, cut in half-inch pieces
1½ cups frozen mixed pepper strips
¾ cup frozen chopped onion
¾ cup Zoned Mushroom Sauce (*see page 83*)
2 cups garden salad mix (lettuce and shredded red cabbage)
1 teaspoon olive oil
⅛ teaspoon Worcestershire Sauce
⅛ teaspoon red wine
Salt and pepper to taste

In a nonstick sauté pan, add oil, beef, pepper, onions, Worcestershire Sauce, and red wine. Cook until beef is browned and pepper and onions are tender, then add Zoned Mushroom Sauce. Cover and simmer for 5 minutes until mixture is hot, stirring occasionally to blend flavors. On a large oval plate arrange garden salad mix. Spoon beef and vegetable mixture onto the center of plate on top of garden salad. Sprinkle with salt and pepper and serve immediately.

LATE AFTERNOON SNACK

CHIPS AND SALSA

1 ounce Cheddar cheese, fat-free shredded
½ ounce, baked tortilla chips
1 tablespoon, salsa*
1 tablespoon, pureed avocado

Place tortilla chips on snack plate. Blend avocado with salsa and pour over tortilla chips, then sprinkle with shredded cheese and serve.

*NOTE: Salsa comes with different levels of heat. Choose one that best fits your taste.

DINNER

PEPPERY STIR-FRY

6 ounces extra-firm tofu, diced
1 teaspoon cornstarch
¾ cup canned tomatoes, chopped
1 cup frozen mixed pepper strips
¼ cup frozen chopped onion
¼ cup chickpeas, rinsed
1 teaspoon olive oil
⅛ teaspoon celery salt
¼ teaspoon Worcestershire Sauce
1 teaspoon garlic, minced
2 teaspoons cider vinegar
Dash hot pepper sauce
⅛ teaspoon paprika
⅓ cup lemon and lime-flavored water
Dash lemon and herb seasoning

In a medium nonstick sauté pan, heat ⅔ teaspoon of oil. Add tofu, celery salt, and Worcestershire Sauce. Stir-fry until browned and crusted on all sides. In second pan heat remaining oil. Add peppers, onion, chickpeas, garlic, vinegar, hot pepper sauce, and paprika. Cook until the vegetables are tender. Add tomatoes, water, and cornstarch.

(Mix cornstarch with water to dissolve it before adding to saute pan.) Combine tofu and vegetable mixture. Spoon onto serving plate and sprinkle with lemon and herb seasoning.

LATE EVENING SNACK

FRUIT AND CHEESE

1 cup strawberries
1 ounce low-fat cheese
3 almonds

DAY 3 FOR THE TYPICAL FEMALE

BREAKFAST

CHEESY WINTER FRUIT COMPOTE

3/4 cup low-fat cottage cheese
1/2 grapefruit, in sections
1/3 cup mandarin orange sections
1/2 Granny Smith apple, cored and chopped
3 teaspoons almonds, slivered and toasted
1/8 teaspoon cinnamon
1/8 teaspoon nutmeg
Paprika

In small mixing bowl combine cottage cheese with cinnamon and nutmeg. Mound onto serving dish. Arrange grapefruit and orange sections around cheese. Combine almonds and apple pieces, spoon onto cheese. Sprinkle paprika over cheese and serve.

LUNCH

BARBECUE CHICKEN SALAD

3 ounces chicken tenderloins, diced (or skinless chicken breast)
1½ cups frozen mixed pepper strips

½ cup frozen chopped onions
¼ cup, Zoned Barbecue Sauce (*see page 84*)
1 cup garden salad mix (lettuce and shredded red cabbage)
1 cup shredded cabbage (or cole slaw mix)
1 teaspoon olive oil
⅛ teaspoon cider vinegar
⅛ teaspoon Worcestershire Sauce
1 teaspoon minced garlic
Salt and pepper to taste

In a nonstick sauté pan, add oil, chicken tenderloins, peppers, onion, vinegar, Worcestershire Sauce, and garlic. Cook until chicken is browned and vegetables are tender, then add Zoned Barbecue Sauce. Cover and simmer for 5 minutes until mixture is hot, stirring occasionally to blend flavors. Blend together garden salad mix and shredded cabbage, then place blended salad-cabbage mixture on a large oval plate. Spoon chicken and vegetable mixture onto the center of plate on top of salad-cabbage mixture. Sprinkle with salt and pepper and serve immediately.

LATE AFTERNOON SNACK

TOMATO SALAD

1 ounce Cheddar cheese, fat-free shredded
2 tomatoes, diced
⅓ teaspoon, olive oil
1 garlic clove, minced
½ teaspoon, fresh basil leaf, chopped
Paprika
Salt and pepper

Using a knife, cut tomatoes in half, then carefully cut out the insides of the tomatoes to create tomato shells. Sprinkle insides of tomatoes with salt and pepper. Dice tomato pulp into small chunks. In a mixing bowl combine diced tomato chunks, garlic, basil, oil, and cheese. Place tomato shells on snack plate, then stuff tomatoes with cheese mixture and let any excess mixture overflow tomato shells onto snack plate. Sprinkle with paprika and serve.

DINNER

SALMON WITH ASIAN FRUITY SALSA

4½ ounces salmon steak
½ cup blackberries
½ cup salsa*
½ cup canned pineapple cubes
½ Granny Smith apple, cored and diced
⅔ teaspoon olive oil
2 teaspoons soy sauce
1 teaspoon gingerroot, chopped
½ teaspoon dill
Dash hot pepper sauce

Brush baking dish with oil, place salmon steak in baking dish. Sprinkle with soy sauce, gingerroot, dill, and hot pepper sauce. Cover and bake in a preheated 350-degree oven for 30 to 35 minutes. In a medium bowl, combine salsa and fruit. Place fish on one side of a serving plate and salsa beside it.

*We use a medium salsa; use whatever heat you prefer.

LATE EVENING SNACK

HUMMUS DEVILED EGGS

2 hard-boiled eggs
1 ounce hummus

Cut the hard-boiled eggs in half, and discard the egg yolks. Fill each half of the hard-boiled egg-white with the hummus.

DAY 1 FOR THE TYPICAL MALE

BREAKFAST

SMOTHERED VEGETABLE CHEESE OMELETTE

¾ cup egg substitute
1 ounce low-fat shredded Cheddar cheese

¼ cup canned mushrooms, chopped
½ cup frozen bell peppers, chopped
½ cup frozen pearl onions
1 cup tomatoes, seeded and diced
¼ cup salsa*
1 teaspoon cornstarch
1 orange, quartered
1⅓ teaspoons olive oil, divided
¼ teaspoon garlic, minced
⅛ teaspoon celery salt
⅛ teaspoon Worcestershire Sauce
1 teaspoon cider vinegar
Salt and pepper to taste

In a medium nonstick sauté pan heat ⅔ teaspoon oil. Add mushrooms and sauté for 3 minutes. Stir in peppers and cook an additional 3 minutes. Add onions, tomatoes salsa, and cornstarch to form a sauce. (Mix cornstarch with a little water to dissolve it before adding to pan.) Heat remaining oil in a second sauté pan. In a small bowl combine egg substitute, garlic, celery salt, Worcestershire Sauce, cider vinegar, salt and pepper. Pour into second sauté pan. Cook until almost set. Spoon vegetable mixture onto half of omelette. Fold over and cook for an additional 3 to 5 minutes. Lift with spatula onto serving dish. Top with shredded cheese and serve. Garnish with quartered orange.

*NOTE: Salsa comes with different levels of heat. Choose one that best fits your taste.

LUNCH

SAUTÉED STEAK WITH VEGETABLE MEDLEY

4 ounces sirloin steak, ¾" thick
1½ cups tomatoes, chopped
1 cup frozen pearl onions
1 cup frozen green beans
2½ cups frozen chopped spinach
¼ cup cooked kidney beans
1 kiwi, sliced
1⅓ teaspoons olive oil, divided

2 teaspoons garlic, minced
¼ teaspoon Worcestershire Sauce
⅛ teaspoon celery salt
1 tablespoon cider vinegar
1 teaspoon parsley, chopped
Salt and pepper to taste

In a medium nonstick sauté pan, heat ⅓ teaspoon oil. Combine all vegetables and seasonings and sauté 5 to 7 minutes until crisp-tender. In a second sauté pan heat remaining oil and saute steak until cooked to the desired degree. Place steak on one side of serving dish, vegetables on the other side of serving dish; garnish with kiwi slices.

LATE AFTERNOON SNACK

GRANNY SMITH APPLE WRAPPED IN HAM

1½ ounces, deli-style ham, diced
½ Granny Smith apple, cored and diced*
1 macadamia nut, finely diced

Wrap ham around diced apple pieces and secure with a toothpick. Arrange on serving dish and garnish with diced macadamia nut.

   *NOTE: Dip diced apple pieces in lemon juice to prevent browning (oxidation) from occurring.

DINNER

NEW ORLEANS CREOLE-STYLE CHICKEN

4 ounces chicken tenderloins, ½" cubes
½ cup frozen chopped onion
¾ cup Zoned Barbecue Sauce (*see page 84*)
½ cup canned mushrooms, sliced
1½ cups celery, sliced
2 cups frozen red and green pepper strips
1⅓ teaspoons olive oil
1 teaspoon chili powder

½ teaspoon dry red wine
2 teaspoons garlic, minced

Heat oil in medium nonstick sauté pan, add chicken, onion, mushrooms, celery, pepper strips, chili powder, wine and garlic. Stir-fry
until chicken is cooked and vegetables are tender. Stir in Zoned Barbecue Sauce and cook an additional 3 minutes. Spoon onto heated
plate and serve.

LATE EVENING SNACK

WINE AND CHEESE

4 ounces of wine
1 ounce of cheese

DAY 2 FOR THE TYPICAL MALE

BREAKFAST

OMELETTE FLORENTINE

½ cup egg substitute
1 ounce Cheddar cheese, fat-free shredded
1½ ounces deli-style ham, diced
¾ cup, frozen onion, diced
2½ cups frozen chopped spinach
1½ cups tomatoes, chopped
¼ cup, salsa*
¼ cup cooked kidney beans, rinsed
2 teaspoons cornstarch
1⅓ teaspoons olive oil, divided
½ teaspoon garlic, minced
⅛ teaspoon chili powder
2 teaspoons apple cider vinegar

½ teaspoon cilantro, chopped
⅛ teaspoon celery salt
Salt and pepper to taste

In a medium nonstick sauté pan, heat ⅓ teaspoon of oil. Combine onion, spinach, tomato, salsa, kidney beans, and seasonings. (Mix cornstarch with a little water to dissolve it before adding to pan.) Cook for 5 to 8 minutes, stirring occasionally. In a second sauté pan, heat remaining oil. Using a medium bowl blend egg substitute, ham, salt, and pepper. Pour egg mixture into pan and stir to distribute ham evenly. Cook until set. Flip omelette over with spatula and cook another 2 minutes. Place omelette on serving plate and spoon spinach mixture onto half of omelette. Fold omelette over and sprinkle with cheese and serve.

*NOTE: Salsa comes with different levels of heat. Choose one that best fits your taste.

LUNCH

MEDITERRANEAN BEEF SALAD

4 ounces beef eye of round, ⅛" slices, cut in half-inch pieces
2 cups frozen mixed pepper strips
1 cup frozen chopped onion
1 cup Zoned Mushroom Sauce (*see page 83*)
2½ cups garden salad mix (lettuce and shredded red cabbage)
1⅓ teaspoons olive oil
⅛ teaspoon Worcestershire sauce
⅛ teaspoon red wine
Salt and pepper to taste

In a nonstick sauté pan, add oil, beef, pepper, onions, Worcestershire sauce, and red wine. Cook until beef is browned and pepper and onions are tender, then add Zoned Mushroom Sauce. Cover and simmer for 5 minutes until mixture is hot, stirring occasionally to blend flavors. On a large oval plate arrange garden salad mix. Spoon beef and vegetable mixture onto the center of plate on top of garden salad. Sprinkle with salt and pepper and serve immediately.

LATE AFTERNOON SNACK

CHIPS AND SALSA

1 ounce Cheddar cheese, fat-free shredded
1/2 ounce, baked tortilla chips
1 tablespoon, salsa*
1 tablespoon, pureed avocado

Place tortilla chips on snack plate. Blend avocado with salsa and pour over tortilla chips, then sprinkle with shredded cheese and serve.

*NOTE: Salsa comes with different levels of heat. Choose one that best fits your taste.

DINNER

PEPPERY STIR-FRY

8 ounces extra-firm tofu, diced
2 teaspoons cornstarch
3/4 cup canned tomatoes, chopped
1 1/2 cups frozen mixed pepper strips
1/2 cup frozen chopped onion
1/4 cup chickpeas, rinsed
1 1/3 teaspoons olive oil
1/8 teaspoon celery salt
1/4 teaspoon Worcestershire Sauce
1 teaspoon garlic, minced
1 tablespoon cider vinegar
Dash hot pepper sauce
1/8 teaspoon paprika
1/3 cup lemon and lime-flavored water
Dash lemon and herb seasoning

In a medium nonstick sauté pan, heat 2/3 teaspoon of oil. Add tofu, celery salt, and Worcestershire Sauce. Stir-fry until browned and crusted on all sides. In second pan heat remaining oil. Add peppers, onion, chickpeas, garlic, vinegar, hot pepper sauce, and paprika. Cook until the vegetables are tender. Add tomatoes, water and cornstarch. (Mix cornstarch with water to dissolve it before adding to sauté pan.) Combine tofu and vegetable mixture. Spoon onto serving plate and sprinkle with lemon and herb seasoning.

LATE EVENING SNACK

FRUIT AND CHEESE

1 cup strawberries
1 ounce low-fat cheese
3 almonds

DAY 3 FOR THE TYPICAL MALE

BREAKFAST

CHEESY WINTER FRUIT COMPOTE

1 cup low-fat cottage cheese
½ grapefruit, in sections
⅓ cup mandarin orange sections
1 Granny Smith apple, cored and chopped
4 teaspoons almonds, slivered and toasted
⅛ teaspoon cinnamon
⅛ teaspoon nutmeg
Paprika

In small mixing bowl combine cottage cheese with cinnamon and nutmeg. Mound onto serving dish. Arrange grapefruit and orange sections around cheese. Combine almonds and apple pieces, spoon onto cheese. Sprinkle paprika over cheese and serve.

LUNCH

BARBECUE CHICKEN SALAD

4 ounces chicken tenderloins, diced (or skinless chicken breast)
2¼ cups frozen mixed pepper strips

1 cup frozen chopped onions
½ cup, Zoned Barbecue Sauce (*see page 84*)
1½ cups garden salad mix (lettuce and shredded red cabbage)
1½ cups shredded cabbage (or cole slaw mix)
1⅓ teaspoons olive oil
⅛ teaspoon cider vinegar
⅛ teaspoon Worcestershire Sauce
1 teaspoon minced garlic
Salt and pepper to taste

In a nonstick sauté pan, add oil, chicken tenderloins, peppers, onion, vinegar, Worcestershire Sauce, and garlic. Cook until chicken is browned and vegetables are tender, then add Zoned Barbecue Sauce. Cover and simmer for 5 minutes until mixture is hot, stirring occasionally to blend flavors. Blend together garden salad mix and shredded cabbage, then place blended salad-cabbage mixture on a large oval plate. Spoon chicken and vegetable mixture onto the center of plate on top of salad-cabbage mixture. Sprinkle with salt and pepper and serve immediately.

LATE AFTERNOON SNACK

TOMATO SALAD

1 ounce Cheddar cheese, fat-free shredded
2 tomatoes, diced
⅓ teaspoon, olive oil
1 garlic clove, minced
½ teaspoon, fresh basil leaf, chopped
Paprika
Salt and pepper

Using a knife, cut tomatoes in half, then carefully cut out the insides of the tomatoes to create tomato shells. Sprinkle insides of tomatoes with salt and pepper. Dice tomato pulp into small chunks. In a mixing bowl combine diced tomato chunks, garlic, basil, oil, and cheese. Place tomato shells on snack plate, then stuff tomatoes with cheese mixture and let any excess mixture overflow tomato shells onto snack plate. Sprinkle with paprika and serve.

DINNER

SALMON WITH ASIAN FRUITY SALSA

6 ounces salmon steak
³/₄ cup blackberries
¹/₂ cup salsa*
¹/₂ cup canned pineapple cubes
¹/₂ Granny Smith apple, cored and diced
1 teaspoon olive oil
2 teaspoons soy sauce
1 teaspoon gingerroot, chopped
¹/₂ teaspoon dill
Dash hot pepper sauce

Brush baking dish with oil, place salmon steak in baking dish. Sprinkle with soy sauce, gingerroot, dill, and hot pepper sauce. Cover and bake in a preheated 350-degree oven for 30 to 35 minutes. In a medium bowl, combine salsa and fruit. Place fish on one side of a serving plate and salsa beside it.

LATE EVENING SNACK

HUMMUS DEVILED EGGS

2 hard-boiled eggs
1 ounce hummus

Cut the hard-boiled eggs in half, and discard the egg yolks. Fill each half of the hard-boiled egg-white with the hummus.

ZONED MUSHROOM SAUCE

SERVINGS: 4—1 cup (carbohydrate) serving each**

4¹/₂ cups mushrooms, sliced
10 teaspoons cornstarch
3 cups strong beef stock
¹/₈ teaspoon Worcestershire Sauce

*We use a medium salsa; use whatever heat you prefer.
**NOTE: Each cup of Zoned Mushroom Sauce contains no protein or fat. This recipe is used as a component of other Zone recipes.

1 tablespoon red wine
1/8 teaspoon chili powder
1/2 teaspoon garlic, chopped
1 tablespoon dried parsley flakes
Salt and pepper to taste

Combine all ingredients in a small saucepan to form a sauce. (Mix cornstarch with a little cold water to dissolve it before adding to saucepan.) Heat sauce to a light simmer, constantly stirring until mixture thickens. Transfer sauce mixture to a storage container, let cool and refrigerate.*

*NOTE: This sauce may be refrigerated for up to 5 days, or if you prefer the sauce may be frozen and defrosted for later use. Although the sauce is freeze-thaw stable, after sauce has been frozen and defrosted it may need to be stirred to reincorporate the small amount of moisture that forms on the sauce during the freezing and thawing process.

ZONED BARBECUE SAUCE

SERVINGS: 4—1/2 cup servings each*

4 teaspoons cornstarch
1 cup tomato puree
1/3 cup unsweetened applesauce
1 tablespoon liquid smoke flavoring
4 teaspoons garlic, minced
1 teaspoon Worcestershire sauce
3/4 cup strong chicken stock
3 tablespoons cider vinegar
1/4 teaspoon chili powder

Combine all ingredients in a small saucepan to form a sauce. (Mix cornstarch with a little cold water to dissolve it before adding to saucepan.) Heat sauce to a light simmer, constantly stirring with a whip until mixture thickens. Transfer sauce mixture to a storage container, let cool and refrigerate.**

*NOTE: Each 1/2 cup of Zoned Barbecue Sauce contains no protein or fat. This recipe is used as a component of other Zone recipes.
**NOTE: This sauce may be refrigerated for up to 5 days, or if you prefer the sauce may be frozen and defrosted for later use. Although the sauce is freeze-thaw stable, after sauce has been frozen and defrosted it may need to be stirred to reincorporate the small amount of moisture that forms on the sauce during the freezing and thawing process.

After seeing the volume of these anti-aging Zone meals, I now trust you realize that once you switch to low-density carbohydrates, you will neither be deprived on the Zone Diet nor be hungry. Yet at the same time you are guaranteed all the anti-aging benefits of calorie restriction. In the Appendix you will find another week of Zone meals for both typical males and females. In addition it includes some very simple methods to make Zone meals and snacks along with meals to eat on the road and even in fast-food restaurants.

Yet how can you possibly function on so few calories? The first reason is that you are using stored body fat for extra energy. By keeping insulin levels in a zone, you are allowing your body to access stored fat more effectively. Second, by eating small meals and snacks throughout the day, you are essentially creating an intravenous drip of nutrients (especially protein which stimulates glucagon) into the body, thus keeping insulin levels in a zone. This maintains a steady level of blood sugar, so that hunger is not present and mental acuity remains at peak levels throughout the day. Finally, you are increasing the efficiency of producing ATP, the actual biochemical fuel that drives your body's metabolism. As discussed earlier, initially with calorie restriction there is a transient decrease in metabolic rate. But within a short period of time, it actually increases to become equal, if not exceed, the metabolism of the animals who are not calorie restricted (when based on the lean body mass of each animal).

Let me return to the hunger problem since it is often assumed that intense hunger will accompany calorie restriction. That will be true on a calorie-restricted diet that doesn't have adequate levels of protein to maintain sufficient glucagon secretion (which will maintain blood glucose levels). But it is not true for the Zone Diet since each meal contains about 30 percent of the total calories in the form of low-fat protein. This amount of protein (usually about 3 ounces of low-fat protein for females and 4 ounces of low-fat protein for males) at each meal is sufficient to maintain both lean body mass and blood glucose levels. No one would seriously suggest that these protein amounts represent excessive protein levels at any one meal. The Zone Diet treats food as if it were an intravenous drug with small amounts of macronutrients delivered into the system over the course of three meals and two small snacks throughout the day. As a result, at no time is the body exposed to large amounts of incoming protein or calories. The end result is stable and controlled insulin levels.

The real power of the Zone Diet is that you don't have to be perfect at every meal since you are building up a hormonal reserve capacity. If you make a mistake at a meal (and everyone does), just make sure your next meal is hormonally correct to get you right back to the Zone. In fact, I always recommend that at least once a month you pig-out on a big carbohydrate meal just to feel miserable the next day. This will reinforce how powerful food is as a "drug."

Although the concept of calorie restriction is at the cutting edge of anti-aging research, in reality it is essentially how your grandmother told you to eat. Her advice consisted of four sound anti-aging principles:

(1) Eat small meals throughout the day.
(2) Have some protein at every meal.
(3) Always eat your fruits and vegetables.
(4) Take your cod-liver oil.

Here's how your grandmother's dietary recommendations parallel the Zone Diet. By eating small meals, you are not overproducing insulin because you are maintaining a low calorie intake and a reduced carbohydrate load. By eating some protein at every meal, you are ensuring adequate production of the hormone glucagon to balance off the insulin increase and maintain adequate blood glucose levels without calling upon backup hormonal systems like cortisol. By eating fruits and vegetables you are again making sure that the carbohydrate load of that meal is as low as possible and also maximizing the intake of vitamins and minerals with the least amount of insulin stimulation. Finally, by taking cod-liver oil (or any other suitable form of fish oils), you are making sure that adequate levels of EPA will counterbalance the levels of omega-6 fatty acids routinely found in low-fat protein sources.

So, how well does the Zone Diet integrate with the mechanisms of aging I outlined earlier? Although the concept of calorie restriction is relatively simple, once you analyze many of the other mechanisms of aging, you find that there is a unifying thread that again leads back to the Zone Diet. First as a calorie-restricted diet, the Zone Diet will reduce the production of free radicals. Second, you maintain a stable level of insulin. By keeping insulin within a stable zone, blood glucose is also stabilized, thus minimizing the production of AGEs. The stabilization of blood glucose levels will also reduce glucose-induced toxicity in the hypothalamus. Simultaneously, there is a decreased need for the activation of increased cortisol synthesis to help maintain blood glucose levels since glucagon is adequately stimulated. As a result of lowered cortisol levels, cortisol-induced neural toxicity in the brain is reduced, and eicosanoid synthesis is not unduly inhibited. The reduction of excess insulin means that there is less cellular turnover, which means less shortening of the telomere lengths of the DNA in each cell. Finally, by preventing the elevation of insulin levels, there are fewer disruptions in hormonal communication as mediated by eicosanoids. All things considered, the Zone Diet is as close to the ideal anti-aging "drug" as possible, since it positively impacts every mechanism of aging.

But does the Zone Diet work for humans in real life? To answer that question, we have to go back to that group of individuals who appear to be aging much faster than the general population. They are Type 2 diabetics.

CHAPTER 8

TYPE 2 DIABETICS:
CANARIES IN THE COAL MINE
OF AGING

In the early days of coal mining, miners would bring canaries with them into the mines. If there was a buildup of toxic gases in the mine, the canaries would die, alerting the miners to impending danger. We are all aging, but clearly there are some people who are aging faster than others. If we could identify these people, they would make the ideal human subjects to conduct dietary experiments using the Zone Diet to determine if the anti-aging benefits of a calorie-restricted diet can be achieved in humans without deprivation or hunger. In essence, they become the canaries in the coal mine of aging. One such population not only exists, but is rapidly growing in America. They are Type 2 diabetics.

These individuals are the proverbial canaries in the coal mine when it comes to aging. Type 2 diabetics age faster than others of the same age; they suffer from more chronic diseases than others of the same age; and they cost the health care system more than others of the same age. Why? Because they make more insulin and have higher blood glucose levels than their age-matched peers.

When you think of diabetics, you commonly think of individuals who can't make insulin and therefore need daily injections of this hormone to prevent death. These are Type 1 diabetics. Of the estimated 16 million diabetics in this country, Type 1 diabetics constitute a very small minority. According to the American Diabetes Association, between 90 to 95 percent of all diabetics over the age of 20 are Type 2 diabetics. Type 2 diabetics, unlike Type 1 diabetics, produce more than enough insulin, but their cells are simply just not responsive to it. They have severe insulin resistance. As a result, blood levels of both insulin and glucose build up just as they do in the animals fed *ad libitum* (i.e., eat-at-will) diets. As I discussed earlier, elevated blood glucose will accelerate glycosylation of proteins and induce neurotoxicity in the hypothalamus. As I will discuss later, elevated levels of insulin also increase the likelihood of heart disease and cancer. Therefore, the hallmarks of any successful anti-aging program should focus on the reduction of both insulin and blood glucose as well as the reduction of glycosylated proteins. Since elevated blood glucose, insulin, and glycosylated protein levels are the clinical parameters used to characterize a Type 2 diabetic, then we have the ideal subjects to begin testing the Zone Diet as a practical anti-aging diet.

In addition to being the ideal subject for testing the anti-aging potential of the Zone Diet, the Type 2 diabetic patient is also the most costly group of patients in our health care system. Because of the long-term complications associated with diabetes, such as blindness, amputation, and kidney failure, diabetic patients account for approximately 8% of all health care expenditures in this country, even though diabetics account only for about 3 percent of the population. In 1997, these expenditures were more than $77 billion dollars. That's a lot of money. Furthermore, the typical Type 2 diabetic patient cost HMOs about three to four times more than the average patient. This is because diabetic patients are two to four times more likely to have heart disease than age-matched nondiabetic subjects, they are two to four times more likely to have a stroke compared to age-matched nondiabetic subjects, and if they have a stroke, diabetic patients are two to three times more likely to die than nondiabetic patients. They are about four times more likely to become blind than the nondiabetic population and have nearly eight times the likelihood of developing cataracts and glaucoma. And diabetics are two to four times more likely to have kidney failure than nondiabetics. Add to this nightmare accelerated aging, increased rates of impotence (five times more likely) and increased likelihood of pregnancy complications, and it is clear that diabetics simply don't have what you call a great quality of life. And the final statistic is that their life expectancy is reduced between 5 and 10 years compared to nondiabetics. If there were ever a group of individuals to test out any anti-aging program, it would be Type 2 diabetics. And this is where luck played an important role for me to clinically test my theories on anti-aging.

In early 1997, I got a call from a physician who had read my first book, *The Zone,* and was impressed with the program's potential. Like any good physician, he first tried the Zone Diet himself, promptly lost 25 pounds and observed dramatic changes in his blood chemistry. That in itself was not unusual, but this same physician also happened to be the owner of a major physicians' group that had full economic responsibility for some 60,000 patients, including some 4,000 Type 2 diabetics. In medical terms, full economic responsibility is referred to as "fully capitated," meaning the physicians are paid a fixed rate by the insurance company for each patient. If they treat the patient at lower cost, they make money. If it costs more to treat the patient, they lose money. Basically it's high-stakes poker. If you decide to play this game, where can you really make money? Take those patients who cost you the most (i.e., Type 2 diabetic patients), educate them on proper diet, and presto, you should make money hand over fist since their long-term complications will be significantly reduced.

Based on this logic, the physicians' group previously hired highly trained diabetic educators for a trial program to aggressively instruct about 10 percent of their diabetic patients (or about 400 patients) according to the current treatment gospel as espoused by the American Diabetes Association (ADA). Eat more carbohydrates, eat less fat, and exercise every day. These patients received individualized instruction, attended weekly support meetings, and read lots of beautifully printed documents from the ADA. If the Type 2 diabetic patients were successful on the ADA program, then the physician group would immediately put their other diabetics on the same program, and probably extend it to all of their other patients since what's good for Type 2 diabetic patients is probably good for everyone. Unfortunately, when they analyzed their one-year costs for the pilot group of 400, they found that instead of decreasing their costs, their expenses had actually increased by some one million dollars. Rather than making money by stressing prevention, they were losing money!

This didn't make a lot of sense until the physician-owner read *The Zone*. In my book I had included a small pilot study conducted with elderly overweight Type 2 diabetic patients to show that the Zone Diet could produce clinically important benefits compared to the American Diabetes Association diet—the same diet that had just cost his physicians' group an extra million dollars in expenses for 400 patients.

Now let's go back to that eventful phone call. The physician had no question about whether or not the Zone Diet worked. Rather, his only concern was whether or not his patients would follow it. His patients had on average a seventh-grade education and for many of them, English was not their first language. Could the Zone Diet work for them? "Of course," I replied, "no problem." Hanging up the phone, I figured I had about three weeks to put together a patient educational program based on the Zone Diet to see if it could reverse a disease that had resisted the best efforts of the medical establishment for the past 30 years. Ironically, it is also during those same 30 years that Type 2 diabetes became such a major medical problem with its incidence increasing by some 600 percent. Furthermore, the chance to work with a large group of Type 2 diabetic patients at virtually no cost was a once-in-a-lifetime opportunity. What better way to put all the cards on the table and demonstrate the power of the Zone Diet to not only treat Type 2 diabetes, but also demonstrate its potential as an anti-aging program in an ideal population that is aging at an accelerated rate.

I consulted with my medical staff of one, Dr. Paul Kahl, who was one of the early believers in the Zone Diet when I first proposed it nearly a decade ago. I burst into his office and told him the news. The good news was we had our opportunity to prove the therapeutic potential of the Zone Diet. The bad news was that he was going to have to spend 6 weeks in the middle of summer in Texas to educate these patients. Meanwhile, the owner of the physician group was so convinced that the program would succeed, he wanted all 4,000 of his diabetic patients on it. (Actually he wanted all 60,000 of his patients on the program.) At this point, better judgment prevailed. I suggested that we take a quarter of those patients who had already been aggressively educated according to the American Diabetes Association guidelines for the past year and work with them as a test group. This gave us a group of approximately 100 Type 2 patients.

Paul arrived in Texas anticipating a celebration reminiscent of American troops liberating Europe in World War II. After all, he had the tool—the Zone Diet—to finally treat this growing epidemic of Type 2 diabetes and in the process make this physician group very rich. Unfortunately, reality quickly set in. While the owner of the physicians' group was totally committed to this study, let's say that the rest of the nearly 60 other physicians were not so quick to embrace this concept. And just think how the newly hired diabetic educators felt about being told their dietary educational methods were wrong. Paul was initially treated with more disdain than support.

Rather than using one-on-one individualized instruction, we split the patients into groups of 10 and 20. Paul gave four seminars each day, so that by the end of a week all 100 patients received one hour of instruction in a step-by-step approach to the Zone Diet. This was carried out for a total of four weeks. Essentially, four hours of instruction to change a lifetime of poor dietary habits.

Six weeks after the study began, the moment of truth arrived—the blood testing to determine whether or not anything beneficial was actually taking place. In reality, it wasn't a moment of truth, since we knew from the weekly sessions that each of the patients was feeling incredibly better, was more energetic, and was losing excess body fat. More telling, however, was a warning from Paul to the other physicians prior to the study that if they didn't reduce the diabetic and hypertensive medications for their patients once the program began, that within a week they would come in feeling lethargic. This is because the Zone Diet can so quickly normalize their patients' elevated blood glucose levels and high blood pressure that the medications they were currently taking would drive them into low blood glucose (i.e., hypoglycemia) and low blood pressure (i.e., hypotension). Of course, they all laughed at Paul because in a medical culture in which pills are king, they knew that it was impossible for diet to have much importance. Sure enough, within the first week of the program, many patients started complaining of low blood glucose and low blood pressure. Already, Paul was beginning to command a little more respect.

So when the 6-week test results arrived, it was no surprise to us that they were dramatic. Some of these results can be found in Table 8-1.

TABLE 8-1

Trial #1 ($n = 98$)—6-Week Blood Results

PARAMETER	START	6 WEEK	CHANGE	% CHANGE	STATISTICAL SIGNIFICANCE
Blood Glucose	171	148	−23	−13	$p < 0.001$
HgA$_{1C}$	7.8	7.0	− 0.8	−10	$p < 0.0001$
TC/HDL	4.9	4.6	− 0.3	− 6	$p = 0.002$
TG/HDL	4.3	3.4	− 0.9	−21	$p = 0.006$

Every clinical parameter important for the treatment of Type 2 diabetes had improved. This was especially important because this was basically a crossover test. For the previous year, these same patients had been on the ADA diet, with relatively little change, thus remaining at high risk for long-term diabetic complications. Now within 6 weeks, simply by changing to the Zone Diet, dramatic clinical changes were observed. More important, we now had enough patients to determine whether the changes were real.

In any human study, you always have to ask what the likelihood is that any observed change can be repeated. That reproducibility is known as statistical significance. Statistical significance (as measured by the p value) simply gives you an indication of how real the observed changes are and how likely they can be repeated if the same test is repeated. The lower the p value, the more likely the results are real. If the p value is less than 0.05, this means that if you repeat the same experiment 100 times, you are likely to get the same result 95 times. If the p value is 0.0001, this means if you repeat the same experiment 10,000 times, you are likely to get the same result 9,999 times. Considering all the variables at play in free-living humans, it is rare that human experiments ever generate low p values, and any p value of less than 0.05 is considered the gold standard.

One way to overcome this variability in free-living humans is to conduct clinical trials with thousands of very carefully screened patients in the hopes of getting some statistically significant results or place a smaller number of patients on a hospital ward where they can be constantly monitored like lab rats. And here we were trying to get statistically significant data with a relatively small number of patients who had been written off as hopeless in their ability to change their dietary lifestyles. Yet the results were stupendous, and more important, they were achieved using calorie restriction without deprivation or hunger. Their blood glucose levels dropped, their glycosylated hemoglobin levels dropped, and their cardiovascular risk profiles (both the total cholesterol/HDL cholesterol and the total triglycerides/HDL cholesterol) improved. Their biological markers of aging had been reversed. And all of this with a statistical significance rarely, if ever, observed in even the largest clinical trials using thousands of carefully screened patients.

But, the result I was not prepared for was the effect of the Zone Diet on kidney function. In selecting these patients, a couple of the more skeptical physicians included patients in the study who were already spilling protein into their urine. This condition is known as microalbuminuria, and it is the first sign of impending kidney failure. In fact, after it reaches a certain level (about 30 μg/ml), you can almost plot with precision when the patient's kidneys will fail. Kidney dialysis costs about $200,000 per year, and it is one of the reasons why the cost of diabetic health care is so high. Some of these skeptical physicians reasoned what better way to demonstrate that the Zone Diet was one of those dangerous high-protein diets than by showing that these patients would soon have even more protein appearing in their urine, thus accelerating the onset of kidney failure. Unfortunately for these critics of the Zone Diet (but fortunately for the patients), the opposite happened. There was a 56 percent reduction in their urine protein after six weeks on the Zone Diet. Although only six patients were in this subgroup, this trend was very suggestive. Not only was the Zone Diet safe for patients with kidney problems, but there was an indication that it might become the future treatment of choice to prevent kidney failure.

Of course, I was elated, not only because of the cardiovascular benefits, but also the implications for anti-aging. As I will discuss in a later chapter, these clinical changes observed in the Type 2 diabetics are the same clinical parameters that must be met to experience the anti-aging benefits of calorie restriction. But clinical improvement is of little consequence unless this dietary plan could be followed on a lifetime basis.

Although this was a calorie-restricted diet (approximately 1,400 calories for males and 1,100 calories for females), many of the patients said that they couldn't eat all of the food (because of the substitution of low-density carbohydrates, such as vegetables, for high-density carbohydrates, such as rice and pasta). More amazing is the fact that many of these patients still went to Taco Bell for dinner (see the Appendix for the meals they ate at Taco Bell), but thanks to the educational sessions, they were able to do so and still create Zone meals. Is it possible that the concept of calorie restriction and eating at Taco Bell can be mentioned in the same sentence? Yes it can, and the data proves it.

Needless to say, the owner of the physicians' group was overjoyed with the results, and much of the criticism from the other physicians and diabetic educators fell silent. But now the owner of the group challenged us by saying, "Once is great, now repeat the results." This time the physicians chose patients that I call the Type 2 diabetic plus. These patients were selected from the original pool of the 400 diabetic patients who received intensive diabetic education according to the ADA guidelines, but they also had other coexisting disease conditions, such as congestive heart failure, advanced atherosclerosis, etc. This is why I call them the "plus" patients. Compared to the first group of patients, this was a much sicker group.

In working with this group, we made one slight adjustment in the Zone Diet, adding more fish oil to their diet to provide extra amounts of long-chain omega-3 fatty acids (like EPA). As I will explain in a later chapter, this would allow them to produce even more "good" eicosanoids than the first group did. These patients were taking a supplemental dosage consisting of 6 grams of purified fish oil per day. This may sound like a lot, but it would be the same amount of long-chain omega-3 fatty acids found in two teaspoons of cod-liver oil (about 2/3 of the standard dosage that most kids got two generations ago from their grandmother). The results are shown in Table 8-2.

TABLE 8-2

Trial #2 ($n=68$)—Plus Fish Oil

PARAMETER	START	6 WEEK	CHANGE	% CHANGE	STATISTICAL SIGNIFICANCE
Insulin	30	22	− 8	−27	$p < 0.0001$
Blood Glucose	168	153	−15	− 9	$p = 0.02$
HgA$_{1C}$	7.8	7.3	− 0.5	− 6	$p < 0.0001$
TC/HDL	4.5	4.1	− 0.4	− 9	$p < 0.0001$
TG/HDL	4.2	3.1	− 0.9	−21	$p < 0.0001$

If anything, the results were virtually identical in magnitude to those of the first study, but now with an even higher degree of statistical significance. Furthermore, in this group we also measured fasting insulin levels, the hallmark of any successful anti-aging program. Those levels had dropped by some 27 percent in only 6 weeks, which was similar to the drop in the ratio of fasting triglycerides to HDL cholesterol. This is why the fasting triglyceride to HDL cholesterol ratio can be used as a surrogate marker for fasting insulin.

Since that time, we have completed a third study. These results are shown in Table 8-3.

TABLE 8-3

Trial #3 ($n = 38$)—Plus Fish Oil

PARAMETER	START	6 WEEK	CHANGE	% CHANGE	STATISTICAL SIGNIFICANCE
Blood Glucose	166	143	− 23	−14	$p < 0.0001$
HgA$_{1C}$	8.2	7.4	− 0.8	−10	$p < 0.0001$
TC/HDL	4.5	4.2	− 0.3	− 7	$p < 0.05$
TG/HDL	4.7	3.3	− 1.4	−30	$p = 0.0005$

As you might reasonably conclude, the Zone Diet seems to produce remarkably consistent results with Type 2 diabetic patients. In fact, when you average the clinical results of all three trials, you get the results seen in Table 8-4.

TABLE 8-4

Average of Three Combined Studies with Type 2 Diabetic Patients ($n = 204$)

CLINICAL PARAMETER	% CHANGE
Blood Glucose	− 12.0 ± 1.5
HgA$_{1C}$	− 8.7 ± 1.3
TC/HDL	− 7.3 ± 0.8
TG/HDL	− 24.0 ± 3.0

From the standpoint of using the Zone Diet for Type 2 diabetes treatment, these results are remarkable. But from my standpoint of using the Zone Diet as an anti-aging program, they are even more profound. The key to anti-aging using calorie restriction is the normalization of blood glucose levels and the reduction of insulin levels. Drastic calorie restriction can achieve that. But here we had the ideal human subgroup of individuals aging at a faster rate than they should, and within an incredibly short period of time (6 weeks), they had reversed their aging profile simply by making slight adjustments to their current diets without experiencing deprivation or hunger.

But is the Zone Diet only good for Type 2 diabetic patients and not average individuals? To answer that question, we ran simultaneous studies with staff members of the same physician group who were not diabetic and therefore had normal blood glucose levels. If the Zone Diet was to have an effect on them, then we should see that their blood glucose levels would remain constant, and their insulin levels would decrease. Unfortunately, testing for fasting insulin is a difficult and expensive test (that's why we could only get the physicians' group to pay for it with the second group of Type 2 patients). However, as already explained the ratio of fasting triglycerides to HDL cholesterol is a good surrogate marker for fasting insulin levels. The physicians' group routinely used that test, and therefore was willing to pay for it. So if the Zone Diet was applicable to a general population, then we would expect that blood sugar levels would remain normal and the ratio of triglycerides to HDL cholesterol would drop. And that's exactly what happened as there were no statistically significant changes in blood glucose, but significant reductions in the fasting triglyceride/HDL ratio did occur. The results are in Table 8-5.

TABLE 8-5

Studies with non-Type 2 Diabetic Patients

STUDY GROUP	TG/HDL STARTING	TG/HDL AT 6 WEEKS	PER CENT CHANGE AT 6 WEEKS	STATISTICAL SIGNIFICANCE
#1 ($n = 121$)	2.7	2.3	-15%	$p < 0.05$
#2 ($n = 56$)	3.2	2.2	-31	$p < 0.005$
#3 ($n = 38$)	3.2	2.3	-28	$p < 0.01$

The reason for the better results in the second and third studies was that the patients were given extra EPA compared to those in the first study. With the increased EPA supplementation, the percentage drop in the fasting triglyceride/HDL ratio nearly doubled, and the statistical significance of the results was also greatly improved. And as I will explain in greater detail later, results from Harvard Medical School indicate that reductions in the triglyceride/HDL ratio may be the most important factor in determing future heart attacks. This means the non-diabetic individuals decreased their risk of cardiovacular disease just as the Type 2 diabetic patients did. Furthermore, since the fasting triglyceride/HDL cholesterol is a surrogate marker for fasting insulin, these results are strongly suggestive that they have also lowered insulin, the primary pillar of aging.

Yet as impressive as the results are, the most important thing in science is replication by others. Research published in 1996 from Switzerland demonstrated that a diet similar to the Zone Diet produced similar results in insulin reduction with overweight individuals under metabolic ward conditions. Then in 1998 an Australian group reported their results of using another diet similar to the Zone Diet in both overweight and Type 2 diabetics: they were virtually identical to the results that we had obtained. The only difference was that they were taking their blood chemistry at a much earlier stage than we did. They found that their Zone-like diet lowered elevated insulin by nearly 40 percent within four days. Our data with free living Type 2 diabetics (who were still going to Taco Bell) only confirms this already published work.

The Zone Diet is a calorie restriction diet that clinically demonstrates many of the same benefits in humans that calorie-restriction produces in animal studies. The results have been replicated by other researchers in different parts of the world. It is a dietary program that free-living individuals can follow without hunger or deprivation. And there is no controversy in the anti-aging world that if you can achieve calorie restriction, you will reverse aging. But are there any other "drugs" in addition to the Zone Diet that can be used to reverse aging? Yes. The next two chapters will reveal them.

CHAPTER 9

EXERCISE:
ANOTHER "DRUG" TO
ALTER HORMONES

Does exercise make you live longer? The answer is yes and no. If you are purely sedentary, any type of exercise will increase your life span up to a point. How much exercise before you reach a plateau of longevity? Data gathered from studying Harvard graduates gives a clear picture, and it turns out to be approximately 2,000 calories of exercise-related expenditure per week. Since there are seven days in a week, this translates into less than 300 exercise-related calorie expenditure per day. It really doesn't matter much what type of exercise you do as long as you burn about 300 calories per day. Let's put that level of caloric expenditure in perspective as seen in Table 9-1.

TABLE 9-1

Minutes Spent in Various Activities to Burn 300 Calories per Day

ACTIVITY	AVERAGE MALE	AVERAGE FEMALE
Rowing machine	24	32
Bicycling	26	35
Swimming	26	35
Stationary bike	30	40
Jogging slowly	30	40
Walking briskly	35	47
Walking slowly	69	94

A couple of observations come from this table. The first is that men burn more calories than women. This is because of their greater weight and therefore greater muscle mass. The second is that probably the most convenient exercise to get your 300 calories per day is simply walking briskly. It doesn't require a machine or a gym. And it's not boring.

As you can see from this table, that's not a lot of exercise, and for most individuals a brisk walk for a little more than a half hour per day will more than meet their requirements. Not surprisingly, this simple form of exercise also generates nearly a 70 percent reduction in the incidence of breast cancer in women.

From the perspective of the four pillars of aging, moderate exercise is an exceptionally useful "drug." First, it lowers excess blood glucose (although the mechanism is still not clear). Second, it lowers excess insulin since exercise requires the use of stored energy, not its continued storage. And at moderate exercise intensities, most of that stored energy will come from fat.

If some exercise is good, isn't more better? Unfortunately not. A more careful inspection of the longevity curve and exercise indicates that after about 2,000 calories per week, the curve simply flattens out. Part of the reason is that as you increase exercise intensity, you also increase the levels of oxidative stress on the body. You are making more free radicals because your muscles require more ATP. Although you will be fitter, you probably won't live longer. Apparently, the increased production of free radicals at the molecular level counterbalances the increase in fitness, so that the net effect on the longevity curve is nil. The second reason is that the more intense the exercise, the greater the production of cortisol in response to that stress. So higher exercise intensity actually can increase two pillars of aging: free radicals and cortisol. If your goal is longevity, then moderate exercise is your best course of action. The more intense the exercise, the faster the oxidative candle burns.

However, there is data that suggests that while overall life span may not be increased by more intense exercise (especially weight training), functionality later in life can. This is especially true for the maintenance of muscle mass and strength. Your functionality in later years will be strongly dependent on your ability to preserve muscular strength. So while overall longevity may not be enhanced by more intense exercise, quality of life is. And what's the good of an anti-aging program if the quality of life (i.e., functionality) is not enhanced? Can you still maintain muscle mass with moderate exercise? The answer is yes, and in a later chapter I'll show you how.

The anti-aging benefits of exercise are mediated through two different hormone systems. Each one requires a specific type of exercise. The first hormonal system directly affects one of the four pillars of aging: excess insulin. The reduction of insulin will be achieved primarily by aerobic exercise. Aerobic exercise simply means exercising at an intensity at which sufficient oxygen is delivered to the muscle to do the required work. As you age, your aerobic capacity decreases. This usually means you have to lower your intensity of exercise to maintain sufficient oxygen transfer to the muscles. The longer you exercise aerobically, the more you lower insulin.

While lowering excess insulin has great benefits for increased longevity, increased functionality requires the maintenance of muscle mass. The building of muscle mass can be accomplished through the other hormones affected by exercise: growth hormone and testosterone. The secretion of these hormones will be increased by anaerobic exercise. Anaerobic exercise is any exercise whose intensity causes insufficient oxygen transfer to the muscle cells. This rapidly produces lactic acid as a breakdown product of glucose, which causes the burning sensation in the muscles. Needless to say, aerobic exercise is a lot easier, but as you will shortly see, there is a need for coupling it with anaerobic exercise.

Two different hormonal systems, two different types of exercise. You choose which hormone system you want to alter. But since excess insulin is one of the four pillars of aging, let's talk about it first.

Remember from an earlier chapter that insulin is a storage hormone that stores incoming calories as fuel for future use. As a storage hormone, high levels of insulin prevent the release of stored energy, such as carbohydrates from the liver and fat from the adipose tissue into the bloodstream, so that they can be used by the muscle cells for additional energy. This forces the muscle to use its relatively limited amounts of stored carbohydrate for additional ATP synthesis during exercise. Without continued access to this stored fuel in the fat cells and liver to make more ATP, your muscle cells will soon be running on empty.

What normally happens during aerobic exercise? In the beginning, actively exercising muscles take up blood glucose for their increased energy needs. In fact, actively exercising muscles take up nearly 30 times more glucose than they do when they are at rest. This uptake of blood glucose is a noninsulin-driven event, and to this day, it is not well understood exactly how this process takes place. The very intricate and elegant pathways using the insulin receptor and various proteins involved in the insulin-mediated entry of glucose into the cell are simply bypassed during exercise. In an ideal situation, as blood glucose levels fall, glucagon levels should rise in order to replenish blood sugar. If this rise in glucagon isn't sufficient, then secondary hormonal systems come into play to help replenish blood sugar. One of these systems is the increased secretion of cortisol from the adrenal glands. During short-term acute stress (i.e., fight or flight response), the hormone adrenaline is released from the adrenal glands, whereas in longer-term stress situations (like intensive exercise), the cortisol system predominates. Obviously, the more effective the glucagon system is working to maintain blood glucose levels, the less other backup systems are called into play. This is why lower-intensity aerobic exercise ensures that adequate blood glucose levels are maintained for the brain, thereby keeping these backup hormonal systems of adrenaline and especially cortisol in reserve.

Different events occur during anaerobic exercise where you are trying to enhance the release of human growth hormone and testosterone. Actually, the release of these hormones (growth hormone in particular) doesn't occur during exercise, but in a window 15 to 30 minutes after exercise. The more intense the exercise, the more growth hormone and testosterone are released. This is why anaerobic training, like weight-lifting and wind sprints, is ideally suited for maximizing new muscle mass development.

Growth hormone release is primarily needed to repair the micro-tears in the muscles that occur during intense anaerobic exercise. The more intense the training, the more damage to the muscle tissue. Growth hormone not only repairs the damaged muscle tissue, but also increases the size of the existing tissue. In addition, weight training also causes the increase of testosterone that works in concert with growth hormone to form new muscle mass.

Unfortunately, the more insulin in the bloodstream, the less growth hormone will be released regardless of the intensity of your anaerobic training. This means that all of the hormonal benefits of anaerobic exercise can be quickly undone by a high-carbohydrate sports "energy" drink consumed just after exercise.

And like aerobic exercise, it is possible to overtrain with anaerobic exercise. Anaerobic exercise produces far more stress than aerobic exercise. After approximately 45 minutes of weight-lifting, the levels of cortisol have increased to such an extent that diminishing hormonal returns take place. In addition, testosterone levels begin to drop as more precursors of testosterone are diverted to facilitate increased cortisol production in response to exercise-related stress.

The question might be: "Why weight train at all when you could possibly get all of the benefits by injections of growth hormone? Carefully controlled studies have indicated that strength in elderly men is not enhanced with growth hormone injections compared to placebo injections if both groups are following the same weight-training program. On the other hand, it is known that strength in elderly individuals can be increased nearly 100 percent by weight-training alone.

Although exercise is important, it will not have nearly the effect on longevity as the Zone Diet will. The reason why your diet can impart a far greater effect on your anti-aging program than exercise alone, is that you will probably only exercise one hour per day, but you can eat 24 hours per day. As a consequence, all of the hormonal benefits of exercise can be offset by your diet. This is why I am a strong advocate of the 80/20 rule when it comes to lowering insulin. Eighty percent of your ability to lower insulin levels will come from the Zone Diet. Only 20 percent will come from exercise. But use the two together, and you have a formidable "drug" combination to lower insulin levels. On the other hand, trying to increase your exercise to counterbalance the increase in insulin induced by a high-carbohydrate diet is ultimately self-defeating for the following reasons. First, you are consuming too many calories, which will increase the production of free radicals. Second, the increased exercise levels will further increase free radical production. Finally, there will be an increased cortisol output to maintain blood glucose levels since there isn't enough protein in the diet to stimulate your primary blood glucose restoration hormone (i.e., glucagon).

If you want to combine diet and exercise maximally, there are three windows of opportunity for applying the diet to enhance both types of hormonal changes induced by exercise. The first window is approximately 30 to 45 minutes before exercise. The muscles are not being stressed so demands on blood glucose levels are minimal. But that situation will soon be altered by your workout. Your primary hormonal system for maintaining blood glucose levels during exercise is glucagon. This becomes an excellent time to begin increasing its levels. Since protein is the primary stimulator of glucagon release, you should ingest a small amount of protein (about 7 grams or 1 ounce of low-fat protein) 30 to 45 minutes before working out. Since demands on blood glucose will soon be increased greatly, you also want to simultaneously consume about 9 grams of a low-glycemic carbohydrate to make sure it enters the bloodstream slowly. Finally, to ensure that carbohydrate will enter the bloodstream at a rate slow enough not to spike insulin, you also want to consume about 1–2 grams of fat at the same time. This hormonal touchup (i.e., Zone snack) prior to exercise contains about 100 calories. Not enough calories to divert significant energy or blood flow toward digestion, but enough calories in the correct macronutrient proportion to ensure you are already changing the hormonal environment of the bloodstream before you exercise.

The second window of opportunity occurs right after exercise stops. Insulin levels that are depressed during exercise (unless you are drinking a lot of high-carbohydrate sports "energy" drinks) will begin to rise back to their pre-exercise levels. If you have done anaerobic training, this increase in insulin will inhibit the release of growth hormone. Therefore to moderate this increase in insulin, have another Zone snack as described above right after you finish your exercise. This sets the stage for maximum growth hormone release that occurs 15 to 30 minutes after ending anaerobic exercise.

The final window occurs within 2 hours after the end of any exercise. Insulin levels continue to return to baseline, and this is the best time to eat a larger Zone meal to ensure that both protein and carbohydrate are present to replenish the muscle cells. However, you want to balance these two macronutrients to make sure that you don't overspike insulin. It has been shown that when protein and carbohydrate are given together, muscle glycogen is replenished at a faster rate and to a greater extent than when carbohydrate is given alone. For the average male this means consuming about 30 grams of low-fat protein and 40 grams of low-glycemic carbohydrates along with about 6 grams of extra fat. Any more protein can't be used by the body and will be converted to fat. Any more carbohydrate will cause insulin to overspike, and the fat ensures the slowest possible entry of the carbohydrate into the bloodstream to moderate insulin response.

Using moderate exercise, you have another "drug" to reduce two of the four pillars of aging (excess insulin and excess blood glucose). Combine moderate exercise with the Zone Diet and you have an exceptionally powerful way to lower all four pillars of aging and improve hormonal communication. In the next chapter, I will discuss another way to reduce cortisol. It isn't as powerful as the Zone Diet or moderate exercise for increasing longevity, but it has been used for thousands of years with great success. It's called meditation, and it's a key for brain longevity.

CHAPTER 10

THE BRAIN:
IT'S A TERRIBLE THING
TO WASTE

What good is a successful anti-aging program if the mind fails before the body does? The loss of mental capacity is the greatest fear of aging. It is estimated that more than 50 percent of all individuals over age 85 have some degree of mental impairment. And if you want to increase your functional life span, preservation of mental capacity should be a top priority.

Aging takes a heavy toll on the brain. The brain reaches its maximum weight of about 3 pounds at age 20 and can lose 10 percent of that mass by age 90. The brain contains more than 100 billion nerve cells and billions more other cells, such as glia cells that are involved in a variety of housekeeping activities. With an estimated loss of 100,000 nerve cells per day, this would only account for an overall loss of 2 billion nerve cells by age 50, but more than 40 percent of the loss comes from the neocortex where rational thought is concentrated.

The four pillars that accelerate aging in the body also accelerate the aging of the brain. The brain is the most vulnerable part of the body. As I have already shown, the Zone Diet is the primary "drug" to address each of the four pillars, and moderate exercise can also reduce two of the same pillars (insulin and blood glucose). But is there any "drug" for the brain that can be used to promote its longevity? Before I explore this concept, let's see how the brain works.

The brain is the central information-gathering center for any organism. The less advanced the species, the less information that must be processed. Most of this backroom processing is done within the limbic system, which represents the most primitive part of the brain. The hypothalamus and the hippocampus are located in the limbic system. Although the hypothalamus is the site that sends out various releasing hormones to the pituitary to start various hormonal cascades, it does so only after the hippocampus has integrated enough information to tell it to do so. This is why the hormonal responses I have discussed have been highly conserved throughout evolution. However, what distinguishes man from animal is rational thought. The potential loss of that ability is the greatest fear of aging.

Thinking is a combination of two parts. The rational mind is centered in the neocortex, and memory is located primarily in the hippocampus. When you need to recall memories in order to act on them or compare new information with stored information to make an appropriate decision, different parts of the brain are called into action. Decisions are ultimately made by the neocortex, but the information needed to make that decision is stored in the hippocampus. Memory is stored in two ways. Short-term memory gets put into kind of a holding tank that if properly reinforced, becomes encoded in long-term memory. As I will explain later, much of this reinforcement comes from a proto-hormone known as nitric oxide. If for some reason this short-term memory doesn't get transported to long-term memory, it is gone forever.

The first sign of brain aging is the disruption of this translation process for turning short-term memory into more stable long-term memory. You tend to forget items of very recent memory (like where did I put the keys), but still retain long-term memories with great clarity. Either neural pathways are not reinforced due to a lack of nitric oxide formation or neural death has taken place that disrupts the formation of the more stable pathways that we call memory. Neurons are very sensitive to their environment, and controlling this environment is your primary tool to prevent brain aging.

First and foremost, the brain must have glucose to survive. This is why more than 25 percent of the blood supply goes to the brain even though it only accounts for 2 percent of the body's mass. The blood-brain barrier that separates the brain from the circulatory system (and everything else in the bloodstream) is largely composed of endothelial cells. While the blood-brain barrier is very effective in keeping blood components from your brain, glucose has no trouble crossing it. However, any breaks in this blood-brain barrier allow molecules to leak into the brain that shouldn't be there, and this sets off an immunological response with your nerve being caught in a cross-fire. The glucose contained in the constant river of blood circulating around the brain is needed to maintain adequate ATP levels in the mitochondria of the brain cells to continually pump out excitory neurotransmitters (like glutamate and aspartate) into surrounding glia cells for storage. If there is a lack of glucose to make ATP, then the glia cells are unable to remove these neurotransmitters. They remain in the synaptic junctions between nerves for a longer period of time. By continuing to excite the nerve, these excitatory neurotransmitters can eventually lead to its destruction through a cascade of hormonally driven events that start with a continuing influx of calcium into the nerve endings. Essentially, the channel door of the nerve is constantly turned on. Unless it is turned off by pulling these excitory neurotransmitters out of the synaptic junction (which is done by the glia cells), nerve death is the result. Like the muscles of the heart, once a nerve dies, it can never be replaced.

Lack of glucose to drive ATP generation in the glia cells is not the only thing that can kill nerve cells. Overexposure to glucose can do the same. As I mentioned earlier, the glucoreceptors in the ventromedial nucleus (VMN) of the hypothalamus are exceptionally sensitive to glucose levels. Too high a level of glucose in the brain, and these nerves also die. Considering the importance of blood glucose, it is surprising that the entry of glucose into the brain does not require insulin or its receptor. Since there is no hormone receptor for controlling the entry of glucose into the brain, the only way to prevent glucose-induced toxicity in the brain is to maintain stable blood glucose levels on the other side of the blood-brain barrier (i.e., the bloodstream). This is why 40 million years of evolution has yielded some very complex hormonal control systems to help maintain stable glucose levels in the bloodstream. Obviously the most important of these control systems is the insulin-glucagon axis. Insulin drives nutrients into cells, which reduces blood glucose levels. This is great for the body, but bad for the brain. Glucagon restores blood glucose levels. This is great for the brain. However, if glucagon is not doing its job correctly (and that is quite likely if you are on a high-carbohydrate diet), then the brain will call up other backup hormonal systems to help restore blood glucose levels. The primary backup system is cortisol. Cortisol does a reasonably effective job of increasing blood sugar levels, but excess cortisol is perhaps the brain's greatest enemy.

Just as there are gluco-sensitive neurons in the brain, there are also cortisol-sensitive ones that have receptors for cortisol. The vast majority of the cortisol-sensitive neurons receptors in the brain are located in the hippocampus. These are easily damaged, if not outright killed, in the presence of excess cortisol. Any significant loss of the hippocampal neurons by exposure to excess cortisol makes it difficult to provide the necessary feedback mechanism for maintaining information flow to the hypothalamus in order to effectively operate your biological Internet. And to add insult to injury, cortisol also reduces the uptake of glucose into the hippocampal neurons, which also decreases their viability.

The loss of these hippocampal neurons also makes it very difficult to send short-term memories into long-term storage. The recall of long-term memory is assisted by a process known as long-term potentiation that requires the excitatory neurotransmitter, glutamate. Unfortunately, excess cortisol prevents the uptake of glutamate by glia cells (the housekeeping cells that surround the synaptic junctions), so that glutamate levels rise in the synaptic junction. Just as described above, when the glia cells can't make enough ATP, this excess glutamate causes neural death by overexciting the neuron with excess calcium inflow. So, while excess cortisol produces a short-term benefit of improved glucose delivery to the brain to prevent neural death, it generates a long-term problem of cortisol-induced nerve death. It is a no-win situation.

The other thing the brain needs to survive is oxygen. Without adequate blood flow, not only is not enough glucose supplied to the brain, but neither is enough oxygen. Excess insulin not only increases the likelihood of cardiovascular disease, but also increases the likelihood of stroke by its adverse effects on eicosanoids that ultimately control blood flow to the brain. This is why Type 2 diabetic patients have two to four times the likelihood of both heart attacks and strokes. Reduce insulin levels, and you get an increase in the production of "good" eicosanoids that increase blood flow. As blood flow is increased, the chances of transient blockage of the cerebral arteries is decreased. Much of our memory loss as we age is due to the accumulation of ministrokes, known as transient ischemic attacks (TIA). No one ministroke is sufficient to cause total loss of capacity, but with each ministroke enough nerves die, so that over time the accumulated damage is just as severe as a major stroke.

Of course, the most frightening word in aging is Alzheimer's. Cancer has a more optimistic outcome than Alzheimer's because at least there is a chance. More devastating is that there is no dignity with Alzheimer's disease. Alzheimer's disease is characterized by the accumulation of amyloid plaques. The amyloid protein is a natural constituent of the brain, but it appears that the increasing glycosylation of this protein accelerates its accumulation and precipitation. In many ways, Alzheimer's disease can be viewed as the equivalent of heart disease inside the central nervous system. This is reinforced by the fact that it appears that the incidence of Alzheimer's disease is highly correlated with the ε-4 form of the ApoE gene. This is the same mutation of the ApoE gene that is associated with increased heart attack risk. Therefore, if any approach is useful in reducing the likelihood of heart disease, it should also have benefits in preventing Alzheimer's. Basically what's good for the heart is good for the brain.

Finally, the brain is exceptionally vulnerable to free radical attack. Fifty per cent of the dry weight of the brain is lipid and about one-third of the lipid is composed of polyunsaturated essential fatty acids making it the most likely target for free radical attack. Any strategy that reduces free radical formation will benefit eicosanoid formation and that can pay great dividends to increase the longevity of the brain.

Whether nerves die from lack of glucose, increases in cortisol, decreased oxygen, development of Alzheimer's, or free radical damage, once they are dead, they are dead forever. As more of your neurons fail, brain function begins a downward spiral. Thus the key to brain longevity is maintaining nerve viability for as long as possible. And this is one of the greatest challenges for any anti-aging program to address.

This is where the Zone Diet comes into play. The Zone Diet was designed to keep insulin in a zone, and by doing so maintains a constant level of blood glucose. Since the Zone Diet provides adequate protein in small amounts throughout the day, glucagon levels are maintained ensuring that the insulin-glucagon axis is working efficiently. As a consequence, there is no need to call into play the extra production of cortisol. The Zone Diet is also a calorie-restricted diet that makes sure that excess free radical production is minimized. It has been convincingly shown in mice on calorie-restricted diets that damage to the brain mitochondria DNA is significantly less, plus there are increases in the levels of antioxidant enzymes in the brain that otherwise decrease with age.

However, the key reason the Zone Diet is your best protection against brain aging is its ability to alter eicosanoid levels. By making more "good" eicosanoids (i.e., vasodilators) and less "bad" ones (i.e., vasoconstrictors), cerebral arteries can maximize oxygen transfer to the brain, thus minimizing the likelihood of a TIA. In addition, the uptake and release of brain neurotransmitters are also related to eicosanoid levels in the brain. Finally "good" eicosanoids represent the ultimate backup systems for the hypothalamus and pituitary to ensure that proper endocrine hormone communication is maintained by boosting the levels of certain biological response modifiers within the cell (the importance of this will be shown later).

Is the Zone Diet the only step you can take to ensure maximum brain function as you age? Although it is the most important, there are two other critical components. The first is exercise. In the last chapter I discussed the role of exercise in reducing insulin levels. Couple a consistent moderate exercise program with the Zone Diet and you have a formidable tool to maximize brain function. The other tool has been known for thousands of years, but is only now beginning to be understood. This is stress-reduction through meditation.

Meditation is not simply sitting back and thinking good thoughts or daydreaming. It is a very precise way to control cortisol. This use of meditation for a specific physiological purpose (i.e., cortisol reduction) is a key for your brain longevity program. This is not to say that the use of meditation to achieve spiritual goals is not a higher purpose, but that requires a far greater commitment. Here we are simply looking at meditation as another anti-aging tool. This is a very Western (i.e., goal-orientated) approach. In essence, it is practical meditation.

Herbert Benson, a cardiologist at Harvard Medical School, has done a great deal of research to demystify meditation. Practical meditation is not some purely mystical technique known only to a few gurus. Practical meditation is a series of defined actions, as Benson has pointed out in his many works on the physiology of meditation. There appear to be common themes that run throughout recorded history on how to meditate. There is usually a constant chanting of a word or phrase or a focus on a physiological action (such as breathing)—and always a return to one's focus on a word, phrase, or physiological function when your thoughts begin to wander (i.e., day-dreaming). In essence, you are trying to clear the decks mentally.

Here is a thumbnail sketch of practical meditation. Find a quiet place with a comfortable chair. Close your eyes and repeat a word (the word *one* is a good choice) or phrase continually. At the same time, focus on your breathing. Always try to expand your stomach when you inhale. By focusing on the word (or phrase) and your breathing, you are trying to keep random thoughts from coming into your consciousness. If such random thoughts do appear, simply refocus your attention on the word and your breathing until they pass. Do this for 20 minutes a day—and there you have it, practical meditation.

Meditation (even practical meditation) takes practice (just like diet and exercise), but with increasing skill, significant physiological changes related to reduction of cortisol levels can be achieved. These include the reduction of blood pressure and heart rate, and plus improved immune function. Yet all these changes are also associated with improved eicosanoid balance. That should not be too surprising since cortisol is a very powerful inhibitor of eicosanoid formation; thus reduction of cortisol should improve eicosanoid synthesis.

Do practical mediation for 20 minutes a day and you have a proven "drug" to reduce cortisol levels. It's a simple technique that helps alter hormonal response and in the process improves brain longevity. As you become more skilled in meditation, it is then worth learning how to use meditation to achieve its spiritual benefits: establishing a sense of oneness with the universe.

The same three "drugs" (the Zone Diet, moderate exercise, and practical meditation) that can alter the pillars of aging for your body can also alter the hormonal environment in which the brain must function. Your ability to use these "drugs" correctly will determine whether your mind outlasts your body in the anti-aging game. If you win, the quest for anti-aging is well worth it. If you lose, the years gained through anti-aging will be shallow without the mind to enjoy them.

How to put these three "drugs" together is the key to the Anti-aging Zone Lifestyle.

CHAPTER 11

THE ANTI-AGING ZONE LIFESTYLE:
THE SELF-CARE PYRAMID

Asking Americans to change their lifestyle to prevent disease has not been a workable strategy in recent years. Look around and ask yourself if Americans are healthier now than they were 15 years ago. Asking Americans to change their lifestyle to treat disease also has a very low likelihood of success, because everyone seems convinced there is a pill or surgical intervention that will save them. As a country we have been romanced by the idea that whatever our medical problem, there is, or soon will be, a pill to take care of it. The successful marketing of this idea by the pharmaceutical companies has taken individuals off the hook for taking responsibility for their future. At least they think so.

However, I believe if Americans are convinced that a change in their lifestyle can reverse the aging process, then there is an outside chance they may make a change to reach that goal.

Reversal of the aging process can never be put into a two-piece capsule. However, the aging process can be reversed if you are willing to incorporate the basic components of a lifelong hormonal control strategy into your daily activities. These include calorie restriction using the Zone Diet, moderate exercise, and stress reduction through meditation. Unfortunately, they are not all equal in their ability to reverse aging. In fact, what you get is a pyramid of anti-aging interventions as shown in Figure 11-1 on page 114.

The base of this pyramid is occupied by far and away the most important component of any anti-aging lifestyle: a calorie-restricted diet, in particular the Zone Diet. Calorie restriction is the only proven way to reverse aging. There is no controversy about that. The Zone Diet is simply a more advanced version of calorie restriction diets that provides far greater hormonal benefits. Thus without the Zone Diet

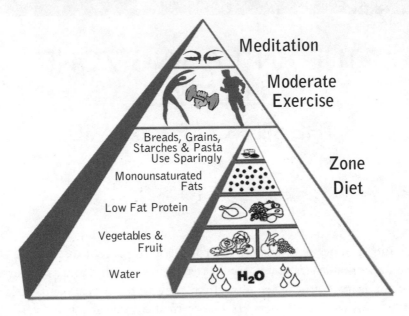

Figure 11-1   Anti-aging Zone Lifestyle Pyramid

as the foundation of your anti-aging program, it will be very difficult to achieve the maximum benefits of age reversal.

The next step of the Zone Lifestyle Anti-aging Pyramid, which has a lesser impact on anti-aging, is moderate exercise. The data on exercise and longevity is mixed. It is quite clear that lack of exercise increases the aging process. However, higher levels of exercise intensity will also increase free radical formation and cortisol levels: two of the four pillars of aging. So the key is moderate, but consistent, exercise. But as you can see from the Pyramid, even the best exercise program can be obliterated by the wrong diet.

Finally, at the top of the Zone Anti-aging Lifestyle Pyramid is stress reduction, particularly through meditation. Meditation can have profound hormonal effects, especially on cortisol levels. Unfortunately, we have no data on the impact that meditation has on overall longevity. Furthermore, only one of the pillars of aging (i.e., excess cortisol) can be lowered by meditation. Nonetheless, we know from an intuitive viewpoint that stress reduction can only help any anti-aging program because of its benefits for brain longevity. However, just like exercise, the cortisol-lowering benefits of meditation can be destroyed by a hormonally incorrect diet.

If you choose to engage in only one of the three components of the Anti-aging Zone Lifestyle Pyramid, you will obviously get the most anti-aging bang for the buck from following the Zone Diet. Conversely, you will get the least benefit through meditation if you ignore diet and exercise. On the other hand, put all three components together, and you have adopted a warrior's code for anti-aging. I say warrior's code because there are rules and regulations you have to follow on a lifetime basis for successful anti-aging. When it comes to aging, you are either reversing it or accelerating it. Each day, and in fact with each meal, you want to ask yourself the following question: Did I accelerate the aging process or did I reverse it? You might be very surprised (or disappointed) by the answers at the end of each day.

From a practical standpoint, just what does it take to follow the Anti-aging Zone Lifestyle? First and foremost, a calorie-restricted diet like the Zone Diet requires a little advance planning. You have to ensure that adequate levels of low-fat protein are available at every meal along with copious amounts of vegetables and moderate amounts of fruits. If you are using fresh sources of fruits and vegetables, neither has a very long shelf-life. Therefore you may have to go shopping two or three times a week. On the other hand, if time is your enemy, new technology is making frozen foods taste significantly better, and the variety of frozen foods (especially precut vegetables) has never been greater. This allows for great flexibility in putting together Zone meals and snacks in a very short period of time. Alternatively, one could prepare a week's worth of Zone meals on the weekend, then freeze them and microwave just prior to a meal. The secret to maintaining the Zone Diet is (1) eating all the food you are supposed to, and (2) never letting more than five hours go by without eating a Zone meal or snack. Again this is no different than taking a drug. Be consistent with the dosage and the timing.

The power of the Zone Diet is that all four pillars of aging are reduced simultaneously. Because the Zone Diet is a calorie-restricted diet, you are also reducing excess free radical formation. At the same time, you are reducing excess blood glucose because you are not consuming excess amounts of carbohydrates. Likewise, you are also reducing excess insulin, which is stimulated by excess carbohydrate consumption. Finally, you are reducing the likelihood of any excess cortisol production to maintain blood glucose levels since at every meal you are eating adequate levels of low-fat protein that stimulate glucagon secretion (the primary hormonal system to restore blood glucose levels). This is why the Zone Diet is the base of the Anti-aging Zone Lifestyle Pyramid.

The next level of the Anti-aging Zone Lifestyle Pyramid is moderate exercise. With the exercise component you want to have a cross-training program to affect as many hormonal systems as possible. To reduce insulin, you should plan to do 30 minutes of aerobic exercise every day, with brisk walking one of the best. In addition, for increasing growth hormone release, you want to spend 5 to 10 minutes a day on a strength-training program.

Strength training is not thought of fondly by most people, but it is the only form of exercise that will build and maintain the muscle mass necessary for maximal functionality in the future. For upper body strength, the best exercise is push-ups. The word *push-up* conveys dread to most individuals. Therefore, if you are not physically fit, start your daily anaerobic exercise with push-aways from a wall. Stand two to three feet from a wall and extend your hands in a direct line from your shoulders until they reach the wall. Make sure the placement of the hands is low enough on the wall so that when you lower yourself your shoulders will be just above your hands. Lower your body toward the wall, and then push away to return to the original position. Do three sets of 10 to 15 repetitions with a minute's rest between sets.

If you can do this easily, then graduate to counter push-backs. Stand two to three feet from a counter top (again positioning your hands in a direct line from the shoulder) and extend your hands to reach the top of the counter. (When lowering yourself to the counter, your shoulders should be directly over your hands). Lower your body to the counter and then push back to the original position. As you originally did with the push-aways from the wall, do three sets of counter-top push-backs each with 10 to 15 repetitions.

Once these are mastered, then move on to the knee push-up. Here you kneel on the floor with your arms extended to the floor (again in a direct line from your shoulder). Lower yourself until your chest (not your stomach) touches the floor, and then raise yourself back up to the original position. Once you have mastered this exercise for 10 to 15 repetitions in three sets, then you are ready to graduate to the dreaded push-up in which only your toes are touching the ground and your arms are totally extended (again so the hands and shoulders are in a direct line). Lower yourself to the floor until your chest reaches it and then return to the original position. Once you can achieve 10 to 15 repetitions for three sets, then you have two additional options. One is to simply do more repetitions in each set. The other is to raise your feet off the floor (like on a chair) and then do your push-ups. Of the two, the first (more repetitions) is easier and probably safer. Don't be disappointed if you have to start with the wall push-aways due to lack of current upper body strength. It just means you have greater potential for improvement.

The best exercise for developing lower body strength is the squat. In earlier days it was known as a deep-knee bend. Just like the push-up, you start this exercise slowly, depending on your initial fitness level. As a start, just stand in front of a chair that has side-arms. Place your hands on the arms of the chair, and then slowly lower yourself to the seat of the chair. Still using the arms of the chair for support, raise yourself back up to a standing position. Do three sets of 10 to 15 repetitions with a minute rest between each set.

The next step is to do the same exercise, but now not using the arms of the chair for support (however the arms are always there to be used for support if needed, like a safety net). Again, your goal is to achieve 10 to 15 repetitions in three sets.

The next level still uses the chair, but now your arms are crossed over your chest as you do your squat. As you did with the push-ups, simply increase your repetitions once you exceed 15 per set.

This strength-training program will take less than 10 minutes per day. Regardless of your fitness level, these exercises for upper and lower body strength should be done every day. Since they don't require any equipment, they can be done at home or on the road. There is simply no excuse not to make them part of your Anti-aging Zone Lifestyle.

These exercises (brisk walking and simple weight-bearing exercises) should be the core of your moderate exercise program. But this doesn't mean that more exercises can't be added. For more aerobic intensity, think about walking on a hilly terrain as opposed to a flat landscape. When you travel, this might mean walking up and down the stairs of your hotel. Alternatively, you may want to invest in a home exercise machine, like a rower, a stationary bicycle, or a treadmill to increase the intensity of the workout or decrease the time spent exercising aerobically so that you get your 300 calories of daily energy expenditure. For additional anaerobic training, you might want to get a set of adjustable dumbbells because they are easily stored and they provide maximum flexibility in the number of weight-training exercises you can do. If you do any additional strength training, never do more than 45 minutes of strength training because beyond that point, cortisol levels begin to rise and testosterone levels will drop. Extended strength training beyond this time frame in a single session will start to accelerate the aging process.

Since maintaining strength is one of your most important components of functionality, you would like to have some measure of how you are progressing on this component of your Anti-aging Zone Lifestyle. Here's how you can measure your strength at home.

For determining your upper body strength, males will do standard push-ups and females will do knee push-ups. Always make sure that your back is not sagging (just pull your abdominals in) and that you are touching the floor with your chest and not your chin. Remember no one is watching you, so you want to get a true test of your current upper body strength.

Push-ups: Men

	AGE				
	20–29	*30–39*	*40–49*	*50–59*	*>60*
Excellent	>55	>45	>40	>35	>30
Good	45–54	35–44	30–39	25–34	20–29
Average	35–44	25–34	20–29	15–24	10–19
Fair	20–34	15–24	12–19	8–14	5–9
Low	0–19	0–14	0–11	0–7	0–4

Knee Push-ups: Women

	AGE				
	20–29	*30–39*	*40–49*	*50–59*	*>60*
Excellent	>49	>40	>35	>30	>20
Good	34–48	25–39	20–34	15–29	5–19
Average	17–33	12–24	8–9	6–14	3–4
Fair	6–16	4–11	3–7	2–5	1–2
Low	0–5	0–3	0–2	0–1	0

Don't be dismayed if you have a low score. Most Americans will. In fact, the average male teenager can't do 10 push-ups. But with consistent exercise, your upper body strength will increase.

Lower body strength is measured by the number of times you can do a squat with weights. Use a chair of standard height without arms. Males should hold 15-pound dumbbells in each hand (a total of 30 pounds), and females should hold 5-pound dumbbells in each hand (a total of 10 pounds). Keeping your legs as wide as your hips, do a standard squat until you touch the seat of the chair and then return to your starting position. Do as many standard squats as you can while maintaining good form. Then check out how you rate in lower body strength.

30-Pound Squats: Men

	AGE				
	20–39	30–39	40–49	50–59	>60
Excellent	>55	>45	>40	>35	>30
Good	45–54	35–44	30–39	25–34	20–29
Average	35–44	25–34	20–29	15–24	10–19
Fair	20–34	15–24	12–19	8–14	5–9
Low	0–19	0–14	0–11	0–7	0–4

10-Pound Squats: Women

	AGE				
	20–39	30–39	40–49	50–59	>60
Excellent	>49	>40	>35	>30	>20
Good	34–48	25–39	20–34	15–29	5–19
Average	17–33	12–24	8–19	6–14	3–4
Fair	6–16	4–11	3–7	2–5	1–2
Low	0–5	0–3	0–2	0–1	0

Finally your cross-training program should include flexibility exercises. In addition to 5 minutes of stretching to warm up and cool down before and after more intensive exercises, you should plan to do at least 20 minutes every other day of continuous stretching. It doesn't matter if it's basic sports stretching or yoga, both are great.

So here is your basic Anti-aging Zone exercise program:

1. 30 minutes of brisk walking every day.
2. 5 to 10 minutes of basic strength-building exercises (push-ups and squats) every day.

So far not too hard. Try to do this every day, but if you do these basic exercises at least 5 days a week, you will be making progress in your anti-aging program. Then if you want to add to this basic program, consider the following:

1. Replace the brisk daily walking with slightly higher intensity aerobic exercise (rowing, bicycling, or walking on a treadmill) until you have burned 300 calories.
2. Do no more than 45 minutes of strength-training with dumbbells (or free weights and exercise machines) every other day.
3. Do 20 minutes of flexibility exercises on the days that you don't do any strength-training.

The moderate exercise component of the Anti-aging Zone Lifestyle Pyramid will reduce excess insulin and excess blood sugar, two of the four pillars of aging without increasing cortisol or free radicals. Not quite as good as reducing all four pillars of aging as with the Zone Diet, but by increasing strength and aerobic fitness, you will increase your functionality in later life.

The final component of the Anti-aging Zone Lifestyle Pyramid is meditation because it can lower at least one pillar of aging: excess cortisol production, which is important for promoting brain longevity. Since we are dealing with practical meditation (that is directed at cortisol reduction, not at the improvement of spirituality) as detailed in the previous chapter, a reasonable time expenditure is 20 minutes per day.

So there is the total Anti-aging Zone Lifestyle Pyramid. You will probably spend one to two hours per day on food preparation and eating, another 40 minutes per day on exercise, and 20 minutes in daily meditation. Two to three hours per day to reverse the aging process. That's all it takes if you are consistent.

Obviously, there needs to be a commitment, but then anti-aging is not a short-term program like a diet—it's a lifetime endeavor. It requires constant diligence. Is it worth it? It depends on your faith in unproven technologies, like taking supplements found in the local health foodstore or who-knows-what new pharmaceutical "discoveries" are yet to be marketed. The Anti-aging Zone Lifestyle Pyramid is proven to work. It has no side effects. And it's free. But that is still not enough for most people. They need to see hard evidence that they are indeed turning back the aging process. They want to see numbers. Such verification exists, and it's in your blood. It is what I call your Anti-aging Zone Report Card.

Your blood has no political agenda when it comes to aging. Your Anti-aging Zone Report Card allows you to chart your progress in reversing the aging process and to maintain your commitment to the Anti-aging Zone Lifestyle Pyramid. What those blood parameters are can be found in the next chapter.

CHAPTER 12

YOUR ANTI-AGING ZONE
REPORT CARD:
THE TESTS YOU WANT TO PASS

Your blood is the key to determining how successful you are with your anti-aging efforts. Your blood is a harsh critic, and it tells no lies. Can your blood tell you whether you are aging faster or slower than your chronological age would suggest? The answer is yes, but you have to know what parameters to look at. Once you do, you can use the Anti-aging Zone Report Card to chart your progress in reversing the aging process. This is one report card that should have passing grades every time you take the test.

What blood parameters do you want to test? The important test you want to pass is the level of insulin in your bloodstream. As I have already discussed, the elevated levels of insulin in Type 2 diabetics are strongly correlated with increased heart disease, stroke, obesity, blindness, kidney failure, amputation, and impotence. Measurement of fasting insulin is a great starting point since it is a direct measure of the primary pillar of aging, and it is also the risk factor most highly correlated with the development of heart disease. Unfortunately the test is relatively expensive and requires careful sample preparation to give reliable results. If you do have this test, then ideally your levels of fasting insulin should be less than 10 μU/ml. If your fasting insulin levels are above 15 μU/ml, you are definitely aging at a faster rate than you should be.

Your ability to control blood glucose on a long-term basis (and therefore minimize cortisol production) is best measured by glycosylated hemoglobin levels. Since excess blood glucose and excess cortisol are also pillars of aging, this test gives an insight into how well you are making an impact on aging. Glycosylated hemoglobin is an AGE product. The higher the level of glycosylated hemoglobin, the more

AGEs you are producing throughout the body. This is also a relatively expensive test, but sample preparation of the blood is not nearly as critical. Your glycosylated hemoglobin should be less than 5 percent. The typical levels of glycosylated hemoglobin in Type 2 diabetics are between 8 and 11 percent. Once their glycosylated hemoglobin is under 7 percent, they can almost be assured that long-term complications associated with diabetes will not occur. One of these long-term complications is impotence. If you're a male and you're really worried about impotence, before reaching for a pill like Viagra, try lowering your glycosylated hemoglobin levels.

Measuring fasting insulin and glycosylated hemoglobin are not standard tests and because of their expense, it is unlikely they will be used to screen large populations. However, there is one other blood marker that is very accessible. This is the ratio of fasting triglycerides to HDL cholesterol. This lipid ratio is very sensitive to insulin and thus becomes a surrogate marker for fasting insulin. In work done at Harvard Medical School, it was clearly demonstrated that the higher the fasting triglyceride/HDL cholesterol ratio, the more likely you are to have a heart attack. In this study, the researchers compared individuals who had just survived their first heart attack with age-matched, weight-matched, and socio-economic matched controls. When they compared the fasting triglyceride/HDL cholesterol ratios, they found that those patients who had the highest ratios were 16 times more likely to have a heart attack than those who had lower ratios. A 16-fold greater risk is a pretty significant number, considering that smoking increases the likelihood of a heart attack by a factor of four, and high cholesterol increases the likelihood for a heart attack by a mere factor of two. We have made the campaigns to lower cholesterol and eliminate smoking national priorities in order to decrease the deaths from the number-one killer: heart disease. But we may have been fighting the wrong enemy all the time. The real villain in heart disease is excess insulin, which can be tracked by the fasting triglyceride/HDL cholesterol ratio.

One reason the higher the fasting triglyceride/HDL cholesterol ratio is so strongly correlated with heart disease is due to a greater predominance of small dense atherogeneic LDL particles. These are the type of LDL particles that are highly associated with heart disease. The higher the fasting triglyceride/HDL cholesterol ratio, the greater the percentage of the small dense atherogenic LDL particles. The second reason is that a high fasting triglyceride/HDL cholesterol ratio is indicative of elevated insulin levels, which in turn increases the production of "bad" eicosanoids, such as thromboxane A_2, that are the underlying hormonal factor in heart attacks. It is this subgroup of eicosanoids that promotes platelet aggregation and the vasoconstriction of arteries. About 25 percent of people who die of heart disease have few, if any, arterial lesions upon autopsy. These people died of vaso-spasms in the artery that caused a temporary blockage of blood flow. After death the arteries relax, and the physician scratches his or her head wondering why the person died of a heart attack. Obviously, one of the best ways to prevent a heart attack is to prevent the production of thromboxane A_2, a particularly nasty "bad" eicosanoid. There is one standard drug that does a very effective job of that. That drug is called aspirin. So, if you have a high triglyceride/HDL cholesterol ratio, either start taking aspirin or begin following the Anti-aging Zone Lifestyle. Aspirin may reduce heart attacks, but it has no effect on the aging process.

Bottom line, if you want to slow down—if not reverse—the aging process, then lower your ratio of fasting triglyceride/HDL cholesterol. The ratio should be below 2, and ideally less than 1. If the fasting triglyceride/HDL cholesterol ratio is greater than 4, you are aging faster than you should. Not surprisingly, in virtually all the Type 2 diabetics we have studied, their fasting triglyceride/HDL cholesterol ratio is always greater than four.

Finally, there is your percentage of body fat. Currently about 75 percent of Americans over 50 are overweight, and more than 50 percent of the adult population is overweight. What should your weight be? Well it doesn't matter, because the important parameter is not your weight, but your percentage of body fat because it is directly related to your insulin levels. Your body fat should be less than 15 percent for males and less than 22 percent for females. If your current body fat is above these percentages, you are accelerating aging. Unfortunately, the body fat for the average American male is 25 percent and for the average American female is 33 percent. No wonder half of America is obese.

Here is a quick way to determine whether or not you are close to these desired levels of body fat. If you are a male and have love handles, you probably have more than 15 percent body fat. If you are a female and have cellulite, then you probably have more than 22 percent body fat. For more precison in determining your body fat percentage refer to the methods using your body measurements described in detail in the *The Zone* and *Mastering the Zone* to determine what your current percentage body fat is in order to know how far you have to go to enter the Anti-aging Zone.

Table 12.1 is the summary of your Anti-aging Zone Report Card.

TABLE 12.1

Anti-aging Zone Report Card

PARAMETER	AGING SLOWER THAN NORMAL	AGING FASTER THAN NORMAL
Fasting insulin	less than 10 μU/ml	more than 15 μU/ml
Glycosylated hemoglobin	less than 5%	more than 8%
Triglyceride/HDL	less than 2	more than 4
Percent Body Fat		
Males	less than 15%	more than 25%
Females	less than 22%	more than 33%

If your test results indicate that you are aging at a slower than normal rate, then by all means keep on doing whatever you are doing. On the other hand, if your Anti-aging Zone Report Card indicates that you are aging faster than you should, what can you do about it? The first answer is to follow the Zone Diet, because it will lower the blood parameters while simultaneously reducing excess body fat. As I have shown previously with Type 2 diabetic patients, each of these blood parameters can be lowered within six weeks. These individuals were literally turning back the hands of time with the food they were eating. But is the Zone Diet only useful for individuals, such as Type 2 diabetics, who are aging at a faster rate than they should or is it applicable to the general population as well? As I pointed out in the chapter on Type 2 diabetics, in simultaneous studies with normal individuals, the fasting triglyceride to HDL cholesterol levels were dramatically lowered by the same Zone Diet that was so effective for Type 2 diabetics.

If you are only following one component of the Anti-aging Zone Lifestyle Pyramid, you have to work harder to get a passing grade on the Anti-aging Zone Report Card. The more components of the Anti-aging Zone Lifestyle Pyramid you add to your daily activities, the less work you must do to get a passing grade. And if you are not following the Zone Diet, then you are probably working much too hard on the other components of the Anti-aging Zone Lifestyle Pyramid in order to get a passing grade.

An example of how a hormonally incorrect diet can overwhelm exercise and meditation as an anti-aging intervention was the famous Lifestyle Heart Trial, in which cardiovascular patients with high triglycerides/HDL cholesterol ratios were enrolled in a 5-year trial emphasizing meditation, exercise, and a low-fat, high-carbohydrate vegetarian diet. Unfortunately, most of the Anti-aging Zone Report Card testing parameters were not reported, except for the triglyceride/HDL cholesterol ratio, which is a surrogate marker for fasting insulin levels.

These patients started out with a very high triglyceride/HDL cholesterol ratio of 5.7. And according to Harvard Medical School, these patients should be considered at high risk for a heart attack. Yet after 5 years on this program, their triglyceride/HDL cholesterol ratio had increased to an even more dangerous level of 7.1. In fact, one year after the results of this trial were published, the lead author of Lifestyle Heart Trial, K. Lance Gould, one of the country's leading cardiologists, made this statement in a letter to the *Journal of the American Medical Association*:

> Frequently, triglyceride levels increase and HDL-cholesterol levels decrease for individuals on vegetarian, high-carbohydrate diets. Since low HDL-cholesterol, particularly with high triglycerides incurs substantial risk of coronary events, I do not recommend a high-carbohydrate strict vegetarian diet.

Hardly a ringing endorsement of the low-fat vegetarian diet used during the Lifestyle Heart Trial.

Recently new research has examined the role of diet alone (excluding the confounding factors of exercise and stress reduction, of both which are known to lower insulin) in cardiovascular patients. These patients were put on isocaloric diets of increasing carbohydrate content that represented moderate calorie restriction compared to their previous diets. This one-year study, published in 1997, demonstrated that as the percentage of fat in these isocaloric diets was decreased below 26 percent (which means an increase in the amount of carbohydrates to keep the calories constant), the worse the triglyceride/HDL ratio became. Furthermore even though these were calorie-restricted diets, with each slight decrease in fat content (and thus increase in the carbo-hydrate content of the diet), the levels of insulin also increased as shown in Figure 12-1.

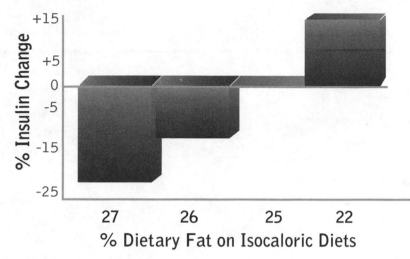

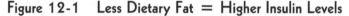

% Dietary Fat on Isocaloric Diets

Figure 12-1   Less Dietary Fat = Higher Insulin Levels

As the authors of this study stated in a 1998 issue of the *Journal of the American Medical Association:*

> Thus there is no proof that the Lifestyle Heart Trial diet per se is responsible for the reported benefit or that the observed reductions in HDL or increases in triglycerides are without harm.

This would strongly suggest that the recommendations of exercise and stress reduction make great sense to everyone (because they reduce insulin), but maybe a low-fat, high-carbohydrate diet should be considered highly experimental and perhaps even dangerous in certain individuals because of the demonstrated increase in insulin levels and its surrogate marker (the ratio of triglyceride to HDL cholesterol). And if your goal is to reverse aging, then decreasing, not increasing insulin (which is the primary pillar of aging) should be your goal.

Just as you should change the oil in your car every 3 to 6 months, you should check on your aging progress as measured by the Anti-aging Zone Report Card parameters every 3 to 6 months. Knowledge is power, especially when it comes to successful anti-aging. These are the tests you don't want to fail.

PART III

WHY THE ANTI-AGING ZONE LIFESTYLE PYRAMID WORKS

CHAPTER 13

HORMONES:
THE LONG COURSE

I believe the underlying molecular basis of aging is due to increasing hormonal miscommunication. To understand what causes an otherwise efficient communication system to lose fidelity with age, you have to better understand hormonal complexity and how hormones exchange information. In the earlier chapter on hormones, I described different routes that hormones take to deliver information to their target cells. Endocrine hormones are made in a discrete gland and are then secreted into the bloodstream to seek their target cells and specific receptors on those target cells. Paracrine hormones are secreted over very short distances and usually through a defined pathway, like a nerve or duct. Finally, autocrine hormones either act on the secreting cell or its nearest neighbor.

Aside from being classified by the way they are delivered to the target tissue, hormones can be further subdivided into groups based upon the dietary precursors of which they are derived. While polypeptide hormones, neuropeptides, and neurotransmitters are made from amino acids (the building blocks of protein), steroid hormones are derived from cholesterol, and eicosanoids are generated from fat. As you can begin to see, your diet will have a major impact on providing the building blocks for making these critical signaling agents. The dietary precursors of various hormones are shown in Table 13-1 on page 132.

A further distinguishing characteristic of hormones is their great variation in size. Obviously the larger the hormone, the more difficulty it will have reaching its target tissue. The polypeptide hormones are relatively large, like giant beach balls. Steroid and thyroid hormones are very small in comparison. Some paracrine hormones (like melato-

TABLE 13-1

Types of Hormones

Amino acid based hormones
   Polypeptide endocrine hormones
      Insulin
      Glucagon
      Insulinlike growth factor (IGF)
      Growth hormone
   Amino acid-endocrine hormones
      Thyroid
   Amino acid-paracrine hormones
      Serotonin
      Melatonin

Cholesterol based hormones
   Steroid endocrine hormones
      DHEA
      Estrogen
      Progesterone
      Testosterone
      Cortisol

Fat based hormones
   Autocrine hormones
      Eicosanoids

nin) and especially autocrine hormones (like eicosanoids) are lipid soluble because they do not circulate over wide distances and are very small, allowing them to easily diffuse between cell membranes.

Now to add even more complexity, many of the hormones that circulate in the bloodstream are associated with binding proteins specific for that particular hormone. Once bound to these much larger binding proteins, the hormone is inactive but is constantly cycling through the body like a circulating reservoir. By doing so, the lifetime of the hormone in the bloodstream is substantially increased so that it is ready for action once released from its carrier protein. Once the hormone is released from the binding protein, it can then exert its biological action. This eliminates the need (and time) for synthesis of the hormone in a distant gland, thus providing even better regulatory control of hormone communication. Virtually all steroid and thyroid hormones circulate in this manner. So do a few polypeptide endocrine hormones (e.g., insulin-like growth factor or IGF), but most polypeptide hormones (e.g., insulin, glucagon, or growth hormone) don't have specific binding proteins and thus have very short lifetimes in the bloodstream. Paracrine and autocrine hormones don't require binding proteins because they travel over very short distances and aren't meant to circulate in the bloodstream.

Getting to a target cell is no easy task for a hormone since most cells (muscles, heart tissue, lungs, and especially the brain are protected from the bloodstream by a group of cells called endothelial cells (see Figure 13-1). These cells act as a potent barrier to prevent many things (based primarily on size) passing from the bloodstream into the space (known as the interstitial space) between the endothelial cells and the actual target tissues of the hormones.

If the endothelial cell barrier is functioning well, hormones are not impeded from reaching the target cell. As you might imagine, any dysfunction in the endothelial cells will raise havoc with ultimate hormonal action by decreasing the concentration of the active hormone in the interstitial space. The integrity of the endothelial cell barrier therefore becomes another underlying factor in the aging process. If the hormone can't get to its target site, it's as if it weren't there in the first place, even though there may be higher than normal levels of that

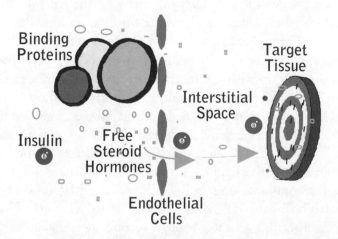

Figure 13-1   Endothelial Cells Separating Hormones from Target Tissues

hormone in the bloodstream. This inability to reach the target cell coupled with elevated levels of the hormone in the bloodstream is known as resistance. I have already discussed that the most common form of hormone resistance is insulin resistance, which is readily observed in Type 2 diabetics.

And now, we can finally talk about hormone action because it is the concentration of the active hormone within this interstitial space between the bloodstream and the target cell that starts the process of hormonal communication.

Even if you have adequate hormone levels in the interstitial space, the hormones still have to find their appropriate receptors on the cell surface. Receptors are the equivalent of a locking mechanism in which the hormone key must fit with precision. If you have the right key fitting the correct lock, then the door opens, and the biochemical message initially carried by the hormone can exert its action in the target cell. However, this lock on the cell membrane is in a fluid environment. The fluidity of a membrane depends on its fatty acid composition. The more fluid the plasma membrane (the outer membrane of a cell), the easier it is for the lock and key mechanism to make the right fit. The less fluid the membrane environment in which the receptor sits, the more difficult it becomes to get the two to come together. This is why saturated fats are minimized on the Zone Diet, since they would decrease membrane fluidity, making it more difficult for hormones to interact with their receptors.

Many hormones never get beyond this external contact with the receptor on the cell surface. They interact with the receptor that spans the membrane but never actually enter the cell. So how do they exert their action? Through molecules known as second messengers. Second messengers are molecules formed within the cell in response to the hormone linking up with the receptor on the outer surface of the cell. These are the actual agents that induce the hormonal messenger within the cell. The most widely studied second messenger is cyclic AMP (cAMP). The enzyme adenylate cyclase catalyzes the synthesis of cyclic AMP from ATP. In fact, the 1971 Nobel Prize in medicine was awarded to Earl Sutherland for his research on this second messenger.

Other second messengers include cyclic GMP (cGMP), 1,4,5-inositol triphosphate (IP_3), and diacylgylcerol (DAG). Hormones, such as insulin, that operate through second messengers, such as IP_3 and DAG, decrease cyclic AMP levels. This means that if a cell has multiple hormone receptors and is being bombarded by different hormones, then the final biological response of the cell depends on which second messenger system (cAMP or IP$_3$/DAG) predominates at that point in time. This is why the second messengers (IP$_3$/DAG) produced by insulin are antagonistic to the second messengers (cAMP) produced by "good" eicosanoids.

These second messengers are made in response to hormonal signals on the outer surface of the cell. Once synthesized inside the cell, they start a cascade of events that leads to the final biological response in the cell, which was originally signaled by the hypothalamus. It is the level of these second messengers within the target cell that actually controls hormonal communication. This is why "good" eicosanoids play such a prominent role in aging, they are able to increase the levels of cyclic AMP in the target cell, thereby ensuring better transmission of the biological information delivered by endocrine hormones. And maintaining threshold concentrations of these second messengers (especially cyclic AMP) is the key to anti-aging since second messengers represent the final phase of hormonal communication.

However, not all hormones act through receptors on the outer surface of the cell to generate second messengers. A few, like insulin, enter into the cell through a very complex transport system; once inside the cell, they promote the synthesis of second messengers. Still other hormones, like steroid and thyroid hormones enter into the cell by diffusion (after being released from their binding proteins in the bloodstream) and then find their target receptors either in the cytoplasma of the cell or on the membrane of the cell's nucleus. Once bound to these receptors, they are transported into the nucleus where they generate the synthesis of new proteins to exert the biological action originally signaled by the hypothalamus.

You can already appreciate that endocrine hormones rely upon a very complex series of steps to communicate information. Before these very complex endocrine hormone systems evolved, seemingly less complex hormones were already operational. The first hormones developed by living organisms are called autocrine hormones because they are secreted and either come back to act on the original secreting cell or on its immediate neighboring cell via discrete receptors. In essence, autocrine hormones act like scouts, sampling the immediate environment and then reporting back to the fort (the cell) about what it's like out there.

These first hormones didn't need (nor do they need now) a complex highway system like the bloodstream to travel upon to reach their target cell. Nor did they require a hypothalamus to direct hormonal traffic flow or the complex feedback control systems found in endocrine hormonal axis systems. Yet in many ways these autocrine hormones may be the most powerful hormones in your body, controlling the microenvironment of each of the 60 trillion cells in the human body, including the glands that synthesize endocrine hormones. In essence, autocrine hormones are your master hormones. They are the hormones that affect all other hormones. Like the Intel computer chip that controls your personal computer, these autocrine hormones control your hormonal communication system acting as a backup system to generate the necessary second messengers should the primary endocrine hormone system become dysfunctional. As a result, many of the hormonal axis systems that human life is based on depend upon these autocrine backup systems as a fail-safe mechanism to make sure that a threshold level of second messengers are present within a target cell. The more this baseline level of the appropriate second messenger is maintained, the less of that endocrine hormone is required to exert its biological action. So even if endocrine hormone levels decrease with aging, if you are maintaining adequate levels of autocrine hormones (which can raise the levels of second messengers, especially cyclic AMP), then hormonal communication is preserved, and you have reversed aging.

As part of evolutionary development, between these two groups of hormones (endocrine and autocrine) are the paracrine hormones. Paracrine hormones diffuse from one neighboring cell to another and don't travel the superhighway of the bloodstream like endocrine hormones. The best example of these hormones are neurotransmitters, like serotonin, that travel in discrete paths from one cell to another. Other examples are the releasing hormones that travel short distances through the hypophyseal duct from the hypothalamus directly to the pituitary gland.

It is useful to return to the analogy of the telephone system to visualize the interrelationships of these three hormone groups. Endocrine hormones are equivalent to a long-distance service using microwave towers to carry their message over distant areas. Paracrine hormones are like the local phone line that feeds directly to your telephone. Autocrine hormones are like the receiver of the phone that actually communicates the message to you. All three components must work in unison, but a dysfunction in the receiver (i.e., autocrine system) can wipe out the entire message. Hormonal miscommunication is primarily an autocrine hormone failure.

But hormones are far more complex than a phone system because they don't simply have to communicate, but must exert biological actions as well. As I have stated earlier, they are more like the Internet with complex information-filtering systems and redundant backup systems to make sure the message gets to the correct location at the correct time. The better this communication system works, the better the living organism functions. On the other hand, any degradation of this sophisticated communication system will give rise to systemwide information breakdowns. Since this would represent a general deterioration with time, breakdowns in hormonal communication can be viewed as the molecular definition of aging.

The molecular foundation of aging is not due to a lack of hormones, as much as it is due to increasing hormonal miscommunication. And the supports for the foundation of hormonal miscommunication are the four pillars of aging. Therefore, the most important hormones you want to modify in a successful anti-aging program are those that can directly affect each pillar of aging. Fortunately, each of those key hormones can all be directly influenced by the Anti-aging Zone Lifestyle Pyramid.

CHAPTER 14

INSULIN:
YOUR PASSPORT TO ACCELERATED AGING

Excess insulin is the primary pillar of aging. There is no better way to accelerate aging than to produce too much insulin (the result of excess calorie consumption). However, not all calories are equivalent when it comes to stimulating insulin production. Carbohydrates are the most powerful stimulators of insulin, followed to a much lesser extent by proteins, whereas fat has no effect on insulin.

While too much insulin accelerates aging, bear in mind that without enough insulin your cells will starve to death. This is why the levels of insulin in your bloodstream must be maintained within a zone. For example, recently published research indicates that cardiovascular mortality follows a U-shaped curve based on insulin levels. At low levels of insulin, mortality increased. At high levels of insulin, mortality also increases. Between these insulin extremes, mortality is the lowest. If anti-aging is your goal, then insulin moderation is critical.

As I mentioned earlier, without insulin, your cells essentially starve to death. This is what happens to Type 1 diabetics who can't make any insulin. Can you push insulin too low? Of course you can. This is what happens when you eat a high-protein, low-carbohydrate diet. Fasting insulin levels drop rapidly (often within days on these diets). Unfortunately, you develop a whole new series of problems. One is ketosis.

Your liver has a very limited supply of stored glucose in the form of glycogen (a polymer of glucose) that can be used to replenish blood sugar levels (the glycogen stored in muscles can't be used for this purpose). This glucose reserve can be used up very rapidly within 12 to 24 hours. Without adequate carbohydrate reserves in the liver, the body can't break down fats effectively, leaving behind what are known as ketone bodies. In a pinch, the brain can use these as a poor man's glucose. However, your body will go to great lengths to get rid of these ketone bodies through increased urination, and much of the actual weight loss on these high-protein diets is only water loss. When that happens, you also lose electrolytes, causing hypotension (low blood pressure) and fatigue.

But your brain didn't fall off the turnip truck. The body will start breaking down muscle protein to make glucose. This is known as gluconeogenesis. It's not very efficient, but if the brain requires carbohydrate, it will get it somewhere. In addition, without adequate supplies of glucose, you will become irritable and mental cognition decreases. In addition, research has indicated that the longer you stay in ketosis, the more your fat cells adapt so that they are transformed into "fat magnets," becoming 10 times more active in accumulating fat.

A high-protein, low-carbohydrate diet drives insulin levels too low, thereby causing hypotension, fatigue, irritability, lack of mental clarity, loss of muscle mass, increased hunger, and rapid fat regain when carbohydrates are reintroduced into the diet. Not exactly a prescription for anti-aging. This coupled with the increase in cardiovascular mortality because insulin levels are too low, simply reinforces the need to maintain insulin within a zone: not too high, not too low.

Why insulin is so critical to the aging process has to do with how your body handles food. The two key hormones that direct the utilization of food are insulin and glucagon. Insulin drives nutrients into cells for either immediate use or future storage. Glucagon mobilizes stored energy (primarily carbohydrate) to circulate in the bloodstream as a source of energy, especially for the brain, between meals. From a pictorial viewpoint, insulin can be viewed as a storage hormone and glucagon as a mobilization hormone as shown in Figure 14-1 on page 141.

These two hormones have to work in close cooperation. This is why they form an axis that controls blood sugar levels with incredible precision. Should anything upset this axis of insulin and glucagon, especially increased insulin, then the result is accelerated aging.

Insulin is very efficient at removing nutrients (especially glucose) from circulation and storing them for future use. In an earlier time when you didn't know where your next meal was coming from, producing a strong insulin response to incoming calories was a powerful survival mechanism. Today, in America that ancient survival mechanism has turned into a potent accelerator of aging because we are con-

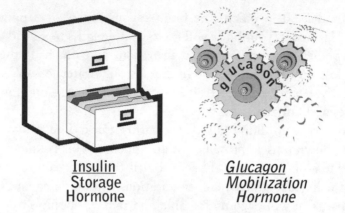

Insulin
Storage
Hormone

Glucagon
Mobilization
Hormone

Figure 14-1   **Insulin and Glucagon Work Together as Storage and Mobilization Hormones**

stantly surrounded by accessible calories. The more calories we eat (especially if they are carbohydrates), the more our insulin levels increase. This trend has accelerated rapidly in the last 15 years in America.

Unlike most hormones, insulin levels increase with aging. First, we know that two of the biological markers of aging are (1) increasing insulin resistance and (2) decreasing glucose tolerance. From the earlier chapter on biological markers of aging, you know these markers are two sides of the same coin—the inability of insulin to communicate with its target cells.

At the molecular level, insulin resistance (and glucose intolerance) just means that target cells in the muscles don't respond well to the amount of insulin in the bloodstream, forcing the pancreas to make more insulin. What is the molecular basis of insulin resistance? No one knows for sure, but a very likely candidate is the cellular barrier that separates target cells from the bloodstream. This is known as the endothelial cell barrier, and any dysfunction in this barrier will prevent insulin (or other hormones of that size or greater) from gaining access to its receptors. Endothelial cell dsyfunction is common in Type 2 diabetics, and the insulin levels in the interstitial space (the space between the bloodstream and the target cell surface) is low compared to the amount of insulin in the bloodstream. This means you might have adequate hormone levels in the blood, but as far as the target cells are concerned there simply isn't enough. As far as the target cell is concerned, there appears to be a *de facto* insulin deficiency. As a result, the pancreas secretes even more insulin, which accelerates aging.

What happens if insulin resistance continues for an extended period of time? Since blood glucose is not being taken up by the target cells, it begins to pile up in the bloodstream. The pancreas, which is constantly sensing blood glucose levels, realizes an unhappy situation is developing and immediately secretes more insulin. Eventually, by brute force, blood glucose levels are brought down, but now you have an excess of insulin floating in the bloodstream. This is called hyperinsulinemia (elevated blood insulin), and it is your worst aging nightmare.

How is it, that this needed ability to store extra calories for a rainy day results in accelerated aging when insulin levels are too high? It turns out there are a whole host of reasons:

1. Excess insulin is indicative of excess calorie consumption. The more calories you eat, the more free radicals you make.
2. Excess insulin inhibits the release of glucagon, whose primary responsibility is restoration of blood glucose levels for optimal brain function. If glucagon secretion is inhibited, you will increase cortisol secretion as a backup hormonal system to restore blood glucose levels. This leads to excess cortisol in the bloodstream.
3. Excess insulin is a powerful growth factor. It causes cellular DNA to turn over more frequently, thereby shortening the telomere length of the DNA.
4. Excess insulin distorts other hormonal systems (in particular eicosanoids) so that the hormonal miscommunication begins to cause chaos within your biological Internet. In addition, excess insulin can decrease the levels of cyclic AMP, the primary second messenger that many endocrine hormones use to generate their biological action.
5. Excess insulin increases insulin resistance, so that insulin levels become more elevated in the bloodstream, which accelerates aging even faster.
6. Excess insulin increases the accumulation of stored fat. This increase in adipose tissue can have negative consequences on the metabolism of sex hormones and increase the likelihood of cardiovascular disease.

These factors explain why your Anti-aging Zone Report Card is so closely correlated with excess insulin. Measurement of fasting insulin gives you a direct insight on your insulin levels. The fasting trigylceride/HDL cholesterol ratio is a surrogate marker of your insulin levels. Likewise, any increase in your percentage body fat is also an indication of increasing insulin levels. Finally, the glycosylated hemoglobin measurement indicates your degree of glucose intolerance.

So, if excess insulin levels should be avoided, how do you do it? The explanation requires some knowledge of how this unique hormone works.

Insulin was the first polypeptide hormone to be isolated and commercially produced. Discovered in 1921, it represented an early triumph for endocrinology because it saved Type 1 diabetics from a certain early death. Commercially, because of its relatively small size and ease of extraction from beef and pork pancreas, it became possible to purify very large amounts of it. And best of all from a drug company's perspective, these patients had to take it for the rest of their life. Because of insulin's early commercial success, we probably know more about this hormone than any other. And the more you know about insulin, the more complex the picture becomes.

Insulin is produced in the pancreas. Unlike other endocrine hormones, there is no direct signal from the pituitary that alerts the pancreas to start making insulin. Some insulin is prestored in granules, which can be released rapidly. This gives rise to what is known as the first-phase response. Anything that interacts with the sweet receptors in the mouth (including artificial sweeteners) will signal for the early release of this stored insulin into the bloodstream in anticipation that carbohydrates will shortly enter the system. The second-phase response consists of the continuing release of newly synthesized insulin in response to changes in the circulating levels of glucose caused by incoming carbohydrates.

But this doesn't mean that insulin is not subject to some indirect control by the hypothalamus. In the hypothalamus, the balance of two neurotransmitters (serotonin and dopamine) have a significant impact on insulin secretion. As serotonin levels rise, insulin secretion is increased. If dopamine levels rise, insulin levels decrease. Since serotonin levels in the hypothalamus rise at night, this means that the later you eat a large meal, the more insulin will be secreted and those late-night calories will be stored as fat.

Insulin levels can also be controlled by other hormones, particularly its axis partner glucagon. Glucagon was discovered at nearly the same time as insulin. Unlike insulin, which is needed to drive nutrients into cells, glucagon's primary purpose is to release stored carbohydrates from the liver into the bloodstream to restore and maintain blood glucose levels. As glucagon levels rise, insulin levels drop. Thus, one of the best ways to control excess insulin is to maintain adequate glucagon levels.

Glucagon levels are largely determined by the amount of incoming dietary protein, just as insulin levels are strongly related to the amount of incoming carbohydrate. Although, incoming protein has a slight stimulatory effect on insulin, it has a much more powerful effect on glucagon secretion. Protein must be consumed at every meal and snack because it is the primary stimulator of glucagon, whose main biochemical function is to release stored carbohydrate from the liver into the bloodstream to maintain adequate levels of blood glucose for the brain. Unlike insulin, glucagon uses a different second messenger to achieve its task. That second messenger is the same one used by most other endocrine hormones, cyclic AMP. This is also the second messenger that can be increased by making more "good" eicosanoids. (As I stated earlier, the second messenger used by insulin (IP_3/DAG) will depress cyclic AMP levels). So by increasing the levels of "good" eicosanoids, you make the biological response of glucagon more effective.

One last factor can affect insulin levels: other hormones. The most important are two of the primary players in aging—cortisol and eicosanoids. Although cortisol raises blood glucose levels, as does glucagon, it also can increase insulin levels. Whereas glucagon lowers insulin secretion directly, cortisol increases insulin resistance, thereby indirectly increasing insulin levels. As levels of insulin increase in the bloodstream, glucagon secretion is further inhibited. This forces the increased secretion of even more cortisol to help increase blood glucose levels. This increase in cortisol further increases insulin resistance, forcing the pancreas to pump out even more insulin to overcome the growing inability of glucose to get into its target cells. The end result is increasing cortisol secretion, which can cause the death of cortisol-sensitive cells in the thymus (which profoundly affects your immune status) and in the hippocampus of the brain (which controls memory and helps with the integration of incoming signals to the hypothalamus). Neither event is beneficial for any anti-aging program.

An even more complex situation arises in the case of eicosanoids. Some eicosanoids inhibit insulin secretion, others increase it. In particular, insulin stimulates the production of "bad" eicosanoids that generate even greater insulin output. Again, as with cortisol, a positive feedback loop for insulin is developed. As more insulin is secreted, greater amounts of more "bad" eicosanoids are synthesized, which in turn cause the secretion of more insulin. The eicosanoids that increase insulin secretion are the same ones that increase the likelihood of heart disease, cancer, and arthritis.

Insulin levels are really controlled by a combination of factors, ranging from diet, the balance of neurotransmitters in the hypothalamus, and other hormones in the system that are affected by insulin. As you might expect, with all of these factors in play, it's easy for something to go wrong with this insulin control system. And when that happens, insulin levels increase and aging accelerates.

To understand the role that insulin has on the aging process at the molecular level, you have to understand how insulin delivers information to its target cells. Although insulin is a polypeptide hormone, it doesn't use a binding protein to maintain its circulatory levels. As a result, the half-life of insulin in the bloodstream is about 4 to 6 minutes. In this time period, insulin has to reach the target cell, find its receptor, and then (unlike most other hormones) be taken into the cell by a process known as endocytosis. Once inside the cell, insulin activates its second messengers (DAG and IP_3) to tell the cell to allow nutrients (especially glucose) to enter.

Ironically, although the brain is critically dependent on incoming glucose from the bloodstream, there are no insulin receptors on the surface of the brain. Glucose enters the brain by non-insulin mediated transport. The amount of glucose entering the brain is controlled by its levels in the bloodstream. At first glance, excess glucose in the bloodstream should be just fine for the brain as it needs glucose to maintain itself. Unfortunately, excess glucose in the bloodstream also means excess glucose in the brain. This excessive glucose can cause glucose-induced toxicity in the gluco-receptors of the ventromedial nucleus (VMN) in the hypothalamus. And the greater the glucose levels in the bloodstream or the brain, the greater the likelihood of producing damaging AGEs. Thus, maintaining glucose in a very tight zone becomes critical for human life.

There is another important reason why you want to keep insulin within a zone—it is the most important predictor of heart disease. The data on excess insulin levels and heart disease have been accumulating for more than 20 years in the scientific literature. If all of this is known, why is so little discussed about insulin and heart disease? Conversely, why is it that all we hear is "eating fat causes heart disease," since fat has no effect on insulin? The answers to both questions elude me. My first book, *The Zone,* was written purposely to address that point. Four years later, a growing body of new research reinforces my original position that the true villain in heart disease is excess insulin, not dietary fat.

Heart disease at the cellular level is caused by the death of heart muscle cells that don't get enough oxygen. Blocked arteries increase the likelihood of decreased oxygen transfer, but 25 percent of heart disease deaths occur in individuals who have no advanced atheroscleroic lesions in their arteries. These people die because of a spasm (i.e., a cramp) that decreases or even stops blood flow to the muscle cells of the heart. These people also tend to have normal cholesterol levels. This is not to say that reducing cholesterol levels is not important, but only to point out that cholesterol levels are not a gold standard for predicting heart attacks. In fact, it is estimated that nearly 50 percent of patients hospitalized with heart disease have normal cholesterol levels. If cholesterol is not such a great predictor of impending heart disease, then what is?

A study published in 1998 in the *Journal of the American Medical Association* gives some answers. This study looked at traditional risk factors compared to fasting insulin levels to see which was more predictive of developing heart disease over a 5-year period in individuals who had no trace of heart disease at the beginning of the study. The results are shown in Figure 14-2 on page 146.

You can see from this figure that fasting insulin levels are more than twice as predictive for the development of heart disease than LDL cholesterol, which is currently considered the gold standard. Yet, billions of dollars are spent each year on drugs that reduce LDL cholesterol, and yet, the one drug (i.e., the Zone Diet) that can reduce fasting insulin levels is ignored.

Notice also in Figure 14-2 that triglycerides are also more predictive of developing heart disease than LDL cholesterol levels are. One of the first signs of hyperinsulinemia is increased triglycerides. As you have already seen, both insulin and triglycerides drop dramatically on

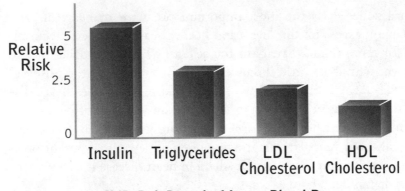

Figure 14-2   CHD Risk Ratio for Various Blood Parameters

the Zone Diet within weeks. Although HDL cholesterol by itself is a less powerful predictor of future risk of heart disease than is LDL cholesterol, when you multiply the increase in risk of elevated triglycerides by the increase in risk of decreased HDL cholesterol, the result is only slightly behind fasting insulin as a predictor of heart attacks. This should not be too surprising since the fasting triglyceride/HDL ratio is a surrogate marker for fasting insulin. One of the reasons why the fasting triglyceride/HDL ratio is very predictive for heart disease may be due to the formation of small dense atherogenic LDL particles that are very prone to oxidation. The higher the fasting triglyceride/HDL ratio, the greater the proportion of the small, dense atherogenic LDL particles, and the greater the risk of heart disease.

This is why any diet recommended for cardiovascular patients (or anyone for that matter) that increases the fasting triglyceride/HDL cholesterol ratio must be considered potentially dangerous. How dangerous? Researchers at Harvard Medical School gave us a clue in a 1997 article in *Circulation*. They took patients who had survived their first heart attack (these are the strong ones, since the others died within the first 6 weeks) and then compared them to matched patients who had no history of heart disease. When they looked at the triglyceride/HDL ratio to see how predictive it was, a dramatic result was observed (see Figure 14-3 on page 147).

The patients with the highest ratio of triglycerides/HDL cholesterol were 16 times more likely to have a heart attack than those with lower ratios. Let's put this in perspective. As I stated earlier, high cholesterol increases the likelihood of a heart attack by a factor of 2. And everyone in medicine recommends lowering excessive cholesterol

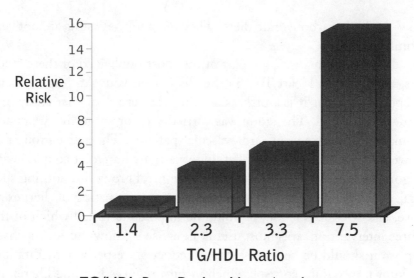

Figure 14-3   TG/HDL Ratio Predicts Heart Attacks

levels. Smoking increases the likelihood of a heart attack by a factor of 4. And everyone in medicine recommends that you stop smoking. Yet a high triglyceride/HDL ratio increases the likelihood of a heart attack by a factor of 16 and no one does anything about it even though the drug is available today to reduce that ratio. What is that drug? It's the Zone Diet.

Much has been said about dietary fat as the cause of heart disease and therefore its implication in accelerated aging. Americans have come to believe that fat intake must be reduced at all costs. But is that really so? No, because fat has no direct effect on insulin.

This is why in 1997, a group of leading nutrition researchers wrote in the *New England Journal of Medicine* that there is no persuasive data supporting the hypothesis that a low-fat, high-carbohydrate diet has any long-term benefit in treating obesity, heart disease, and cancer. Why? Because each of those disease conditions is associated with hyperinsulinemia. Fat has no effect on insulin secretion, whereas carbohydrates have a major stimulatory effect.

Defenders of low-fat, high-carbohydrate diets continue to point to all the epidemiological studies that "prove" these low-fat, high-carbohydrate diets are next to godliness. Unfortunately, epidemiology doesn't prove anything. It only makes associations (which are very different than actual causes) that lay the groundwork for studies under controlled clinical situations. Do such studies exist on the "benefits" of low-fat, high-carbohydrate diets? They do, and the results are not very comforting.

I have already discussed part of the most publicized of these studies, the Lifestyle Heart Trial in the chapter on your Anti-aging Zone Report Card, but it is worth examining the results of that study in a little more detail. The study was carried out for some five years and compared two groups of cardiovascular patients. The active group followed a strict vegetarian low-fat, high-carbohydrate diet coupled with vigorous exercise, and meditation. The control group did nothing special. Since this was a multi-factorial program consisting of diet, exercise, and stress reduction, it would be impossible to tell which of the three interventions was most useful. Exercise is known to reduce insulin, so it should be beneficial. Stress reduction, especially meditation, is known to reduce cortisol, which in turn reduces insulin. Therefore, it should be useful. That's why both meditation and exercise are components of the Anti-aging Zone Lifestyle Pyramid.

This leaves only the diet employed in the Lifestyle Heart Trial, which was a vegetarian, low-fat, high-carbohydrate diet. This is the type of diet that can cause even greater elevations of fasting insulin in susceptible individuals if they have insulin resistance.

Even though we cannot isolate any one of the three simultaneous interventions, a look at the data after 5 years is instructive. Although there was improved blood flow in the active group compared to the control group, it is impossible to tell which of the interventions was responsible. After all, exercise will increase blood flow, as will reduction of cortisol by stress reduction. However, there was a more ominous trend developing in these patients: the increasing ratio of triglycerides/HDL cholesterol in the active group, but not in the control group (see Table 14-1).

In the control group, the ratio of triglycerides to HDL cholesterol

TABLE 14-1

TG/HDL Ratios after 5 Years of the Lifestyle Heart Trial

	TG/HDL AT START	TG/HDL AT 5 YEARS
Active Group	5.7	7.1
Control Group	4.4	3.9

(although still high enough to indicate hyperinsulinemia) decreased slightly after 5 years. On the other hand, the patients in the active group saw their trigylceride to HDL cholesterol increase by some 25 percent to a dangerously high ratio of 7.1. If I am to believe the data from Harvard Medical School, that is not a good sign for aging.

In reality the only statistic that counts is mortality. Since no one died in the control group (whereas one died in the active group), it is hard to say that the Lifestyle Heart Trial based on a vegetarian, low-fat, high-carbohydrate diet represents a major breakthrough in cardiovascular treatment, let alone anti-aging.

As more research is published on the effects of low-fat, high-carbohydrate diets, the results are strikingly consistent, because insulin levels are increased. And that is not good news if you are trying to reverse aging. Published studies on cardiovascular patients with high cholesterol, Type 2 diabetic patients, and post-menopausal women, all demonstrate that low-fat, high-carbohydrate diets consistently increase insulin levels. To reinforce this point, the American Heart Association Nutrition Committee presented an article in the 1998 issue of *Circulation* that includes the following statements about such diets:

> *Very low fat diets in the short term increase triglyceride levels and decrease HDL cholesterol levels without yielding additional decreases in LDL cholesterol levels.*

> *For certain persons, i.e., those with hypertriglyceridema or hyperinsulinemia, the elderly, or the very young, the potential for elevated triglycerides, decreased HDL cholesterol levels, or nutrient inadequacy must be considered.*

> *Because very low fat diets represent a radical departure from current prudent dietary guidelines, such diets must be proved both advantageous and safe before national recommendations can be issued.*

Yet despite all the negative published research evidence, it is as if the popular press (in particular women's magazines) are trying to accelerate aging in this country by constantly stressing the importance of following these same low-fat, high-carbohydrate diets. The success of their campaign can visibly be seen in the growing epidemic of obesity, which is the first consequence of hyperinsulinemia—all this even though Americans are actually eating less fat.

So how do you control hyperinsulinemia? In essence, you have a hormonal carburetor (your diet) that can control the output of insulin and glucagon for a 4-to-6-hour period. Balancing the protein-to-carbohydrate ratio at every meal becomes your primary "drug" to maintain insulin in a zone where sufficient levels are sustained to drive nutrients into cells—but without producing excess insulin (hyperinsulinemia)—and in the process controlling other critical hormonal systems, such as cortisol and eicosanoids.

To determine how well you are controlling insulin, simply use your Anti-aging Zone Report Card. Each of the testing parameters on your report card are related to excess insulin production. If you have passing scores on all the tests, then you know that you are keeping insulin levels under control. If not, then turn to the Anti-aging Zone Lifestyle Pyramid and begin following each of the prescriptions to lower insulin levels. The most powerful of those will be the Zone Diet.

Remember, that the Anti-aging Zone Lifestyle Pyramid contains an exercise component, which can also play a role in insulin control. As mentioned earlier, aerobic exercise is an exceptionally effective drug for lowering both excess blood glucose and increasing insulin sensitivity. Unfortunately, you might exercise only one hour per day, while you can eat 24 hours a day. This is why I use the 80/20 rule for determining the relative importance of the Zone Diet versus exercise for lowering insulin. The Zone Diet will be approximately four times times more beneficial than exercise alone to lower excess insulin. However, combine the Zone Diet and exercise and you have an exceptionally powerful "drug" combination to reduce excess insulin levels, which leads to greater longevity.

CHAPTER 15

CORTISOL:
WONDER DRUG OF THE 50s, MESSENGER OF AGING IN THE 90s

One of the great breakthroughs in twentieth-century medicine was the isolation and synthesis of cortisol, the most important member of a group of hormones known as corticosteroids. These hormones, synthesized in the adrenal glands, are critical to your body's mediation of stress. One potential definition of aging is the deterioration of the body's ability to respond to stress. Therefore, it should not be surprising that an imbalance in your body's levels of adrenal corticosteroids (either too high or too low) can play a significant role in the aging process.

As I mentioned earlier, the most graphic example of how these hormones affect the aging process is observed in Pacific salmon, which undergo rapid corticosteroid-induced aging (due to a virtual shutdown of their immune system) and quick death after spawning. On the other extreme, without sufficient levels of corticosteroids, it becomes impossible to respond, let alone adapt, to changes in long-term stressors whether they are physical (exercise); biological (viral, bacterial, or fungal infections); environmental (temperature), or even social (job, family, etc.).

In humans, there are two graphic examples of what happens when the balance of corticosteroids is disturbed. The first condition is known as Addison's disease, in which adrenal output of cortisol is too low. The other disease condition is known as Cushing's syndrome, in which the output of cortisol is too high. A listing of the characteristics of both diseases in Table 15-1 on page 152, paints a drastic picture of the consequences of poor cortisol control.

It is important to note that too little stress can be just as bad for you as too much stress. Without adequate stress, little adaption takes

TABLE 15-1

Comparison of Clinical Symptoms of Addison's Disease and Cushing's Syndrome

ADDISON'S DISEASE	CUSHING'S SYNDROME
Hypotension	Hypertension
Hypoglycemia	Hyperglycemia
Sodium loss	Sodium retention
Potassium elevation	Potassium loss
	Poor wound healing
	Bone loss
	Impaired immunological tolerance
	Thinning skin
	Muscle wasting
	Development of abdominal fat
	Psychosis

place, and your survival is ultimately compromised because the adrenal glands tend to atrophy, thus reducing their ability to produce cortisol. This is why Addison's disease (the lack of cortisol production) is so deadly. With Addison's disease, you have very little adrenal reserve capacity to handle stress when it does occur and, thus, a reduced ability to turn off an overactive response to stress. Reduced cortisol production, however, can also be a consequence of adrenal burnout due to continued exposure to constant stress. The most common experience of this adrenal burnout is constant fatigue. This is the exhaustive phase described by Hans Seyle in his pioneering studies on stress first published in 1937. In either case, you have exhausted your adrenal reserve capacity, and seemingly small stressors can now have devastating physiological consequences.

More striking are the clinical manifestations of cortisol's overproduction seen in Cushing's syndrome. These symptoms read like the who's who of the conditions associated with aging. As an example, one major problem with excess cortisol levels is the wasting of muscle tissue. As I mentioned earlier, gluconeogenesis (glucose production from protein) is a way the brain can produce enough glucose to meet its needs. Cortisol accelerates that process. The fastest way to lose muscle mass and strength is to maintain high levels of cortisol. If you remember, loss of muscle mass and strength are some of the primary biological markers of aging. Another consequence of excess cortisol is the acceleration of bone loss. Osteoporosis is one of the real fears of aging. Yet, nothing speeds up bone loss faster than increased cortisol levels.

How can the excess of just one hormone be involved in so many manifestations of aging? The explanation requires understanding how stress affects the body at the molecular level. A vivid physiological description of stress and how the body adapts to it was first outlined by Seyle. According to Selye's research, the first response to a stressor is an alarm phase, which increases corticosteroid production. This is followed by an adaptation phase during which corticosteroids continue to be produced to address the stressor until the stressful situation resolves itself, thereby allowing the system to return to its normal state or adapt to a new condition. However, there is also an exhaustion phase, in which continued exposure to the stressor eventually wears out the adrenal glands, thus compromising any future ability to respond to long-term stress.

At the molecular level, cortisol controls stress by shutting down the production of eicosanoids. As you remember from an earlier chapter, eicosanoids are autocrine hormones—made by every cell in the body—that respond to changes in the local environment, especially those caused by some form of stress. In essence, eicosanoids are the true molecular mediators of stress, and cortisol works by reducing overly elevated levels of eicosanoids for a short time period. This temporary shutdown of eicosanoids, gives the body time to adjust to the stress and hopefully resolve it. However, if the stress is not resolved, cortisol continues to be secreted. Because of its inhibitory effect on eicosanoid synthesis, this continued secretion begins to shutting down eicosanoid synthesis completely. As a result your biological Internet also shuts down. That's why excess cortisol is also one of the pillars of aging.

The effect of cortisol on eicosanoids explains why cortisol initially was considered the wonder drug of the 1950s. In 1948, Compound E (which was cortisol) was isolated by Edward Kendall and adminstered by Philip Hench to a woman with severe arthritis. Within days her arthritic symptoms virtually disappeared. The miracle drug was finally at hand, or so people thought. The frenzy of this new medical breakthrough led to Hench and Kendall receiving the 1950 Nobel Prize in

Medicine for their discovery. Virtually every disease where cortisol was used as a treatment, there was a sudden, almost miraculous recovery by the patient.

Nor were the drug companies immune from this frenzy. Although natural corticosteroids were available, they were not patentable. This spawned a great deal of activity by pharmaceutical companies in the 1950s to synthesize new (i.e., patentable) and even more powerful analogs of natural corticosteroids. And for a time, the golden age of steroid pharmaceuticals seemed at hand. Virtually every disease condition with an inflammatory component was magically improved using these new patented drugs. Examples of these drugs include prednisone, dexamethesone, and betamethasone. Yet today, these same drugs strike fear into the heart of any patient who uses them.

Why don't corticosteroids have that golden ring to their name today? Because corticosteroids are non-discriminatory. While they shut down the production of pro-inflammatory eicosanoids (i.e., "bad" eicosanoids), they also shut down the production of "good" eicosanoids that the cardiovascular, immune, and central nervous systems require for optimal hormonal communication. This is why within 30 days of high-dose corticosteroid usage, severe immunological problems set in. An example of this is what happens when you give a single intravenous injection of corticosteroids to normal individuals. Within 24 hours, their T-cells (primarily the T-helper cells) are dramatically depleted. To put this in perspective, the same thing happens to AIDS patients over time, but now the same effect can be created within 24 hours by a single injection. This impact on the immune system is why long-term use of corticosteroids is rarely contemplated, and why these former wonder drugs eventually became the drugs of last resort.

Cortisol inhibits eicosanoid production by causing the synthesis of a protein that inhibits the enzyme (phospholipase A_2) required for the release of essential fatty acids from the membrane phospholipids. This inhibitory protein (called lipocortin) is only synthesized if cortisol interacts with its receptor on the nuclear membrane. While cortisol is complexed to its binding protein (corticosteroid binding globulin or CBG) in the bloodstream, it is inactive. However, once released, cortisol can pass into a cell because it is somewhat water insoluble, and eventually seeks out its receptor within the cell (as opposed to the surface of the cell). This receptor-cortisol complex is then translocated into the nucleus where it can search for the right sequence of DNA to be activated, thus causing the production of lipocortin. In the presence of lipocortin, all eicosanoid synthesis stops because the substrate (essential fatty acids) for eicosanoid formation can't be released from the phospholipids in the cell membrane. This state of eicosanoid inhibition continues until the newly synthesized lipocortin protein is degraded in the cell.

Obviously, you don't want eicosanoid synthesis interrupted for a considerable period of time, so cortisol is relatively short-acting. However, that means if cortisol is used as a drug, it must be given every 4 hours or so. That leads to compliance problems, which were neatly solved by drug companies who synthesized analogs of cortisol that could last for days. Unfortunately, this meant that eicosanoid synthesis would also shut down for days, and that's one of the reasons why the wonder drugs of the 1950s became the ex-wonder drugs of today.

As is typical with most endocrine hormones, the starting site for cortisol production begins in the hypothalamus. The hypothalamus responds to a stressor by producing corticotropin releasing hormone (CRH), which travels via the hypophyseal portal duct to the pituitary gland, which causes the synthesis of adrenocorticotropic hormone (ACTH) as seen in Figure 15-1 on page 156.

Actually CRH never enters the pituitary. It stimulates the synthesis of ACTH through the increased synthesis of second messenger cyclic AMP inside the pituitary gland. ACTH is then released from the pituitary into the bloodstream to reach the adrenal glands.

The adrenal glands consist of an outer surface (the cortex) and an inner core (the medulla). In the medulla of the adrenal glands, the acute stress hormones epinephrine and norepinephrine are synthesized, and their release is also stimulated by ACTH. Most people know these hormones by their common names adrenaline and noradrenaline. These are the "flight-or-fight" hormones you need during times of acute stress. It is in the outer cortex of the adrenals that cortisol is made in response to chronic long-term stress. While ACTH interacts with cell receptors in the adrenal medulla to release adrenaline, it also has receptors in the adrenal cortex to begin a complex series of reactions that eventually lead to cortisol formation.

Not surprisingly, the first step in cortisol's synthesis in the cortex of the adrenal gland involves cyclic AMP. The increase in cyclic AMP causes the release of cholesterol from cholesterol ester storage droplets within the cells of the adrenal cortex. The newly released cholesterol

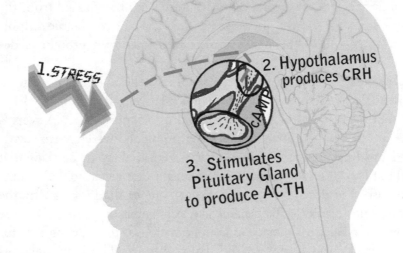

Figure 15-1   Transformation of Stress into Hormonal Action

is acted upon by the mitochondria to form the steroid hormone pregnenolone, which is then converted by a series of reactions to cortisol
(see Figure 15-2 on page 157).

The newly formed cortisol is released into the bloodstream where
it combines with a corticosteroid-binding protein (CBG). This binding protein acts as a controlled release delivery system, allowing small
amounts of cortisol to leach off and circulate freely in the bloodstream.
As free cortisol levels rise, there is a feedback mechanism to the hypothalamus to stop any further release of CRH (see Figure 15-3 on page
158).

This is known as the hypothalamus-pituitary-adrenal axis, which
is a more complex axis system than the insulin-glucagon axis discussed
in the last chapter. Adding to this complexity, cortisol output is also
normally under a circadian rhythm. Cortisol levels are the highest in
the bloodstream between 3 and 6 o'clock in the morning, and then
gradually decrease throughout the day. As you age, this circadian

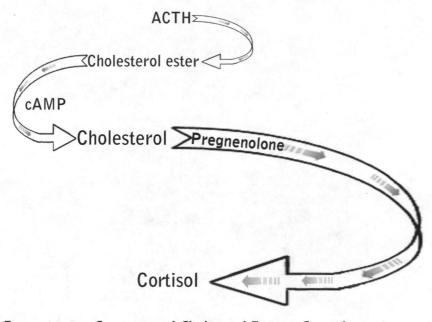

Figure 15-2   Conversion of Cholesterol Ester to Cortisol Requires Cyclic AMP

rhythm is disrupted. However, the primary trouble spot that prevents the hypothalamus-pituitary-adrenal axis from functioning smoothly as you age is the body's constant requirement of cyclic AMP as a second messenger. Cyclic AMP is needed to maintain hormonal communication between the hypothalamus and the pituitary and between ACTH and the adrenal cortex to control cortisol synthesis. If the levels of cyclic AMP drop below a critical threshold level in any of the glands that are part of this axis, then the entire system goes off-kilter. As will be explained in the next chapter, the primary way to maintain a threshold level of cyclic AMP in target cells is to ensure that "good" eicosanoids are constantly being generated.

Besides affecting eicosanoids, excess cortisol has the capacity to kill at the cellular level. In particular, the thymus (which is responsible for making T-lymphocytes) is very sensitive to excess cortisol. This is one reason why the thymus shrinks with age and with a corresponding loss of immune function. Even more important, as I described earlier, is the fact that excess cortisol reduces brain longevity by killing cortisol-sensitive neurons in the hippocampus.

So how do you keep cortisol from becoming too elevated? By following the Anti-aging Zone Lifestyle Pyramid. Of the three compo-

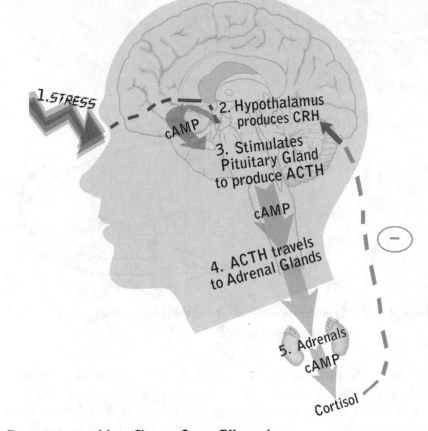

Figure 15-3   How Chronic Stress Effects the Hypothalamus-Pituitary-Adrenal Axis

nents of that pyramid, the Zone Diet will be the most important because it stabilizes blood glucose levels.

As I stated earlier, many physiological functions have numerous backup systems to operate smoothly. Since the brain is the central control system for humans, it is not surprising that at least four different hormonal systems are in place to increase blood glucose levels so that a stable fuel supply for the brain is constantly maintained. The primary hormone responsible for this is glucagon. However, this hormonal system is controlled to a great extent by the protein content of the diet. If the diet is low in protein at any one meal, insufficient levels of glucagon may be generated, forcing the body to move to a secondary backup system. Usually, the increased secretion of cortisol will be that backup system. Since low-protein meals are also usually high-carbohydrate meals, this means that excess insulin will be produced at the same time that glucagon levels are depressed. Excess insulin drives down blood glucose to an even greater extent, forcing the body to produce increasing amounts of cortisol in a valiant effort to maintain blood glucose levels, which should have been the job of glucagon. Unfortunately, the end result will be even greater circulating levels of cortisol, which will have a powerful inhibition on eicosanoid synthesis, thus giving rise not only to immune dysfunction, but to a decrease in cyclic AMP levels. Many of the overt symptoms associated with Cushing's syndrome can be produced on a smaller scale just by continued consumption of a low-protein, high-carbohydrate diet.

The importance of exercise in the Anti-aging Zone Lifestyle Pyramid for controlling cortisol is a little more complex. At low levels of prolonged moderate exercise (like walking), insulin levels are gradually reduced and blood glucose levels rise in response to exercise-related increases in glucagon. With the primary glucose restoration system working smoothly, there is no need for increased cortisol production during moderate exercise. On the other hand, at higher levels of exercise intensity, significant stress is now generated, and cortisol levels begin to rise. Actually the phrase "no pain, no gain" is not true for both exercise and longevity. The more intense the exercise, the fewer benefits it has for longevity. This is why the longevity curve plateaus shortly after moderate exercise is intensified. There is also a corresponding increase in free radical formation with more intense exercise. This fact was recognized by Kenneth Cooper, the father of aerobics, in his book, *The Antioxidant Revolution*, in which he recognizes that a more physically fit individual as a consequence of intense exercise may not be as healthy in the long term as the less physically fit individual who follows a moderate, but consistent exercise program.

The third component of the Anti-aging Zone Lifestyle Pyramid for reducing cortisol levels is stress reduction. It has been shown consistently that any type of stress reduction whether it's meditation, enjoying a hobby, or simply relaxing will lower cortisol levels. However, meditation is the most powerful way to reduce excess cortisol because it is a highly defined system whose benefits in lowering cortisol have been clinically proven.

So, there you have three pretty good hormonal strategies to reduce excess cortisol production: the Zone Diet, moderate exercise, and meditation. That's why they are all components of the Anti-aging Zone Lifestyle Pyramid.

You now know that elevated levels of both insulin and cortisol accelerate the aging process. But how? It's through their adverse effects on eicosanoids. In ancient times, it was said that all roads lead to Rome. I believe it is also correct to say, "all roads to anti-aging lead to eicosanoids."

The story of eicosanoids is really the fundamental story of anti-aging. As you will see in the next chapter, eicosanoids can either make you age faster or slower. More importantly you have the ability to control that outcome.

CHAPTER 16

EICOSANOIDS:
YOUR INTEL COMPUTER CHIP

Now it's time to get to the real hormonal core of anti-aging: eicosa-noids. Ask most physicians and medical researchers what an eicosa-noid is, and you will usually get a blank stare, even though the 1982 Nobel Prize in Medicine was awarded for understanding how eicosa-noids control virtually every aspect of human physiology. As unknown as they are to the vast majority of the medical establishment, eicosa-noids are the hormones that maintain the information fidelity of your biological Internet, which means they become the key to anti-aging.

Eicosanoids are a group of almost mystical, if not magical, hor-mones that are made by every cell in your body. In many ways they are analogous to the Intel microprocessor that transforms your personal computer into an amazing technological marvel. Like the transient flow of electrons that travel through a microprocessor, eicosanoids are also ephemeral. Like electrons in the microprocessor, eicosanoids work in vanishingly low concentrations. And once eicosanoids have done their job, they seem to disappear. But just as the electron flow through a microprocessor controls information traffic for your personal com-puter, all the information that flows through your biological Internet depends on eicosanoids.

If eicosanoids are the key to anti-aging, then why haven't you heard of them? The reason so little is known about these hormones is because they are so complex. Because they are autocrine hormones, eicosanoids don't travel through the bloodstream, they work at incred-ibly minute concentrations and self-destruct in seconds. All of these factors make them virtually impossible to study in the body. This is why most of our knowledge of eicosanoids comes from (a) tissue cul-tures to which you can add eicosanoids, (b) the study of the few stable metabolites of eicosanoids that are found in the urine, or (c) through a greater understanding on the effects of drugs (like aspirin, nonsteroid anti-inflammatories, and corticosteroids) whose primary mode of action is to alter or inhibit eicosanoid formation.

Eicosanoids encompass a wide array of hormones, many of which have never been heard of even by endocrinologists. They are derived from a unique group of polyunsaturated essential fatty acids containing 20 carbon atoms. The different classes of eicosanoids are shown in Table 16-1.

TABLE 16-1

Subgroups of Eicosanoids

Prostaglandins
Thromboxanes
Leukotrienes
Lipoxins
Hydroxylated fatty acids
Isoprostanoids
Epi-isoprostanoids
Isoleukotrienes

Now if you mention prostaglandins to physicians, they are likely to have heard of those particular hormones. But prostaglandins are only a small subgroup of the eicosanoid family, many of which have only recently been discovered. Epi-isoprostanoids, for example, are the eicosanoids that give rise to the anticancer properties attributed to aspirin and were discovered only a few years ago.

But the full story of eicosanoids began more than 60 years ago with the discovery of the most abundant of these hormones: prostaglandins. It turns out that the one organ of the body that has the highest concentration of eicosanoids is the prostate gland. If you collect enough prostrate glands from cattle (like tens of thousands), and then do numerous extractions, you can get an extraordinarily small amount of an eicosanoid-rich fraction that has exceptionally powerful physiological activity. Since it was thought at that time that all hormones had to originate from a discrete gland, it made perfect sense to name this new hormone a prostaglandin. With time it became clear that every living cell in the body could make eicosanoids, and that there was no discrete organ or gland that was the center of eicosanoid synthesis. Continued research led to the discovery of the actual structure of eicosanoids, and an understanding of how the true wonder drug of the twentieth century (aspirin) worked by changing the levels of these hormones. By 1982, enough scientific evidence had been accumulated to award the Nobel Prize in Medicine to John Vane, Sune Bergstrom, and Bengt Samuelsson for their early discoveries on eicosanoid structure and function. Ironically, the scientist who first discovered eicosanoids, Ulf von Euler, did not receive recognition for this Nobel Prize.

The glory days of eicosanoid research lie ahead with new eicosanoids being discovered on almost a yearly basis and with a growing realization of the vast role these hormones play in controlling other hormonal systems. This fact has not been lost upon pharmaceutical companies that have already spent billions of dollars trying to develop eicosanoid-based drugs. Much of this research, however, has gone for naught, because eicosanoids are not orally active, have such a short biological lifetime (measured in seconds), and have to be given interarterially instead of intravenously to be effective. (An interarterial injection requires surgery to get access to the artery, while an intravenous injection is incredibly easy by comparison.) As a result, eicosanoids as drugs have a very limited role in the world of pharmaceuticals. Simply stated they are not only too difficult to work with, but they are also too powerful to be used as a drug.

But, there remains one other way to directly manipulate eicosanoids: your diet. The reason why your diet can be successful where the largest drug companies have been unsuccessful is based on evolution. Eicosanoids were the first hormonal control system developed by living organisms. You can't have organized life unless you have cell membranes separating the internal workings of the cell from its environment. Since all cell membranes contain fatty acids (including the building blocks of eicosanoids, which are known as essential fatty acids), the cell's own membrane became the ideal reservoir for eicosanoid synthesis since you could always be certain that the raw materials for making these hormones were close by.

As autocrine hormones, an eicosanoid's mission is to be secreted by the cell to test the external environment and then report back to the cell what is just outside its boundaries. Based on that information, the cell can take the appropriate biological action to respond to any change in its environment. Any change in the environment of a cell can be considered a stressor. That's why eicosanoids can be viewed as the molecular mediators of stress for a cell. In essence, they are molecular scouts, continually being sent out and then reporting back to the cell about the local environment. If there is any change in the external environment of the cell, then the eicosanoid, by interacting with its receptor on the cell surface, can modify the biological response of that cell.

In biotechnology, one of the hot research areas today is the field of biological response modifiers. Eicosanoids represent the first (and probably the most powerful) biological response modifiers developed by living organisms. In fact, many of the eicosanoids that humans make today are identical to ones made by sponges. Eicosanoids have been around for more than 500 million years, and they have evolved as the control agents for a dazzling array of biological functions.

The reason why eicosanoids play such a central role in anti-aging is due to the second messengers that certain eicosanoids generate. There are a variety of eicosanoid receptors on the surface of the cell, and depending on which eicosanoid interacts with them, a different second messenger is synthesized by the cell. Sometimes cyclic AMP goes up, sometimes cyclic AMP goes down, and sometimes a totally different second messenger (like DAG and IP_3) system is generated. Therefore, not all eicosanoids are created equal when it comes to increasing cyclic AMP levels.

Those eicosanoids that generate increased production of cyclic AMP in the cell are your key to anti-aging. Why? Because cyclic AMP is the same second messenger used by a great number of endocrine hormones in the body to translate their biological information to the appropriate target cell. By maintaining adequate cellular levels of those eicosanoids that increase cyclic AMP levels, you are guaranteed that a certain baseline level of cyclic AMP is always present in a cell. When an additional burst of cyclic AMP is generated by the endocrine hormone interacting with its receptor, it's now far more likely that the overall cyclic AMP levels in the cell will be high enough to ensure that the appropriate biological response (i.e., better hormonal communications) is produced. This is shown in Figure 16-1 on page 165.

In some ways, the levels of cyclic AMP generated by "good" eicosanoids are like a booster signal to ensure that fewer endocrine hor-

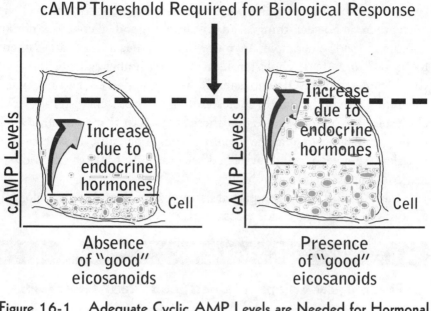

Figure 16-1   Adequate Cyclic AMP Levels are Needed for Hormonal Communication

mones are necesssary to deliver the appropriate biological message. These second messenger boosters are not as important early in life when you have more than adequate levels of endocrine hormones, but they become exceptionally important as you age since the levels of many key endocrine hormones decrease. Thus, even with decreasing levels of endocrine hormones, hormonal communication can be maintained, and that is my molecular definition of anti-aging.

Since there is no discrete eicosanoid "gland", there is no central site that turns "on" or turns "off" eicosanoid action. Nature solved this problem by developing different types of eicosanoids that have diametrically opposed physiological actions. It is the balance of the opposing actions of different eicosanoids that maintain an equilibirum of biological activity. These differences in biological actions are the basis for the eicosanoid "axis."

So in a first approximation, you can view this eicosanoid "axis" as being composed of either "good" or "bad" eicosanoids. In the absence of the evolutionary development of more advanced hormonal systems (like corticosteroids) to control this eicosanoid activity, the balance of "good" and "bad" eicosanoids was the best solution at the time. Obviously, there is no such thing as an absolutely "good" eicosanoid nor an absolutely "bad" eicosanoid, anymore than there is a moral attachment to "good" and "bad" cholesterol. In fact, without adequate levels of "bad" cholesterol (LDL cholesterol), you would die. It's only when the ratio of "good" (HDL cholesterol) and "bad" cholesterol (LDL cholesterol) is out of balance that there is concern that some untoward cardiovascular event may be awaiting you. The same is true of any imbalance between "good" and "bad" eicosanoids. Only the physiological consequences are much higher.

Table 16-2 gives only a partial listing of some of the physiological actions of "good" and "bad" eicosanoids.

TABLE 16-2

Physiological Actions of "Good" and "Bad" Eicosanoids

"GOOD" EICOSANOIDS	"BAD" EICOSANOIDS
Inhibit Platelet Aggregation	Promote platelet aggregation
Vasodilators	Vasoconstrictors
Anti-inflammatory	Pro-inflammatory
Control cellular proliferation	Promote cellular proliferation
Enhance the immune system	Suppress the immune system

An example of a "good" eicosanoid is PGE_1, whereas "bad" eicosanoids include thromboxane A_2 and leukotriene B_4. And there are more than 100 different eicosanoids currently known. The key characteristic property of "good" eicosanoids is that they stimulate cyclic AMP levels when they interact with their appropriate receptors on the cell surface.

As with all other hormonal systems, it is the balancing of opposing actions that determines hormonal communication. Insulin's actions are balanced by those of glucagon. The balance of "good" and "bad" eicosanoids, however, are far more predictive of chronic disease than are imbalances in other hormonal systems. Yet, the balance of these other hormone systems (insulin and cortisol) profoundly influence the dynamic balance of eicosanoids, and that's why all three hormonal systems are so intimately linked together.

What chronic diseases are a consequence of eicosanoid imbalance? They include heart disease, cancer, diabetes, arthritis, and depression among others. The 1982 Nobel Prize in Medicine provided an insight into the molecular nature of chronic disease and redefined it as an imbalance in eicosanoid levels. It also allows us to define wellness and longevity in terms of re-establishing eicosanoid balance. In essence, the more the balance of eicosanoids is tilted toward "bad" eicosanoids, the more likely the development of chronic disease. Conversely, the more the balance is tilted toward "good" eicosanoids, the greater one's wellness and longevity.

For example, if you are having a heart attack, you are making more "bad" eicosanoids (that promote platelet aggregation and vasoconstriction) and not enough "good" ones (that prevent platelet aggregation and promote vasodilation). If you have high blood pressure, you are making more "bad" eicosanoids (vasoconstrictors) and not enough "good" ones (vasodilators). If you have arthritic pain, you are making more "bad" eicosanoids (pro-inflammatory) and less "good" ones (anti-inflammatory). If you have cancer, you are making more "bad" eicosanoids (immune depressing) and too few "good" ones (immune stimulating). If you have Type 2 diabetes, you are making more "bad" eicosanoids (that stimulate insulin secretion) and fewer "good" ones (that inhibit insulin secretion). In fact, just about every chronic disease can be redefined in terms of eicosanoid imbalance.

Listed in Table 16-3 are some of the chronic diseases associated with eicosanoid imbalance.

TABLE 16-3

Chronic Disease Conditions Associated with Eicosanoid Imbalances

Heart disease
Hypertension
Type 2 diabetes
Inflammatory diseases
Auto-immune diseases
Cancer
Depression

Not surprisingly, these are the very disease conditions usually associated with an aging population. So, in a sense, I believe that aging can be viewed as a growing eicosanoid imbalance over time.

If you are skeptical about the statement that eicosanoids play such a fundamental role in so many diverse disease conditions, then ask any physician what happens when they give a high dose of corticosteroids to a patient for more than 30 days. Their answer will be physiological devastation if not death (similar to the Pacific salmon after spawning). As already described, this happens because corticosteroids have only one mode of action, they knock out all eicosanoid production—"good" and "bad."

Unlike corticosteroids that knock out all eicosanoids, some anti-inflammatory drugs, such as aspirin and other nonsteroidal anti-inflammatory drugs (NSAIDs), can only affect those eicosanoids that are synthesized via the cyclo-oxygenase enzyme or COX. It was recently discovered there are two forms of this enzyme known as COX-1 and COX-2. COX-1 enzymes are a constant fixture of the vascular cells that line the bloodstream or in stomach cells that secrete bicarbonate to neutralize stomach acid. COX-2 appears to a be an enzyme that is synthesized only in response to inflammation. Current drugs like aspirin and NSAIDs don't discriminate between these specific forms of the COX enzyme, which is why they have many side effects associated with their long-term use. For example, it appears that the anticancer benefits of aspirin come from its inhibition of COX-2, whereas the side effects come from its simultaneous inhibition of COX-1 (and thus an increase in the likelihood of internal bleeding). However, the cardiovascular benefits of aspirin appear to come from its inhibition of COX-1. This dilemma is indicative of the so-called risk-benefit ratio typical of all drugs.

Once again drug companies are racing (just as they did in the 1950s to make new corticosteroids) to develop new patentable drugs— this time ones that affect only the COX-2 enzyme and not COX-1, thereby reducing the side effects of long-term treatment for inflammation. Overlooked in this frenzy by the drug companies is that an existing "drug" can achieve all of these benefits without any side effects. That "drug" is the Zone Diet.

To understand the importance of diet in controlling these eicosanoids and re-establishing an appropriate eicosanoid balance, we have to understand how the actual precursors of eicosanoids are made. To begin with, all eicosanoids ultimately are produced from essential fatty acids that the body cannot make and, therefore, must be part of the diet. These essential fatty acids are classified as either omega-3 or omega-6 depending upon the position of the double bonds within them. However, typical essential fatty acids are only 18 carbons in length and must be further elongated to 20-carbon fatty acids by the body before eicosanoids can be made. Remember, all eicosanoids come from essential fatty acids that are 20 carbon atoms in length. The Greek word for 20 is *eicosa*, hence the name eicosanoids. It is just not the number of carbon atoms that count, but also their configuration. Eicosanoid precursors must have a certain spatial configuration with at least three conjugated double bonds in order to be converted into an eicosanoid. How your diet controls the formation of dietary essential fatty acids into the actual 20-carbon atom precursors of eicosanoids is a complex story.

The discovery of essential fatty acids was first reported in 1929. At that time essential fatty acids were called vitamin F. But vitamin F was useless unless transformed into an eicosanoid. This began a continuing 70-year journey to understand how the diet affects eicosanoid formation, how it can change eicosanoid balance in the body, and how eicosanoids become the central players in the world of anti-aging.

The metabolism of omega-6 essential fatty acids is shown in Figure 16-2 on page 170. Although the metabolism of omega-3 fatty acids uses the same enzymes and same pathways, the eicosanoids from omega-3 fatty acids are not as important to the aging process as those derived from the omega-6 fatty acids because the physiological actions of the eicosanoids derived from omega-3 fatty acids are much weaker. However, the omega-3 fatty acids have a strong effect on which eicosanoids are made from omega-6 fatty acids because of their influence on the activities of key enzymes.

There are two key steps in this process that determine the amount of eicosanoid building blocks that will be made. These are known in biochemistry as "rate-limiting steps." The first rate-limiting step is controlled by the enzyme, delta-6-desaturase. This enzyme inserts a necessary third double bond in the essential fatty acid in just the right position to begin bending inward and forms gamma linolenic acid (GLA) from linoleic acid.

I define any essential fatty acid that has this new double bond inserted by the delta-6-desaturase enzyme as an activated essential fatty acid, because this new double bond starts bending the essential fatty acid to get the appropriate spatial configuration required to make an eicosanoid. Once this new double bond has been inserted, very

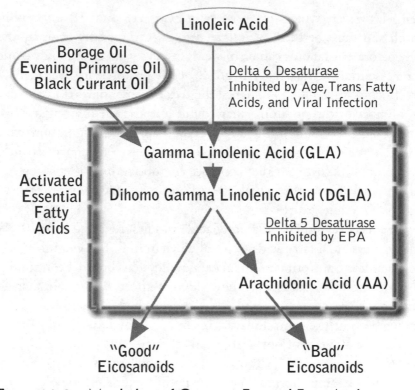

Figure 16-2   Metabolism of Omega-6 Essential Fatty Acids

small amounts of these activated essential fatty acids can profoundly affect eicosanoid balance.

However, there are many factors that can decrease the activity of the delta-6-desaturase enzyme. The most important factor is age itself. There are two times in your life during which this enzyme is relatively inactive. The first is at birth. For the first 6 months of life, the activity of this key enzyme in the newborn is relatively low. But this is also the time when maximum amounts of long-chain essential fatty acids are required by the child since the brain is growing at the fastest possible rate and these long-chain essential fatty acids are the key structural building blocks for the brain. Nature has developed a unique solution to this problem: mother's breast milk. Breast milk is very rich in GLA and other long-chain essential fatty acids, such as the omega-3 essential fatty acid, eicosapentaenoic acid (EPA). By supplying these activated essential fatty acids through the diet, this early inactivity of the delta-6-desaturase enzyme is overcome. The second time in your life during which the activity of this enzyme begins to decrease is after the age of 30. Eicosanoids are critical for successful reproduction. Since the primary child-bearing years for women are between the ages of 18 and 30, it makes good evolutionary sense to start turning down the activity of a key enzyme (in both male and females) needed to make the precursors of eicosanoids required for fertility and conception.

The delta-6-desaturase enzyme can also be inhibited by viral infection. The only known anti-viral agents are "good" eicosanoids, such as PGE_1. If you are a virus, your number-one goal is to inhibit the formation of this type of "good" eicosanoid. By inhibiting the delta-6-desaturase enzyme, the virus has devised an incredibly clever way to circumvent the body's primary anti-viral drug (i.e., PGE_1).

The final factor that can decrease the activity of delta-6-desaturase is the presence of trans fatty acids in your diet. Trans fatty acids don't exist in the real world. They are essential fatty acids that have been transformed by a commercial process (known as hydrogenation) into a new spatial configuration that is more stable to prevent oxidation. The increased stability of these fatty acids makes them ideal for processed foods, but also makes trans fatty acids strong inhibitors of the delta-6-desaturase enzyme. Trans fatty acids occupy the active site of the delta-6-desaturase enzyme, thus preventing the formation of the activated essential fatty acids required for eicosanoid synthesis. In essence, trans fatty acids can be viewed as "anti"-essential fatty acids due to their inhibition of eicosanoid synthesis. As further proof, recent studies strongly implicate these trans fatty acids in the development of heart disease. How do you know if a food product you're consuming contains trans fatty acids? Look for the words "partially hydrogenated vegetable oil" on the label, and if it is there, then you know it contains trans fatty acids.

The journey toward becoming an eicosanoid is still far from over after passing this first hurdle of making GLA. Once GLA is formed, it is rapidly elongated into dihomo gamma linolenic acid (DGLA), which is the precursor to most of the "good" eicosanoids. However, DGLA is also the substrate for the other rate-limiting enzyme in the essential fatty acid cascade (see Figure 16-2 on page 170). That enzyme is called delta-5-desaturase. From an aging perspective, the dietary factors that control this enzyme, becomes one of the keys that ultimately controls the balance of "good" and "bad" eicosanoids.

This is because the end product that the delta-5-desaturase enzyme produces from DGLA is arachidonic acid (AA). DGLA is the building block of "good" eicosanoids, whereas AA is the building block of "bad" eicosanoids. Thus, excess amounts of AA can be one of your worst hormonal nightmares. Ultimately, it is the balance between DGLA and AA in every one of your 60 trillion cells that determines your longevity. You need some AA to produce some "bad" eicosanoids, but in the case of the excess production of AA, the balance of eicosanoids will shift toward accelerated aging and chronic disease.

So how do you help your body block excess AA formation and tilt the balance back toward a favorable DGLA/AA ratio? By making sure your diet has adequate amounts of EPA. EPA is an omega-3 essential fatty acid containing 20-carbon atoms. Although EPA can be made into an eicosanoid, from a physiological perspective the eicosanoids derived from EPA don't do much. The importance of EPA is that it acts as a feedback inhibitor of the delta-5-desaturase enzyme. The higher the concentration of EPA in the cell, the more the delta-5-desaturase enzyme is inhibited, and the less AA is produced. As a result, the presence of EPA in the diet allows you to control the rate of AA production derived from DGLA, and thus generate a favorable DGLA to AA ratio in each cell membrane.

My own odyssey into eicosanoid modulation began some 17 years ago when I was studying the early eicosanoid research on which the 1982 Nobel Prize in Medicine was awarded. When I looked at the metabolic pathways about essential fatty acids, it became apparent to me that the answer of how to treat those chronic diseases mediated by eicosanoid imbalances was obvious. Simply have the body make more "good" eicosanoids and fewer "bad" ones by changing the ratio of DGLA to AA at the cellular level. All I needed (or so I thought) was access to two activated essential fatty acids: EPA and GLA.

Getting enough EPA for this task proved easy. There are lots of fish in the sea. It turns out that fish can't make EPA, but they are at the end of the food chain that starts with plankton, which can. Extract the fish oil and you have a very rich source of EPA. The most common fish oil that contains large amounts of EPA is cod-liver oil, without doubt the worst-tasting food known to man. However, the first documented medicinal use of cod-liver oil for the treatment of arthritis was reported more than 200 years ago. Arthritis is an inflammatory condition characterized by an overproduction of "bad" (i.e., pro-inflammatory) eicosanoids. Supplementation of the diet with cod-liver oil provides the necessary EPA to inhibit the formation of AA, the precursor of pro-inflammatory eicosanoids. The treatment worked 200 years ago, and it still works today. Until recently, a daily dose of cod-liver oil was the standard dietary supplement for every American child before he or she left the house. Without knowing so, every grandmother who gave her children cod-liver oil was manipulating eicosanoid synthesis.

While EPA is easy to obtain, finding activated omega-6 essential fatty acids, such as GLA, is not, because it is contained in very few seeds. To find out which ones, I went to the bowels of the MIT library to begin my search. Of the more than 250,000 known seed types, only about 50 contained GLA. Of that 50, only about 5 had any significant levels of GLA. Of that 5, only 1 in my opinion had great potential for industrial production. That seed was borage.

So in 1983, my brother, Doug, and I set out to the corner the world's borage seed market. Actually, at the time it wasn't too difficult since all the seeds in the world could fit easily into the corner of a small room. By the end of 1983, we owned virtually every borage seed in the world.

We did some pilot experiments and developed an extraction process that gave us a very high-quality oil suitable for human consumption. Finally, I had a good source of GLA to combine with EPA, so that one could alter the ratio of DGLA to AA in some 60 trillion target cells in the human body. Supplementation with GLA would overcome any age-related decrease in activity of delta-6-desaturase, thus ensuring adequate DGLA levels in the cells. The EPA would inhibit the delta-5-desaturase enzyme so that any increase in DGLA levels would not increase AA levels. The end result would be an improved DGLA to AA ratio in every cell in the body. Frankly, it was a very clever approach to alter eicosanoids.

Only two obstacles remained before going to Stockholm to pick up the Nobel Prize and opening up our Swiss bank account to deposit all the money my brother and I were going to make. The first problem was where to grow the borage? It turned out that the two places in the world that borage grows readily are the upper plains of Saskatchewan and the lower valleys of New Zealand. Canada was closer, so we moved to Canada to grow and extract the oil from borage on an industrial scale. The other problem was what should be the correct ratio of

GLA to EPA in order to modulate eicosanoids? For that we needed human subjects. Fortunately we had several: my brother, my wife, my mother, and I. I thought a group of four should be sufficient for a start.

I wasn't flying blind in choosing the appropriate ratio of EPA to GLA because there was existing literature that estimated the ratio of omega-6 to omega-3 fatty acids consumed by neo-Paleolithic man was about 1:1. At the beginning of this century the ratio had increased slightly to approximately 2:1. Currently in America, the ratio has increased to nearly 20:1, due to the rapid increase in the use of vegetable oils (which are rich in omega-6 fatty acids) and a corresponding decrease in fish consumption (which is rich in omega-3 fatty acids). A quick peek back at Figure 16-2 on page 170 will indicate why this may have been one of the most damaging changes to our dietary habits in the twentieth century. A high intake of omega-6 fatty acids (primarily as linoleic acid) creates a downward pressure on all the essential fatty acid metabolism that end up forcing the increased production of AA. Think of a column of water with a constriction at one end. The flow at the other end is totally dependent on the height of the column. The more water you put in the column, the greater the flow from the constricted end. The same is true of omega-6 fatty acids. The more omega-6 fatty acids you consume, the greater the production of AA. Couple this with a decrease in the intake of omega-3 fatty acids (like those in cod-liver oil), and you get a growing buildup of AA and an increased production of "bad" eicosanoids. While we have significantly decreased early childhood mortality, the diseases associated with an overproduction of "bad" eicosanoids (see Table 16–3 on page 167), are the primary causes of mortality associated with an aging population. To a great extent these diseases are all diet related because of their association with eicosanoid imbalance.

This is why long-chain omega-3 fatty acids, like EPA, are so important in the Zone Diet. They inhibit the delta-5-desaturase enzyme, thereby restricting the flow of any omega-6 fatty acids into AA, which therefore decreases the production of "bad" eicosanoids. As long as you are consuming very moderate amounts of omega-6 fatty acids with equal amounts of EPA, then those dietary omega-6 fatty acids in your diet tend to acculumate at the level of DGLA (because of the inhibition of delta-5-desaturase by the EPA), which increases the production of "good" eicosanoids. However, the total amount of omega-3 and omega-6 fatty acids you need is relatively low, which means you still have to add some extra fat to your diet to help slow the entry rate of dietary carbohydrate to control insulin secretion. This is why if any fat is added to the Zone Diet, it should be primarily monounsaturated fat. Monounsaturated fats can't be made into cicosanoids ("good" or "bad"). Thus by having no effect on eicosanoids nor insulin, monounsaturated fats can provide the amount of fat necessary for controlling the entry rate of carbohydrates into the bloodstream without disturbing the overall omega-3 to omega-6 balance that you are trying to achieve with the Zone Diet. The reason for the need of long-chain omega-3 fatty acids in the human diet may be evolutionary. The primary reason for man's dominance on earth is his brain. The brain is the richest source of long-chain omega-3 fatty acids in the body. Since fishing didn't evolve until 20,000 years ago, how did man obtain these relatively rare fats needed for brain development if he wasn't eating fish? The answer may be because (1) there were other sources of EPA besides fish and (2) he was a real weakling.

Compared to other predators a million years ago, man was a loser. He was no match for other animals who had superior strength and hunting skills. However, man was a pretty good scavenger. By the time he arrived at the carcass, there wasn't much left. Probably the one thing left were bones that the predators and stronger scavengers (like hyenas) just didn't have the time to chew on or get their jaws around. And the biggest bone was the skull of the dead animal. But man had one significant advantage, he had tools. Tools (like stones) that could break into the skull of the dead animal and access the brain, which was very rich in long-chain omega-3 fatty acids. Here was a classic case of you are what you eat. By eating scavenged brains rich in long-chain omega-3 essential fatty acids, man stumbled upon the molecular building blocks for more rapid development of his brain. With more brain power, he could make better tools and develop better hunting strategies. By the neo-Paleolithic era, about 10,000 years ago, man had become the most deadly hunter on the face of the earth. Now neo-Paleolithic man could eat whatever part of the carcass he wanted, including the protein-rich muscle.

The meat from wild game contains nearly six times more long-chain omega-3 fatty acids than today's grain-fed beef. So whatever neo-Paleolithic man ate (brains or meat), he was getting a lot of long-chain omega-3 fatty acids, such as EPA. As I mentioned earlier, in the last 50 years there has been a dramatic decrease in the amount of omega-3 fatty acids consumed by Americans. In fact, nearly 20% of the American population today have such low levels of EPA in their blood that it can't be detected. Without sufficient levels of EPA, it is difficult to shut down the activity of the delta-5-desaturase enzyme, which leads to an increased production of AA and the generation of larger amounts of "bad" eicosanoids.

So, let's get back to the story of how I went about determining the correct ratio of EPA to GLA to correct all of these problems. Taking all the data into account, including the increasingly massive overconsumption of omega-6 fatty acids in general, I believed that a 4:1 ratio of EPA to GLA should do the trick. One ratio for everyone: why not? Obviously silly thinking in retrospect, but since I was coming from my background in pharmaceutical drug delivery, it seemed logical at the time. So I started out with this ratio, made some soft gelatin capsules containing both fish oil (i.e., EPA) and borage oil (i.e., GLA), and found some other willing friends (i.e., guinea pigs) outside of my family. I gave them the standard phrase, "Trust me." Fortunately, I had good friends who actually did trust me.

Since I was only working with changing fatty acid levels during this early phase of my research, my initial observations on eicosanoids were not confounded by other potential hormonal modulating approaches, like controlling insulin or restoring endocrine hormone levels. I had a very targeted approach to focus solely on manipulating eicosanoid levels through dietary supplementation with defined amounts of activated essential fatty acids. And many of the physiological changes I observed occurred within weeks, if not days.

The time frame for these physiological actions was important because it was much faster than the reported responses for treatments that focus on the restoration of endocrine hormones. Those changes usually take weeks, if not months, to see measurable effects.

Over time (often several months), however, I noticed that strange things seemed to be happening. Virtually everyone who took the combinations of EPA and GLA felt much better initially. After all, they were now making more "good" and fewer "bad" eicosanoids. But with time, some individuals mentioned that they seemed to have stabilized, or that they even saw a drop-off in the early benefits they first experienced. Nonetheless, they still felt better than before they started. However, there was another group, who saw their initial benefits erode completely and actually began to feel worse than when they started. Some of my friends were no longer quite so friendly—until I figured out what was happening. I called it the spillover effect.

Initially, as the ratio of DGLA to AA improves, the person begins making more "good" eicosanoids and fewer "bad" ones. Everything just keeps getting better. But there will be some point in time, depending on the biochemistry and sex of the person, that the DGLA to AA ratio begins to degrade. They still feel better than when they started, but not quite as good as they first did. For some individuals, this degradation of the DGLA/AA ratio continued and it is possible that they even began to feel worse than when they first started the program, because they were now making many more "bad" eicosanoids. This is shown in Figure 16-3.

What was happening was that they were building up DGLA in their cells. The increased levels of DGLA were providing more substrate for the delta-5-desaturase enzyme to make more AA. The increase in DGLA was overwhelming the amount of EPA supplied to inhibit the delta-5-desaturase enzyme. And this spillover effect seemed to occur more often in females than males. So much for one

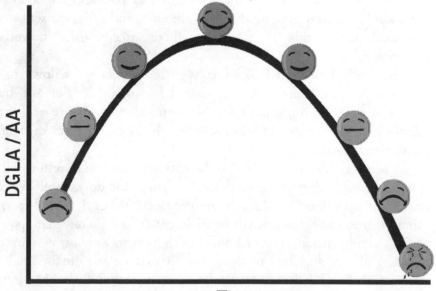

Figure 16-3   Spillover Effect from Overconsupmtion of GLA

ratio of GLA and EPA for all, the Nobel Prize, and the Swiss bank account.

Upon reflection, the answer was obvious. Not everyone is exactly the same biochemically. It is the concept of individualism: any dietary program or supplementation pattern must fit the person's own biochemistry, not vice versa. This is especially true of hormone modulation where biological changes happen very quickly. And supplementing with combinations of EPA and GLA was definitely a hormone modulation program with results seen within a week or two at most. Even most hormone replacement therapies require much more time to see physiological differences.

So, I decided that if one size does not fit all, I had better start making a wide array of different EPA and GLA combinations and fine-tune them for each individual. But how to do this? There was no test for eicosanoid levels, since they don't travel in the bloodstream and very few eicosanoids have stable urine metabolites. Furthermore, the one eicosanoid (PGE_1) that I was trying to increase has no urine metabolites whatsoever. But eicosanoids do leave a biochemical audit trail that gives an insight into their actual balance in different organs in the body. Later in this chapter I will describe the diagnostic chart that not only lets you determine your current eicosanoid status, but I will also show you how to alter the amounts and ratios of activated essential fatty acids to fine-tune these exceptionally powerful hormones.

By 1989, I thought I had finally gotten this concept down to a science. A more complex science than I had originally thought, but one still governed by some basic biochemical rules. However, what finally gave me the insight for developing the Zone Diet was my work with elite athletes.

I began to notice that some of the elite athletes I was working with would have great training sessions, but then not do as well during competition. Others would do extremely well. When I started to ask them if they were doing anything different from a dietary standpoint prior to competition, it turned out that those who were carbohydrate-loading always appeared to do worse than those who maintained a consistent diet. I racked my brain trying to understand what had gone wrong, or what had changed, to explain this sudden shift in their eicosanoid status. Then it struck me. It was carbohydrate-loading that was increasing their insulin levels.

A trip back to the bowels of the MIT library confirmed my suspicion. There I found previously published research that demonstrated high levels of insulin activated the delta-5-desaturase enzyme, whereas glucagon inhibited its activity. All the hormonal benefits I had carefully crafted for each athlete to manipulate their ratios of DGLA to AA were being undermined by the surge of insulin caused by their precompetition carbo-loading. That increase in insulin stimulated the delta-5-desaturase enzyme to increase the production of AA at the expense of DGLA. For those athletes, the result was that a highly favorable DGLA to AA ratio created during training quickly became a very undesirable ratio at the time of competition. It was the same spillover effect that I had observed in the early days of learning how to fine-tune eicosanoid levels. It was at that point I knew that I would never be able to control eicosanoid levels without controlling insulin first. Back to the drawing board.

Was there any confirming evidence that high levels of insulin would affect the DGLA to AA ratio in humans? Such information was published in 1991. The goal of that research was to maintain a high level of insulin for 6 hours in both normal subjects and patients with Type 2 diabetes (who are characterized by excessive insulin levels). The results are shown in Figure 16-4.

After only six hours of exposure to elevated insulin levels, the ratio of DGLA to AA in the bloodstream in both normals and Type 2 diabetics had dropped by nearly 50 percent. The elite athletes who were carbo-loading prior to competition were suffering the same decrease in DGLA/AA ratios by eating more high-density carbohydrates (grains, pasta, and starches), thus increasing insulin, which caused a rapid deterioration of their DGLA/AA ratios.

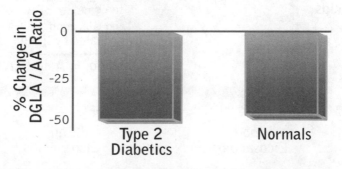

Figure 16-4   Hyperinsulinemia Can Alter DGLA/AA Ratio

So, now the metabolism of activated essential fatty acids had to be modified to take into account the role of insulin and glucagon on the delta-5-desaturase enzyme. This is shown in Figure 16-5.

Insulin was an activator of the delta-5-desaturase enzyme, whereas glucagon was an inhibitor of the same enzyme. The role of excess insulin in negatively affecting eicosanoid balance also finally began to explain why excess insulin was such an excellent predictor of heart disease. The more "bad" eicosanoids you make, the more likely you will promote platelet aggregation and increased vasoconstriction, the underlying factors for a heart attack.

I knew the only way to control insulin required controlling the protein-to-carbohydrate ratio at every meal. Again I was confronted with determining the optimal ratio of protein-to-carbohydrate should be? A good beginning was to attempt to estimate the protein-to-carbohydrate ratio consumed by neo-Paleolithic man some 10,000 years ago, since our genes haven't changed since then.

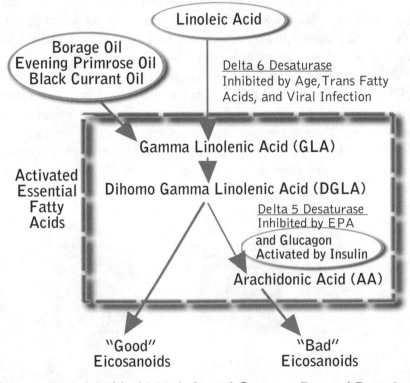

Figure 16-5   Modified Metabolism of Omega-6 Essential Fatty Acids

Fortunately, such an estimate did exist, in of all places the *New England Journal of Medicine*. Using anthropological data and comparing a large number of existing hunter-gatherer tribes, these researchers estimated the average protein-to-carbohydrate ratio in neo-Paleolithic diets to be approximately 3 grams of protein for every 4 grams of carbohydrate, or a protein-to-carbohydrate ratio of 0.75. Using this research as a starting point, I began developing a diet that would control the protein-to-carbohydrate ratio in a range between 0.6 and 1.0 at every meal, so that the balance of insulin and glucagon would be maintained from meal to meal. This diet is the Zone Diet.

Although, I had solved the problem with elite athletes, I still wondered about the probability of compliance by the general population. After all, elite athletes are very disciplined. Could the same discipline be demonstrated by the general population? Fortunately, working with these athletes allowed me to refine my teaching techniques to make the Zone Diet more accessible and easier to follow. It was the invaluable lessons I learned by working with them that let me develop even easier-to-follow instructions for my Type 2 diabetic studies described in an earlier chapter. Essentially, all these educational modules can be found in one of my previous books, *Zone Perfect Meals in Minutes*. If there was ever a "Zone for Beginners," it is that book.

Having described my personal odyssey of learning by hard experience how to control the building blocks of eicosanoids, let me discuss how they are actually made and work. As mentioned earlier, eicosanoids are autocrine hormones. They are not meant to circulate in the bloodstream like endocrine hormones. This is why every cell in the body (all 60 trillion) can make eicosanoids. It's as if you have 60 trillion separate eicosanoid glands each capable of making these exceptionally powerful hormones. Unlike the endocrine hormones, which are under control of the hypothalamus, there is no such central control on eicosanoids. Rather than responding to some master signal, each cell responds to changes in its immediate environment. The first step in generating a cellular response is the actual release of an essential fatty acid from the membrane phospholipids in the cell membrane. The enzyme responsible for the release of the essential fatty acid is called phospholipase A_2. Since there is no feedback loop to stop the production of eicosanoids, the only way to inhibit their continued release from the cell is by making cortisol, which causes the synthesis of a protein (i.e., lipocortin) that inhibits the action of phospholipase A_2.

By inhibiting this enzyme, which releases essential fatty acids from the cell membranes, you choke off the supply of substrate required for eicosanoid synthesis. Obviously, if you are overproducing corticosteroids, especially cortisol, you will bring all eicosanoid synthesis to a crashing halt—including the shut down of the immune system.

Once released from the cell membrane, there are three primary pathways a free 20-carbon essential fatty acid, can follow. The first is via the cyclo-oxygenase system (i.e., COX) that makes prostaglandins. In this pathway the highly contorted essential fatty acid is closed upon itself to form a prostanoid ring. The second is through the 5-lipo-oxygenase (5-LIPO) pathway that makes leukotrienes. There is a third pathway in which the 20-carbon essential fatty acid is simply modified via either the 12- or 15-lipoxygenase (12- or 15-LIPO) enzymes as in the case of hydroxylated essential fatty acids. It is this third pathway that is constantly producing newly discovered eicosanoids. These pathways are shown in Figure 16-6.

Prostaglandins

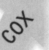

Activated
Essential
Fatty Acids

5-LIPO   Leukotrienes

Hydroxylated
Fatty Acids

Figure 16-6   Various Pathways for Eicosanoid Formation

Certain drugs in addition to corticosteroids can inhibit the cyclo-oxygenase pathway of this eicosanoid formation. The most well known is aspirin, which literally destroys a cyclo-oxygenase enzyme on a one-to-one basis. This is what is known as a suicide inhibitor. When you are suffering from a headache or arthritic pain, you are overproducing "bad" eicosanoids—but in particular, "bad" prostaglandins. The aspirin temporarily shuts down all prostaglandin formation (but not leukotriene or hydroxylated fatty acid formation), until the cell can make more of the cyclo-oxygenase enzyme to replace the ones destroyed by the aspirin. However, you can't use these suicidal soldiers forever, as aspirin also shuts down the synthesis of "good" prostaglandins, especially those that protect the stomach from dissolving itself. When that happens, you get internal bleeding. This is why there are more than 10,000 deaths per year associated with the overuse of aspirin. Other drugs known as nonsteroidal anti-inflammatory drugs (NSAIDs) also inhibit the cyclo-oxygenase enzyme but not the lipo-oxygenase enzyme that makes leukotrienes. The common names for these NSAIDs are Motrin, Advil, Aleve among others. Continued use of these NSAIDs generates the same problems as does long-term aspirin use.

Once an eicosanoid is made in the cell, it is transported outside the cell where it can interact with a receptor on the cell surface of the secreting cell or on a receptor of a neighboring cell. Once that interaction takes place, a second messenger is then synthesized back in the target cell. If a "good" eicosanoid is released, then that second messenger is cyclic AMP. The increased production of cyclic AMP in the target cell will boost any incoming hormonal signal from endocrine hormones that also use cyclic AMP as their second messenger. On the other hand, "bad" eicosanoids (like thromboxane A_2) can actually decrease cyclic AMP levels. The end result of increasing cyclic AMP in cells is that hormonal miscommunication is minimized and aging is reversed as long as you are making more "good" eicosanoids and fewer "bad" ones.

In essence, the "good"eicosanoids act as a cyclic AMP booster system to make sure that biological messages transmitted by endocrine hormones get through to the appropriate cells at the right time and with the appropriate fidelity. The power of this approach to aging is that your diet, and specifically the Zone Diet, can maintain and enhance the production of "good" eicosanoids so that your biological Internet still functions, even with declining endocrine hormone levels.

Although your ability to control insulin will influence the activity of the delta-5-desaturase activity, you still need to pay close attention to the balance of omega-3 to omega-6 fatty acids in the diet. The greater the ratio of omega-6 to omega-3 fatty acids in your diet, the greater the likelihood of overproducing "bad" eicosanoids, regardless of how well you control insulin. You'll get all the omega-6 fatty acids you need from eating adequate levels of low-fat protein. But omega-3 fatty acids, especially long-chain fatty acids like eicosapentaenoic acid (EPA), are a different matter. This is why fish is so important on the Zone Diet. Fish is the only protein source that is rich in EPA. Furthermore, it is the only source of protein that is a relatively poor source of omega-6 fatty acids. Therefore, the increased consumption of fish and/or fish oils becomes your greatest tool to modulate the ratio of your dietary intake of omega-6 to omega-3 essential fatty acids.

However, you don't need a lot of either omega-3 or omega-6 fatty acids every day, probably only 5 to 8 grams of total essential fatty acids (with a ratio of omega-6 to omega-3 fatty acids no higher than 4:1). This amount of dietary fat intake supplies less than 10 to 20 percent of your needed fat, since the average male needs about 40 to 50 grams of fat per day on the Zone Diet. The balance of the dietary fat should come from monounsaturated fats (like olive oil, selected nuts, or avocados) that have no effect on insulin or eicosanoids. The monounsaturated fat provides both improved taste and the ability to slow down carbohydrate entry into the bloodstream, but will have no effect on the balance of "good" and "bad" eicosanoids that you are trying to optimize by controlling insulin and the intake of essential fatty acids.

Therefore, the ideal anti-aging Zone Diet controls both the proper ratio of omega-3 to omega-6 fatty acids as well as the balance of protein-to-carbohydrate at every meal while restricting total calories. This dietary strategy maintains the dynamic balance of eicosanoids by controlling the levels of the actual precursors and the hormones responsible for activating the critical enzymes in essential fatty acid metabolism. By keeping the balance of eicosanoid precursors in an appropriate zone (after all, you need some "bad" eicosanoids to survive), you also control the information flow of your biological Internet. Control that flow and avoid hormonal miscommunication, and you have begun to reverse the aging process.

The development of chronic diseases (heart disease, diabetes, cancer, and arthritis) associated with aging does not occur overnight, but is the result of constant hormonal insults to the body. But by the time they do appear, significant (and potentially irreversible) organ damage may have occurred. So, if eicosanoids act as master hormones that control this complex hormonal communication system, is there some

way we can continue to monitor and fine-tune this ultimate mechanism of aging before chronic disease conditions appear? If the answer
is yes, then you could tell when you are moving out of the appropriate
eicosanoid zone and then you could take immediate dietary steps to
restore that balance. Does such a test exist?

Unfortunately, as I mentioned earlier, there is no simple, direct
diagnostic test for eicosanoids in this century and probably won't be
one in the next either. So, if you can't tell the actual balance of eicosanoids, then maybe the levels of DGLA and AA in the bloodstream
might give a clue? While the bloodstream is easily accessed, unfortunately it is not a very reliable predictor of what the eicosanoid status is
in individual cells. In fact, the blood is not even a good predictor of
the DGLA/AA ratio for different cells in the blood.

Theoretically all the components of the blood should be at equilibrium, therefore the fatty acid composition should be relatively constant
from one cell type to another. But as you see in Figure 16-7, this is
not the case.

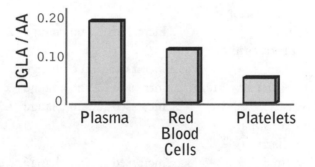

Figure 16-7   DGLA /AA Ratios in Different Blood Components

Depending on the type of cell sampled in the bloodstream, the
ratio of DGLA/AA can be radically different. If you are sampling the
blood, which cell is the best determinant of DGLA/AA balance in the
tissues that you can't sample? I don't know, nor does anyone else at
this time. So, if eicosanoid balance is the key to controlling aging, is
there some other way to determine that balance? Fortunately, eicosanoids leave a biological audit trail based on their physiological actions
that gives a pretty reliable indication of their status in a particular
organ. This biological audit trial, therefore, provides an insight on how
to revise your diet in order to improve your eicosanoid status.

Over the years, I have developed a number of external indicators that predict with a fairly high degree of precision what your eicosanoid status is. These are the same ones that I first developed for the elite athletes I work with. Each week I would have every athlete fill out an eicosanoid status report, and then fax it to me. Within 30 seconds, I could tell whether or not I would have to alter their intake of EPA and GLA to fine-tune their eicosanoid status. When the eicosanoids were perfectly balanced with proper activated essential fatty acid supplementation, the reports would show no change from week to week. What this eicosanoid status report looks like is shown Table 16-4.

TABLE 16-4

Eicosanoid Status Report

1. Daily performance	___increased	___no change	___decreased
2. Appetite for carbohydrates	___increased	___no change	___decreased
3. Length of time of appetite suppression between meals	___increased	___no change	___decreased
4. Fingernail strength or growth	___increased	___no change	___decreased
5. Hair strength and texture	___increased	___no change	___decreased
6. Stool density (sinks or constipation) (loose or diarrhea)	___increased	___no change	___decreased
7. Sleeping time	___increased	___no change	___decreased
8. Grogginess upon waking	___increased	___no change	___decreased
9. Sense of well-being	___increased	___no change	___decreased
10. Mental concentration	___increased	___no change	___decreased
11. Fatigue	___increased	___no change	___decreased
12. Skin condition	___increased	___no change	___decreased
13. Flatulence	___increased	___no change	___decreased
14. Headaches	___increased	___no change	___decreased

At first glance this litany of external signs looks like the pigeon entrails used by Roman soothsayers. Yet, examined from a larger perspective, this report gives a detailed insight into your current eicosanoid status. Now let me explain how this seemingly unscientific way of determining eicosanoid status gives a unique insight into eicosanoid physiology, because with the proper changes in the ratio of EPA and GLA, these physiological parameters can shift dramatically, often within days.

1. **Daily performance.** Increases in daily physical performance (especially increased energy) is indicative that levels of DGLA are increasing and more "good" eicosanoids are being produced, promoting both increased oxygen transfer and better use of stored body fat. Any decrease in daily performance is indicative of a buildup of AA and the corresponding increase in the production of "bad" eicosanoids.

2. **Appetite for carbohydrates.** The craving for carbohydrates will decrease, if not be eliminated, with the decrease of "bad" eicosanoids, especially leukotrienes that tend to stimulate insulin synthesis. However, if you make too many "good" eicosanoids, insulin levels can be depressed too much, leading to an increase in carbohydrate consumption because there is not enough insulin to inhibit the synthesis of neuropeptide Y, which is the most powerful stimulator of appetite.

3. **Length of time of appetite suppression.** Since "good" eicosanoids inhibit insulin secretion, blood glucose levels remain stabilized and hunger is suppressed.

4. **Fingernail strength.** The structural protein keratin is under profound eicosanoid control. "Good" eicosanoids, such as PGE_1, increase its synthesis, leading to rapid fingernail growth with excellent strength. On the other hand, "bad" eicosanoids decrease keratin synthesis leading to brittle fingernails that easily break.

5. **Hair strength.** Keratin is also the principal structural component of the hair. Hair texture can be used as an indicator of eicosanoid status similar to fingernail strength.

6. **Stool density.** The water content of the stool is controlled by the balance of vasodilators to vasoconstrictors in the colon. An overproduction of "good" eicosanoids will lead to too much water flow, producing a very loose stool or diarrhea, whereas an overproduction of "bad" eicosanoids will decrease water flow leading to a very dense stool or constipation. When the stool is isodense with water (i.e., it floats), that becomes a very good indicator of optimal eicosanoid balance.

7. **Sleeping time.** The need for sleep is determined by the amount of time required to reestablish neurotransmitter equilibrium. This process speeds up in the presence of "good" eicosanoids (thereby decreasing sleep needs), and slows in the presence of "bad" eicosanoids (which increase sleep needs).

8. **Grogginess upon waking.** Any increase in grogginess upon waking is indicative that an overproduction of "bad" eicosanoids is taking place inside the central nervous system.

9. **Sense of well-being.** "Good" eicosanoids lead to a state of well-being as opposed to the depression/anxiety/irritability associated with a buildup of "bad" eicosanoids. This is a very sensitive parameter for determing your current eicosanoid balance.

10. **Mental concentration.** This is controlled by the maintenance of blood sugar levels, which are mobilized by glucagon. "Bad" eicosanoid formation will increase insulin secretion that in turn, reduces glucagon secretion. One of the first signs of hypoglycemia is decreased mental concentration.

11. **Fatigue.** This can be the result of either too much vasodilation caused by an overproduction of "good" eicosanoids, leading to electrolyte depletion or to an overproduction of "bad" eicosanoids leading to a decrease in oxygen transfer. If you experience fatigue, try to determine which side of the eicosanoid zone you are in by checking the other parameters, such as grogginess upon waking and stool density.

12. **Skin condition.** An overproduction of "bad" eicosanoids will lead to skin dryness and eczema (caused by increased leukotriene formation). On the other hand, "good" eicosanoids are anti-inflammatory and also stimulate collagen synthesis in addition to improved microcirculation caused by increased vasodilation.

13. **Flatulence.** Flatulence or gas is caused by the metabolism of anaerobic bacteria in the lower part of the intestine. The overproduction of "good" eicosanoids increases the peristaltic action of the intestinal tract, thereby delivering greater amounts of nutrients to these anaerobic bacteria. The end result is greater metabolic activity of these anaerobic bacteria with increased gas formation the end product of their metabolism.

14. **Headaches.** This is similar to fatigue because you can have

either a vasodilation headache (too many "good" eicosanoids) or a vasoconstriction headache (too many "bad" eicosanoids). As with fatigue, you have to look at other parameters to gain a clear picture of eicosanoid status.

The importance of these parameters is that they reflect the overall balance of DGLA to AA in your target organs. If that ratio begins to tilt toward a lower DGLA to AA ratio, then it is very likely that symptoms of chronic diseases associated with a poor eicosanoid balance will soon return. If you begin to see any of these parameters changing, then how do you bring them back into balance? The answer is through the judicious use of essential fatty acids. I say, judicious because when used correctly, combinations of activated omega-3 (like EPA) and omega-6 essential fatty acid (like GLA) are powerful adjuncts to the Zone Diet. On the other hand, used incorrectly, they can actually accelerate disease and aging. Unfortunately, since they are available in every health food store in America, they can be very easily abused.

So, here are some guidelines for using EPA and GLA on the Zone Diet that I have gleaned over the years. If you are making too many "bad" eicosanoids as determined by the eicosanoid status report, then increase your intake of EPA and cut back your intake (no matter how limited) of GLA. If you are making too many "good" eicosanoids, cut back on the intake of EPA. The physiological changes that occur by altering the balance of EPA and GLA (if you are following the Zone Diet) can take place in few days, if not hours. When you deal with activated essential fatty acids, you are dealing with some very powerful biological response modifiers. Treat them with respect.

How much EPA should you take? It is virtually impossible to overdose on EPA, but a good minimum dose would be about 300 to 400 mg per day as long as it has been molecularly distilled to remove any contaminating PCBs. That amount of EPA is equivalent to about two fish-oil capsules per day or one-half teaspoon of the cod-liver oil that your parents or grandparents had you take every day. Of course, they took five to six times that amount of cod-liver oil as children.

However, the amount of GLA to take is a different matter. GLA is a very powerful nutrient, and for some people a potentially dangerous one. At one time I thought I would need thousands of acres of borage to meet the potential demand for GLA. Once I understood the spillover effect, I gained a new respect for this exceptionally powerful hormonal modulator, because it has the potential for increasing the overproduction of "bad" eicosanoids, which can accelerate the aging process.

Furthermore, on the Zone Diet, I have found that the need for GLA falls dramatically and even small amounts over a baseline requirement can give rise to increased AA formation. That's why I rarely recommend more than 1 to 2 mg of GLA per day for most people. Since the standard size of borage-oil capsules sold in a health food store contains 240 mg of GLA, you would have to take a very sharp knife and cut a capsule into 240 equal pieces (good luck) to get the right dosage. A far better way to get 1 to 2 mg per day is to simply eat a small bowl of slow-cooked oatmeal (instant oatmeal will have much less GLA) in the morning. Personally I think the slow-cooked oatmeal is easier, and your grandmother probably did too. However, even this amount of GLA may be too much for many people following the Zone Diet.

As you can see, there is a tremendous variation of biological responses once you start using activated essential fatty acids in combination with the Zone Diet. Most people are not going to be that observant, so I tell them to follow the Zone Diet, take moderate amounts of fish oil, and eat 1 to 2 bowls of oatmeal per week. Not a very racy prescription for eicosanoid modulation and improved longevity, but it works.

PART IV

OTHER HORMONES
AND THE
ANTI-AGING ZONE

CHAPTER 17

SEX AND THE ZONE FOR MEN:
THE SECRET OF VIAGRA

Mention the word *hormone* and most likely the first word association that people make is sex. And it wouldn't be false to say that, since sex at any age is ultimately controlled by hormones. If you want to have better sex, then improving the communication between hormones is your strategy of choice for peak sexual performance.

Male sexual concerns usually focus on one thing: impotence. Impotence is often simply a consequence of lack of blood flow to the male genital area. It occurs in a very high percentage (35 to 75 percent) in males with Type 2 diabetes (characterized by high levels of insulin) and in male hypertensive patients who are taking drugs (diuretics and beta-blockers) that increase insulin. Judged from the increasing number of impotence treatment centers, impotence is a growing problem that no one talked about until very recently, with the introduction of Viagra.

Before I discuss Viagra and impotence, you have to realize what a complex series of events takes place in the male physiology to make intercourse possible. For the male, sex starts in the brain in the hypothalamus. Impulses are sent from the brain via nerves to the penis. This stimulation causes the synthesis of a gaslike proto-hormone, known as nitric oxide (described in greater detail in a later chapter), which causes an increase in the production of a second messenger known as cyclic GMP. Cyclic GMP can cause the relaxation of the smooth muscle cells surrounding two chambers in the penis called the corpora cavernosa. Usually the passages to these chambers are highly constricted by the surrounding smooth muscle cells. Once these muscle cells are relaxed, blood begins flowing into these chambers, and (like a sponge), these chambers become engorged with blood (nearly six times the normal flow) and penile expansion begins. This continued expansion of the corpora cavernosa impinges on the veins that normally carry blood from the penis, and the end result is that the blood is temporarily trapped. As long as the smooth muscle cells are relaxed allowing the filling the corpora cavernosa, and the trapped blood is constricted from leaving, an erection takes place. Some pretty complicated engineering, and that's why a lot of things can lead to erectile dysfunction, or impotence.

It should be obvious from the above description that the major cause of impotence is usually blood flow problems. If you have blocked arteries in the heart, you can bet you probably have blocked arteries in the penis. In fact, the best indicator of an impending heart attack is the development of erectile dysfunction. One study indicated that 25 percent of patients who developed impotence had a heart attack or a stroke within two years.

Besides vascular problems that cause impotence, there can be problems traced to the nervous system. Without impulses from the hypothalamus getting to their target cells in the penis, there is no initiating signal for an erection to take place. Once again male Type 2 diabetics illustrate this problem well because many of them suffer from diabetic neuropathy, in which nerve impulses simply die off faster than they should. Without those nerve impulses operating at full strength, the ability to achieve an erection becomes difficult. Other conditions in which nerve impulses to the genital area are degraded include multiple sclerosis and Parkinson's disease.

Finally, some of the most widely prescribed drugs can cause impotence. It is estimated that some 200 commonly used drugs are strongly associated with increased impotence. In fact, 8 of the 10 most widely prescribed drugs are known to negatively affect sexual performance. Some of the worst offenders are antihypertensive drugs, such as diuretics and beta-blockers. This is why males taking these drugs for hypertension are four times more likely to suffer from erectile dysfunction than age-matched controls who are not taking such drugs.

If hypertensive drugs can interfere with sexual performance, then it should not be surprising that antidepressive drugs also have a negative consequence due to their impact on the generation of nerve impulses. This is especially true of serotonin re-uptake inhibitors, like Prozac, Paxil, and Zoloft, commonly used in the treatment of depression. This list of offending psychopharmacology drugs also includes those commonly used for anxiety, such as tranquilizers. Besides these drugs, there are a number of over-the-counter drugs, such as antihistamines and antacids, such as Tagamet, Pepcid, Axir, and Zantac, that can lead to erectile dysfunction. Who says being a male is easy these days?

We now understand to a far greater degree what is involved in generating and maintaining male erections. Before this knowledge was unlocked, many of the treatments for impotency bordered on the ridiculous. But when it comes to maintaining virility, males will try virtually anything and blame anything other than themselves. This is why impotence is constantly referred to in religious writings. In Genesis, impotency was considered a punishment from God for adultery or even thinking about adultery. The Egyptians believed loss of sexual potency was due to the wrath of one of their many gods. By the Middle Ages, impotency was thought to be caused by witchcraft or demonic possession.

When invocation to God (or gods) was not sufficient to treat the problem, men took over, developing an almost endless array of herbs and potions to treat the problem. Even today, crushed rhinoceros horns are highly prized as virility enhancers. For many centuries, mandrake (which comes from the nightshade family) was an accepted herbal remedy for impotency. Jimsonweed, another member of the nightshade family, is mentioned in both Homer and Shakespeare as a treatment for impotence. Unfortunately, members of the nightshade family (especially jimsonweed) tend to be toxic. If toxic herbs failed to solve impotence, then one could always eat foods that had a phallic shape, such as bananas, carrots, asparagus, or cucumbers.

Now, pharmacology has become the primary weapon in the war against impotence. Actually, the first reports on the use of drugs to treat impotence appeared in 1944 with injections of testosterone, finally vindicating Brown-Séquard. But for the next 35 years, the scientific literature relative to drug treatment for impotence was virtually nonexistent. The use of drug treatment for impotence resumed in 1980 when a physician mistakenly injected a patient in the penis with a drug (papaverine) derived from the opium poppy. This drug is a powerful vasodilator and caused an immediate erection that lasted two hours. Soon afterwards, another drug called phentolamine, which inhibits certain neurotransmitters from constricting blood vessels, was also found to be useful when injected into the penis. Soon combinations of papaverine and phentolamine became the rage. Then it was found that impotence was effectively eliminated by administration of penile injections of an even more powerful vasodilator that was nearly one thousand times more effective than papaverine. That drug was the "good" eicosanoid, PGE_1, which dramatically increased blood flow into the corpora cavernosa by relaxing the surrounding tissue. With injections of PGE_1, erections were virtually guaranteed, no foreplay required. Probably the classic example of this occurred in 1983 when one of the early pioneers in eicosanoid injection therapy, G. S. Brindley, presented a highly scientific discussion of his work at the American Urological Association meeting. At the end of the seminar (always a high-stress situation), he dropped his trousers to demonstrate to his eminent colleagues a very firm erection initiated an hour earlier by an injection of PGE_1. Either giving a very dry, clinical seminar is an aphrodisiac (highly unlikely) or erections can be induced solely by the manipulation of "good" eicosanoids (more likely).

However, given the choice of improving erections prior to intercourse by injections or by a pill, I think most men would wimp out for a pill. And that's what has led to the success of the biggest blockbuster in pharmaceutical history—Viagra.

Ironically, Viagra's discovery as a treatment for erectile dysfunction was a mistake. Viagra was originally developed as a cardiovascular drug to increase blood flow to the heart. It wasn't a very good cardiovascular drug. In fact, Viagra was a failure, so the drug company asked all the participants in their study to return their medications. But for some reason, although all the placebo pills were returned, very few of the pills containing the active ingredient came back. The drug company sent their representatives to find out why. By asking a few personal questions about the side effects of the drug, the answer quickly became apparent. The male subjects were not going to give up their new found virility. So much for "rational" drug delivery. Dumb luck is a better description.

The mechanism of action for Viagra is slightly different than the mechanism of eicosanoid modulation. The increase in blood flow caused by the injection of "good" eicosanoids like PGE_1 came from the increased production of the second messenger, cyclic AMP, which causes vasodilation and greater blood flow. Viagra works by inhibiting the degradation of a similar second messenger called cyclic GMP (caused by the production of nitric oxide) that also causes vasodilation.

Are injections of "good" eicosanoids or Viagra the only ways to alter the levels of these second messengers? Or can many of the benefits of PGE_1 injections or Viagra be achieved by the diet? The answer may be yes.

Let's go back to our prototype individuals who are aging faster than they should: Type 2 diabetics. Not only do they have higher levels of insulin, but also higher rates of heart disease and stroke than age-matched controls. It should also not be too surprising that Type 2 diabetic males also have a higher level of erectile dysfunction. As I stated earlier, it is estimated that 35 to 75 percent of Type 2 diabetic males have some degree of erectile dysfunction. This is nearly five times the levels of age-matched non-diabetics. But why? The answer is excess insulin. This will lead to an overproduction of "bad" eicosanoids, which cause vasoconstriction and neuropathy that decreases the likelihood of the nerve impulses making their way from the sex center in the hypothalamus to the penis. In essence, a double whammy against virility. Remember, Viagra will not work unless adequate nerve impulses are received by the target cells in the penis. Injections of PGE_1, on the other hand, completely bypass the need for nerve stimulation to achieve an erection.

The dietary key for treating erectile dysfunction is (a) to increase cyclic AMP levels (the mechanism of PGE_1), (b) to decrease insulin, or (c) to increase levels of cyclic GMP (the mechanism of Viagra). Since the Zone Diet can simultaneously increase cyclic AMP (by the increased production of "good" eicosanoids like PGE_1) while decreasing insulin, it must be considered the cornerstone of any anti-impotency treatment program. But what about increasing cyclic GMP?

Cyclic GMP is formed in response to increased nitric oxide production. So, how do you make more nitric oxide? The answer: consume protein that is rich in the amino acid arginine. And what foods are rich in arginine? Soybeans and turkey. This is because nitric oxide cannot be formed unless there are adequate levels of arginine present in the bloodstream. Without the adequate intake of arginine-rich foods, it becomes difficult to make enough cyclic GMP to make a difference. Thus, the first step of your dietary strategy to prevent (if not treat) erectile dysfunction is to increase the production of PGE_1 by keeping insulin levels from becoming elevated. How do you achieve that goal? Follow the Zone Diet and take extra EPA to increase PGE_1 formation. The second step is to stimulate cyclic GMP production by providing yourself with adequate levels of protein sources that are rich in arginine, like soybeans and turkey. Do turkeyburgers and soybean hamburgers (in part of the Zone Diet) plus adequate levels of EPA stand as an economic threat to the exploding sales of Viagra? Probably not, but they offer a purely dietary approach to treat erectile dysfunction. Of course, turkey and soybean hamburgers are a lot cheaper and have no side effects.

One of best ways to improve sex for males is to reduce stress. One direct effect of stress is the reduction of testosterone, the hormone required for both libido and sexual performance. Chronic stress will also increase the production of cortisol that, in turn, increases insulin levels. And as I have pointed out, there is no greater turnoff to sexual performance than increased insulin levels because of insulin's ability to alter the balance of "good" and "bad" eicosanoids. One of the best ways to reduce stress prior to sex is to encourage romance.

Sexual dysfunction is clinical and mechanical, whereas romance raises sex to its highest level. Wars have been fought over romance, and great works of literature, art, and music are often based on it. These more noble images of sex are rarely based upon unbridled lust but are far more likely to be based on romance. Romance is not only respect for your partner but it is also based on the development of an atmosphere that encourages the magical aspects of sex. Sex is more than physiology, it is really sharing part of yourself with your partner. So the ultimate aphrodisiac remains romance, not a pill or an injection.

Maintaining male virility is difficult enough as you age. Make it easier on yourself by following the Anti-aging Zone Lifestyle Pyramid because each of its components will immeasurably improve sexual function.

CHAPTER 18

SEX AND THE ZONE FOR WOMEN:
WHERE HAS THE FERTILITY GONE?

The hormonal sexual concerns of women are usually very different than those of men, because their sexual agenda is very different from an evolutionary perspective. Women tend to be concerned about raising families, whereas men are more concerned about making families. Before I am accused of being sexist, I want to say that these generalizations are simply meant to represent a broad spectrum of sex in females that is ultimately controlled by hormones. Therefore, your ability to control hormones will determine your success in achieving your particular sexual goals.

The most pressing sexual problem for premenopausal women today has become fertility. In the 1960s the major problem facing females was how *not* to become pregnant. In the 1990s the problem is now how *to* become pregnant. What has changed so drastically in the last 30 years?

First, women are waiting longer to have children. From a purely evolutionary viewpoint, the primary childbearing years for females are between the ages of 18 and 30. If you recall from the chapter on eicosanoids, after age 30, the average woman's production of the activated essential fatty acids critical for the synthesis of eicosanoids begins to slow down. This is a unique way to decrease fertility in women because without adequate levels of eicosanoids, reproduction is very difficult. Also, remember that women living much beyond the primary childbearing years is a relatively recent phenomenon because of the high mortality rates associated with childbirth in the past. (At the turn of the century, 1 out of 10 women died during childbirth.) Although women are living longer and therefore postponing childbirth to later in life, their genetic makeup and the hormones that control fertility haven't yet been informed of this change.

However, this normal influence of age on childbearing can be altered by the Zone Diet. If you remember, one of the benefits of calorie restriction is the extension of female reproductive functionality. Also remember that eicosanoid production begins to decrease around age 30. These two events are intimately tied together. The Zone Diet is not only a calorie-restricted diet, but also one that improves the production of "good" eicosanoids, which are necessary for successful embryo implantation. This dietary approach can increase the likelihood of fertilization prior to menopause.

Second, this decrease in fertility may also be diet related. In the last 15 years in America, diet has changed dramatically as women have increasingly switched to low-fat, high-carbohydrate diets with a corresponding increase in insulin production. I believe that the increased hyperinsulinemia in women may be responsible for this drastic change for the worse and has spawned a new industry of fertility drugs and fertility centers.

One possible confirmation of this hypothesis may be found in studying a condition known as polycystic ovary syndrome (PCOS). Nearly one-third of all women of childbearing age have polyscytic ovaries. And about 20 to 25 percent of these women have developed PCOS, which is marked by increased insulin levels, increased testosterone (the male sex hormone) production, and decreased fertility. It has been demonstrated clinically that if you can lower insulin, many of the clinical symptoms of PCOS disappear, and fertility returns. It is rather remarkable that such a drastic changeover from infertility to fertility may simply require reducing excessive levels of insulin. Let me explain how that happens:

In women with PCOS, a key enzyme (cytochrome P450c17α) that catalyzes the production of the building block (i.e. androstenedione) for testosterone from progesterone is activated by insulin (see Figure 18-1 on page 201).

Like most key enzymes in the body, rate-limiting enzymes that control important biological activities are often under hormonal control. This is true of the enzyme (3-hydroxyl 3-methyl gluglutaryl-CoA reductase) that controls cholesterol synthesis and the enzyme (delta-5-desaturase) that controls essential fatty acid production. Obviously, making cholesterol and essential fatty acids are important biological functions. And the body's production of sex hormones would likewise be considered an important biological activity. Just as the enzymes

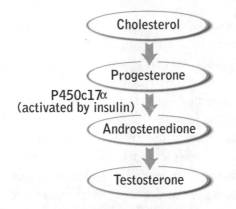

Figure 18-1   Excess of Insulin can Decrease Fertility by Increasing Testosterone

responsible for the increased production of cholesterol and increased production of arachidonic acid are activated by insulin, the enzyme responsible for the precursor of testosterone (at least in women) is also activated by insulin.

With increased testosterone in the bloodstream, fertility drops. As the ratio of testosterone to estrogen increases, not only does fertility decrease, but risk factors for cardiovascular disease increase. This same effect is observed in sex-change operations for females who wish to become males. As they are given larger doses of testosterone, their ratio of testosterone to estrogen increases, with significant increases in their visceral fat mediated by increased insulin levels.

On the other hand, once you reduce insulin levels, then the activity of P450c17α enzyme is inhibited, testosterone levels drop and fertility returns in women with PCOS. For these women, and for perhaps all women experiencing fertility problems, the first "drug" to try is the Zone Diet in order to reduce elevated insulin levels.

The rise of infertility in the past 15 years correlates quite alarmingly with the corresponding increase in obesity and excess consumption of carbohydrates in America. Not surprisingly the average dress size of American women is now a size 14, and many magazines now celebrate the "full-figured" woman. Considering the importance of the diet on insulin levels and fertility, the epidemic of hyperinsulinemia in women of childbearing age should be considered a major factor for decreased fertility in American women.

Another premenopausal condition that impacts a great number of women is premenstrual syndrome (PMS). The typical 30-day cycle that a premenopausal woman faces is a roller coaster ride of changing levels of sex hormones. The ride begins with the release of gonadotropin-releasing hormone (GnRH) from the hypothalamus, which then causes the release of follicle-stimulating hormone (FSH) from the pituitary to prepare the uterine endometrium for a potential fertile egg to be fertilized in mid-cycle. GnRH also causes the increase of another hormone, luteinzing hormone (LH), which causes the release of the egg from the ovary in mid-cycle. At the mid-cycle point, estrogen levels drop slightly and progesterone levels increase. If fertilization has taken place, progesterone stays elevated, thus preventing any more eggs from being delivered. If no fertilization takes place, then there is a rapid decrease in both estrogen and progesterone levels that leads to menstruation to clear out the uterus. Any way you look at it, it is an exceptionally complex series of hormonal events and timing. No wonder that something goes wrong occasionally. And what goes wrong is usually a failure in your "good" eicosanoid booster system because both FSH and LH work by using cyclic AMP as a second messenger. As you might recall, cyclic AMP is produced by "good" eicosanoids, and thus becomes a linkage with PMS.

Approximately 30 percent of the female population has some form of PMS, and of that group approximately one-third (or 5 to 10 percent of the entire childbearing population) has severe and often incapacitating PMS. Research indicates that women with severe PMS also have very low levels of the activated omega-6 essential fatty acid, gamma linolenic acid (GLA). In fact, their levels appear to be nearly 80 percent lower than women without PMS. Without adequate levels of GLA in the pipeline, it becomes difficult to make adequate levels of "good" eicosanoids, the ones that increase the production of cyclic AMP. The obvious solution to the problem would be simply to supplement the diet with extra GLA. And for many women with PMS, this seems to give some relief.

However, as pointed out earlier, GLA supplementation can be a dangerous game to play because much of the supplemental GLA can be converted to AA, thus increasing the overproduction of "bad" eicosanoids that seem to increase the severity of PMS. The increased potential flow of GLA into AA can be prevented by adding back EPA (the inhibitor of the delta-5-desaturase enzyme) while simultaneously controlling insulin levels using the Zone Diet. It has been my experience that PMS can be brought under control within 30 to 60 days by following that dietary prescription. The supplemental GLA fills the pipeline for "good" eicosanoid formation, while the combination of extra EPA and improved insulin control using the Zone Diet prevents the increased levels of GLA from spilling over into arachidonic acid (AA). The end result is a greater increase in DGLA, the building block of "good" eicosanoids, which can increase cyclic AMP levels in the ovary and thus decrease, if not eliminate, the symptoms associated with PMS. That alone will guarantee better sex.

Even after conception, women have to worry about reducing the complications that occur during pregnancy. One of the most worrisome is gestational diabetes caused by excessive insulin levels. As seen with our Type 2 diabetic patients, the Zone Diet coupled with EPA does a very effective job re-establishing insulin control and lowering elevated blood glucose levels. Just as the diet can play a significant role in fertility, during pregnancy it can have a powerful effect on a successful outcome.

Even after birth, the role of diet is not finished. What you feed your newborn will have a dramatic impact on his or her future development. It is now quite clear that breast-feeding is superior to any type of bottle-feeding for young infants. Not only are IQ scores higher, but childhood illness is less. Why? Among the unique characteristics of human breast milk is its fatty acid composition. It is very rich in gamma linolenic acid (GLA) and long-chain omega-3 fatty acids, such as eicosapentaenoic acid (EPA) and docosahexenoic acid (DHA). If you go back to the chapter on eicosanoids, you will understand the importance of these particular fatty acids. Infant formulas are devoid of these unique fatty acids, and this is why newborn children are at greater risk for outright eicosanoid deficiencies. Eicosanoids control the immune system. If you have lower levels of eicosanoids (especially "good" eicosanoids) as a newborn, you will also have a less efficient immune system. The new world is tough enough without having one hand tied behind your back immunologically.

The second reason for breast feeding is even more compelling. In the first two years of life, the brain is the most rapidly growing organ in the newborn child. More than 50 percent of the total brain mass is composed of fat, and much of that is long-chain omega-3 fatty acids, such as EPA and DHA. In fact, your brain is a virtual depository of long-chain omega-3 fatty acids with brain neurons containing more than five times the amount of these activated long-chain omega-3 fatty acids than your red blood cells. Without adequate levels of these long-chain omega-3 fatty acids in the diet of the newborn child, the formation of neurological networks will be compromised. This has been clearly demonstrated in rhesus monkeys in which restriction of long-chain omega-3 fatty acids gives rise to neurological deficiencies.

To add to this problem of getting adequate levels of activated essential fatty acids to the child, the more children a woman has, the lower the levels of long-chain omega-3 fatty acids found in her breast milk with each succeeding child. Maybe the old wives' tale that the firstborn is usually the brightest may have a discrete biological foundation—the first-born child has a greater intake of activated long-chain omega-3 fatty acids than the later siblings.

But before you despair, if you don't breast-feed your child or if you plan to have more than one child, realize that many of the problems can be overcome by your own diet. Breast milk is very sensitive to any dietary increase in omega-3 fatty acids. So by consuming more long-chain omega-3 fats, the breast milk will be fortified correspondingly. If you aren't breast-feeding, then some infant formulas (at least in Europe and Japan) are now being fortified with EPA and DHA. If you don't have access to these more advanced infant formulas, then what do you do? Now you may have to go back to what your grandmother did: add some cod-liver oil (like a fifth of a teaspoon) or some EPA containing fish oil (the equivalent of half a capsule) to the infant formula or mix it into baby food. (Just be sure to use purified fish oil that has been molecularly distilled to remove contaminants such as PCB.)

Bottom line, if you want to increase your chances of fertility, reduce insulin levels by following the Zone Diet. If you want to decrease the likelihood of gestational diabetes, then reduce insulin levels by following the Zone Diet (with a corresponding increase in total protein and total calories because you are eating for two). If you want to optimize your children's immune system and neurological development, breast-feed them and supplement your own Zone Diet with extra EPA and DHA. If you formula-feed your child, then make sure they are getting adequate levels of EPA and DHA in their diet by adding supplemental amounts of purified fish oils.

Toward the end of childbearing years comes menopause when life becomes even more complicated for women. Estrogen levels begin to drop, and that hormonal roller-coaster ride experienced during the normal 30-day premenstrual cycle now seems like a tame merry-go-round. Estrogen has numerous many different biological functions, and its sudden drop upsets the intricate hormonal balance in females. The synthesis of estrogen is orchestrated by FSH through cyclic AMP, whereas progesterone synthesis is stimulated by LH, which also works through cyclic AMP. And here is where the Zone Diet can play an important role to minimize this hormonal roller-coaster. By providing the necessary back-up production of "good" eicosanoids, the production of cyclic AMP is increased. The levels of second messengers generated by FSH and LH can be maintained so that the levels of these hormones will not drop as readily during menopause. As a result, many of the symptoms associated with menopause can be minimized. This is not to say that the Zone Diet will eliminate the symptoms associated with menopause, but it can make the transition much easier.

After menopause, concerns about fertility, PMS, pregnancy, breast feeding and hot flashes become a thing of the past. However, in later life, many women's sexual concerns become more directed to diseases related to lack of sex hormones. In particular, heart attacks (the number 1 cause of death in women), breast cancer (the number 1 fear for women), and osteoporosis. Yet, all three of these diseases are strongly associated with excess insulin levels, excess cortisol, and the resulting eicosanoid imbalance. Although, I will discuss estrogen in greater detail in the next chapter, here is a thumbnail sketch of its role in menopause.

It is well known that within the 10-year period after menopause, the rates of heart attacks in women skyrocket to virtually equal the rates in males. And it is also suggested that estrogen replacement appears to decrease the likelihood of heart attacks and osteoporosis. Because of this, many women in America are being told to take estrogen supplements for the rest of their lives.

Is estrogen the central player in this drama or is something else happening below the surface? As estrogen levels drop, insulin resistance develops insulin levels begin to increase dramatically. The hormonal consequence will be an increase in the production of "bad" eicosanoids. Heart disease can be viewed as simply an overproduction of "bad" eicosanoids. It's not that estrogen protects against heart disease per se, but by controlling insulin (and therefore the balance of eicosanoids) it is instrumental in the reduction of cardiovascular risk.

Why does hormonal replacement therapy (HRT) with estrogen seem to reduce heart attacks? At low doses, estrogen reduces insulin resistance, yet at higher dosages, it increases insulin resistance. This is known as a bimodal effect. At one concentration, a hormone will do one thing, but at a higher concentration it does the opposite. To compound the problem, estrogen is never given in the absence of progesterone (in order to minimize the cancer risk). Unfortunately, progesterone also increases insulin resistance. If insulin resistance increases, then insulin levels also increase. This means the problem is finding the right dose of estrogen and progesterone to keep insulin under control. These differing hormonal effects explain why some women on estrogren replacement therapy experience a sudden weight gain and why many women receiving estrogen replacement therapy still get heart attacks. Both events may be due to increased insulin levels. As always with any hormonal replacement therapy, the key phrase should be "start low and go slow," since a change in any hormone will affect other hormones in ways that most physicians are totally unaware.

Although, women are 10 times more likely to die of heart disease than breast cancer, it is probably safe to say that the number-one health concern of virtually every woman is breast cancer. Why not, as it is consistently reiterated that 1 in 9 women will get breast cancer? But considering the differences in the mortality rates of these two diseases, it is apparent that the breast cancer lobby has a better public relations campaign for the hearts and minds of women in this country.

While estrogen supplementation can apparently decrease the risk of heart disease by lowering insulin, it also increases the likelihood of breast cancer because of its stimulatory effects on breast tissue. What is the best way to reduce the likelihood of breast cancer? Simply by reducing insulin levels. That can be accomplished by following the Anti-aging Zone Lifestyle Pyramid. As mentioned earlier, excess insulin production will increase the production of "bad" eicosanoids that depress the immune system. And that's a pretty good definition of cancer: a depressed immune system. In addition, high levels of insulin also decrease the production of sex hormone binding proteins that bind much of the free estrogen. The levels of these sex hormone binding proteins decrease as insulin levels rise, thus making larger amounts of unbound estrogen available to interact with estrogen receptors in the breast tissue. Even though the total amount of estrogen is declining, there is more free estrogen (because of lower levels of sex hormone binding proteins) to wreak havoc with receptors in the breast tissue. The role of the newest generation of estrogen blockers, such as Tamoxifen, Reflexin, and Elevastin, is to block the binding of estrogen to its receptor sites. Alternatively, raising the levels of sex hormone binding proteins by lowering insulin would achieve the same results, and this can be done through diet. This dietary approach makes more sense than taking some pharmaceutical agent for life.

Finally, what about osteoporosis? Bone loss is promoted by many of the same "bad" eicosanoids (such as PGE_2 and LTB_4) generated by excess insulin and other pro-inflammatory cytokines, such as interleukins (especially interleukin-1 or IL-1) that are also increased by excess insulin. This process, called resorption, is caused by a disturbance in the balance of osteoblasts (bone-building cells) and osteoclasts (bone-resorption cells). The more pro-inflammatory agents you make, the more resorption takes place and the less bone building there is. The net result is bone loss that leads to osteoporosis.

However, the fastest way to speed up bone loss is to promote the production of excess cortisol. Cortisol inhibits progesterone from binding to its receptors in the bones. Since progesterone stimulates new bone synthesis, excess cortisol becomes one of the major factors for developing osteoporosis by blocking the bone-building action of progesterone. And, as explained earlier, the best way to reduce cortisol levels is to make sure that blood sugar levels are stabilized by the Zone Diet. Of course, following the other components of the Anti-aging Zone Lifestyle (exercise and meditation) are also useful in concert with the Zone Diet to reduce excess cortisol levels.

For both women and men, the joy of sex and the fear of the health problems associated with sex hormones are an integral part of their lives. Yet, whatever your sexual concerns, they can be improved by the Zone Diet. This is not about some magic aphrodisiac, but using the Zone Diet can improve the hormonal communication that improves sex while simultaneously decreasing the health problems associated with the changing levels of sex hormones as you age. The end result is that this complex area of humanity becomes something to be enjoyed, not feared.

This is where your dietary strategy to reverse the aging process becomes identical to your hormonal control strategy to improve sex. The Anti-aging Zone Lifestyle Pyramid is the key to better sex for both men and women because of the effects it has on the hormones associated with sex. Better sex with increased longevity—not a bad combination.

Food is truly the way to achieve better sex for both males and females. To reinforce that thought, ask yourself who are considered to be the most romantic people on the earth? Usually the answer is the French. Not surprisingly, the classical French cuisine is very similar to the Zone Diet. Maybe that explains their love of romance and joy of sex.

CHAPTER 19

ESTROGEN:
DOES EVERY WOMAN NEED IT?

To take or not to take. That's the question many women in America are struggling with. Many times they are advised that if they don't want to die of heart disease or get osteoporosis, they have to take estrogen, even if there is a potential increase in breast cancer risk. A truly Faustian bargain.

But before you can come to an answer for yourself, you have to know what estrogen is and what it really does. First of all, there is no single compound known as estrogen, but rather a family of three compounds formed by the body: estrone (E1), estradiol (E2), and estriol (E3). These are shown in Figure 19-1.

All three estrogens are normally made by the body, but at varying concentrations and at varying times. In the absence of pregnancy, estradiol is the primary estrogen produced, and it peaks at midcycle. However, during pregnancy estriol is made in larger quantities and estrone levels also increase to become considerably higher than estradiol. Furthermore, these natural estrogens are not equal in power. Relative to stimulating the growth of breast tissue, estriol is nearly eighty times less powerful than estradiol, and because of this lack of breast tissue stimulation there is evidence that estriol may actually be protec-

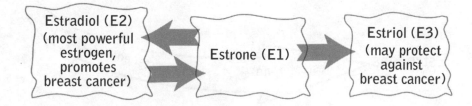

Figure 19-1   Conversion of Estrogens

tive against breast cancer, whereas estradiol is a strong promoter of breast cancer.

The basic building block for all steroid hormones, including estrogen, is cholesterol. To make estrogen, you first have to make testosterone. In fact, without cholesterol, there would be no estrogens or testosterone. The basic pathway of cholesterol to estrogen is shown in Figure 19-2.

The first thing you notice about this pathway is that estrogens are formed from testosterone. This is illustrative of how all sex hormones (both male and female) are made in the body. For all sex hormones, the initiating signal for their synthesis starts in the hypothalamus with the secretion of gonadotropin-releasing hormone (GnRH). This para-

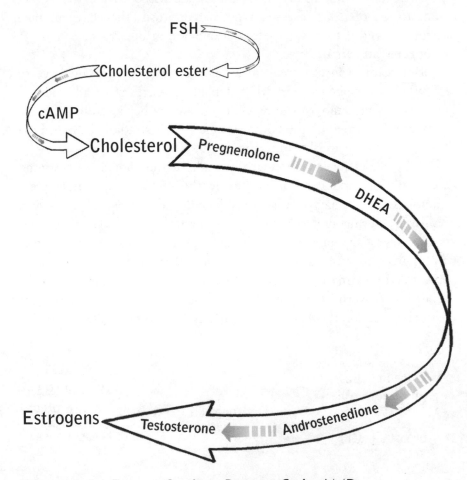

Figure 19-2   Estrogen Synthesis Requires Cyclic AMP

crine hormone then travels to the pituitary to initiate the release of both luteinizing hormone (LH) and follicle-stimulating hormone (FSH). Once secreted from the pituitary, FSH and LH then travel to the ovary and via cyclic AMP cause the synthesis of estrogen and progesterone respectively, through a series of chemical transformations to cholesterol once released from its cholesterol ester storage site in the target cells. The complete pathway is shown in Figure 19-3.

When dealing with female sex hormones, it is often the balance that is more important than the actual levels. This is true of the ratio of estrogen to progesterone, as well as estrogen to testosterone. For females, a higher ratio of testosterone to estrogen is indicative of an increased risk of heart disease. (The opposite is true in males.) In females, as the estrogen to progesterone ratio decreases, it creates an estrogen dominance and an increased risk of breast cancer. As with all endocrine hormones, a unique balancing act must be maintained to generate wellness. An imbalance in opposing hormones, especially sex hormones, usually signals disease.

Bear in mind that estrogens do many things. It is estimated that they have many biological functions, including increasing cell proliferation in the endometrium for fertilization, improving neural connections in the brain, and controlling insulin levels. This is why estrogen

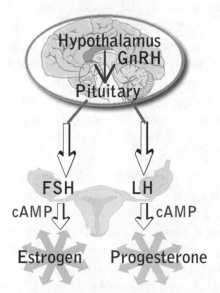

Figure 19-3   Synthesis of Estrogen and Progesterone Requires Cyclic AMP

receptors are found everywhere in the body from the ovary to the pituitary, in the hypothalamus and in various parts of the brain, including the neocortex. Estrogen receptors are also found in the prostrate gland, testes, liver, and kidney. Without estrogen, life becomes very difficult.

On the other hand, too much estrogen, is no picnic either. This is why progesterone is its constant companion. Progesterone works by decreasing the number of estrogen receptor proteins in the nucleus, thus decreasing the likelihood of breast cell proliferation. In addition, progesterone has numerous benefits, including the promotion of new bone growth (estrogen only slows bone loss).

It is the balance of estrogens and progesterone that is the key to sex hormone equilibrium in females, since they exert opposing effects on each other primarily by altering each other's receptor sites. Estrogens increase the number of receptor sites for both estrogen and progesterone, whereas progesterone decreases the number of receptor sites for both hormones. Many of the problems of menopause and post-menopause are caused by an imbalance of estrogen and progesterone, leading to estrogen dominance. It is a very exquisite balancing act, not unlike the axis of insulin and glucagon and "good" and "bad" eicosanoids.

All steroid hormones, including estrogens, are very water insoluble, therefore, they travel in the bloodstream complexed to binding proteins. Estrogen uses the sex hormone binding globulin (SHBG), whereas progesterone uses the corticoid binding globulin (CBG) for transport in the bloodstream. When bound to a circulating binding protein, a steroid hormone is totally inactive. Only when a hormone is released from a circulating binding protein, that it can pass through the membrane of the target cell into the nucleus. Once inside the nucleus, it binds to a receptor protein and becomes activated allowing it to interact with selected genes. This will cause either an induction or repression of new protein synthesis that generates the ultimate biological response initiated by the estrogen or progesterone. As you can see, this is a very different mechanism of hormonal communication than that found in the case of polypeptide endocrine hormones that use cyclic AMP as a second messenger.

Since there is no receptor on the surface of the target cell to control the entry of the steroid hormone into the cell, much of the control of the biological actions of estrogen is mediated by the amount of its binding protein that circulates in the bloodstream. This is where excess insulin comes in. The more elevated the insulin levels, the lower the levels of sex hormone binding proteins in the bloodstream. This means more free hormone can interact with its nuclear receptors than would normally be the case. In essence, excess insulin has decreased one of the primary control points (i.e., levels of binding proteins) for sex hormones.

The same problem can occur after menopause. Although, estrogen levels have decreased (by about 50 percent), estrogens are not totally absent since the adrenal glands and even the fat cells can make estrogens. But if insulin is elevated, sex hormone binding proteins will be depressed to such an extent that excess free estrogen is now a problem because of its potential to cause proliferation of breast tissue. If that proliferation becomes malignant, then it is called breast cancer.

This unique link between estrogen and insulin begins to explain some of the chronic diseases that occur in women after menopause. Recent research indicates that estrogen seems to be a profound governor on the secretion of insulin. As total estrogen levels decrease, insulin resistance and insulin levels begin to rise. Knowing the impact of increasing insulin levels on other hormonal systems, such as the overproduction of "bad" eicosanoids and cortisol, it is not surprising that after menopause heart disease (increased production of "bad"eicosanoids that promote platelet aggregation), breast cancer (increased production of "bad" eicosanoids that depress the immune system), and osteoporosis (increased production of pro-inflammatory "bad" eicosanoids and cortisol) all become significant female health problems.

This understanding of the link between estrogen and insulin also begins to explain many of the benefits of estrogen replacement therapy and also why it doesn't work for every woman. At low doses of estrogen, insulin resistance is reduced. Unfortunately, at higher estrogen levels, insulin resistance is increased. This is a bimodal response because at one concentration the effect of a hormone is totally opposite of what it is at a higher concentration. Compounding the problem, progesterone is usually always given with estrogen replacement therapy. Progesterone also increases insulin resistance. Insulin resistance increases circulating levels of insulin that results in an increased rate of aging and the increased likelihood of chronic diseases specific to women after menopause.

To make a complex problem even more complicated is the fact that natural estrogens (and natural progesterone) can't be patented.

The reason why and the resulting confusion for women is one of the more interesting stories in the history of hormones.

While you can't patent a natural compound, you can patent a novel synthetic pathway to manufacture such a compound. This is commonly done with genetically engineered proteins. Unfortunately, the man who made this synthesis of natural estrogens possible never patented any of the processes in the hope that his scientific breakthroughs would benefit all. That man was Russell Marker and his story has massive implications for all women today.

Russell Marker was truly a scientific genius, which meant he was also more than a bit eccentric. As a professor at Penn State in the 1930s, he developed the method for octane rating that is still used today. But the 1930s was also the heyday of steroid research, and the race to synthesize steroids was as intense as the race to the moon would be 30 years later. The reason was obvious, there was a lot of money to be made. Marker, however, was purely an academic. He wondered if some plant might contain the appropriate starting raw material to make steroid hormone synthesis more efficient. He discovered that the Mexican yam contained that material, and with relatively little effort, he was able to synthetically make progesterone and from then testosterone, and finally estrogen.

With a potential gold mine in hand, he went back to his sponsor, the drug company Parke-Davis, and asked for more funds to scale up his synthetic efforts in Mexico since that was where the yams grew in abundance. Parke-Davis turned him down cold since it was obvious to them that no respectable research could ever be done in Mexico. Of course, another reason for Marker's research being abandoned may have been that the leading chemist of the day, Louis Feiser of Harvard, said such steroid synthesis was impossible, despite the fact Marker had already done it. Maybe this is why they say you can always tell a Harvard man, you just can't tell him much.

But, Russell Marker was not a person to take no for an answer. He moved to Mexico City, looked for the first laboratory listed in the phone book, made them his partners and produced more than one million dollars worth of progesterone. Unfortunately, Marker never took out any patents on the process since he felt that his research should be free for all to use. After many trials and tribulations, Marker quit science in 1950 and became a dealer in pre-Columbian antiquities. And the fate of his partners in Mexico? They re-formed the company that became Syntex, one of the world's major drug companies before it was acquired by another drug giant a few years ago.

How did this tiny Mexican laboratory picked out of a phone book become a pharmaceutical powerhouse? By making patented compounds based on Marker's early research. And here the implication for women today comes into focus. The natural steroids that Marker synthesized in the 1930s are the natural ones the body knows how to use and metabolize. The unnatural, but patentable sex hormone analogs currently used today represent alien chemicals in the body that mimic many of the functions of natural estrogen and progesterone, but with a side-effect profile that the natural steroids don't have.

The first real commercial use of sex hormones was not for treating menopause, but for use as oral contraceptives. There are two types of oral contraceptives. One is the combination pill that contains synthetic analogs of estrogen and progesterone; the other is a pill containing only synthetic analogs of progesterone. Both types of birth-control pills were developed based on the ability of high levels of progesterone to prevent the release of eggs from the ovary or make the environment inhospitable for the implanting of eggs. But why use synthetic analogs of progesterone, when natural progesterone was available? Unfortunately, natural progesterone besides being nonpatentable (thanks to Russell Marker's generosity to mankind), also has a short half-life (like estriol) so that it would have had to be taken several times a day to maintain adequate blood levels. Both problems were solved by the synthesis of new progesterone analogs called progestins (like Provera). These unnatural, but patentable compounds have a longer lifetime which means that they only have to be taken once a day. Good news for drug companies, but bad news for the females taking them because these progestins have their own unique side effects. Nonetheless, these side effects were tolerated since birth control was the primary women's issue of the 1960s and the "pill" represented the first time in history that women could control pregnancy. Perhaps not surprisingly, it was Syntex, Russell Marker's old company, that was the leader in developing birth-control pills.

The nonpatentability of natural estrogens also led to a great amount of work by drug companies to develop and successfully market patentable analogs of estrogens. Yet, as far as the body is concerned, these are fake hormones. The most famous example is Premarin, which consists of different types of estrogens of which only about half are found in the human body. The name, Premarin is a contraction of the actual source of this drug: *Pregnant mare urine.* So successful has the marketing of Premarin been that virtually every woman thinks of estrogen as exactly equivalent to Premarin, while nothing could be further from the truth.

In the early 1960s, menopause was not considered to be a lucrative market to exploit since birth-control pills wouldn't be needed after this change in life. Then, along came Robert Wilson, with his blockbuster book, *Feminine Forever.* This book (written with the backing of the drug company Ayerst Laboratories) promoted the concept that by taking estrogen, women could stay young forever. It just so happened that Ayerst had the patents on Premarin. Within 10 years, nearly 6 million women were taking Premarin to stay feminine forever. Unfortunately, science reared its ugly head in 1975 when an article in the *New England Journal of Medicine* announced that women who had taken Premarin on a long-term basis had nearly an eight times greater risk of breast cancer. My grandmother was among them, and she died of breast cancer in 1976, some 10 years after beginning high-dose Premarin.

This made the drug companies scramble to save their synthetic estrogen franchise. The answer was to use some form of progesterone to counteract the breast cell proliferation properties of Premarin. But which form? You could choose the natural progesterone synthesized by Russell Marker nearly 40 years earlier or use the unnatural, but patentable, synthetic analogs of progesterone known as progestins, which had been used for years as birth control agents. The obvious choice went to progestins (as if you would have thought otherwise).

Just to ensure complete recovery from the Premarin scare, it was pointed out that Premarin also protected against osteoporosis. In reality, while estrogen does slow down bone loss, only progesterone can increase bone mass. Nonetheless, it was a public relations triumph. Sales of Premarin skyrocketed now that it was combined with enough progestins (despite their numerous side effects) to reduce its inherent cancer-promoting effects. Because of the side effects (including PMS, bloating, irritability and depression) associated with progestins, it is estimated that nearly two-thirds of the women who started taking progestins to prevent cancer, stopped taking it, and just use the Premarin.

If a woman is considering estrogen replacement therapy, then what type of estrogen should she use? The original data on increased breast cancer incidence with estrogen replacement used patients taking Premarin. Less than 50 percent of the estrogens in Premarin are human estrogens. Of those only estrone and estradiol are present as there is no estriol in Premarin. Although, estriol is routinely used in Europe for treatment of menopause and post menopausal conditions, it is rarely mentioned in America. Part of the reason, as mentioned earlier, is that it is considered to be a "weaker" estrogen (it is 80 times weaker than estradiol in promoting breast tissue proliferation). Of course, that might be considered to be a real plus if you are worried about the increased risk of breast cancer. In addition, estriol has a shorter half-life in the bloodstream than estradiol, so that you need to take more of it, and more frequently, to maintain adequate blood levels. This extra effort appears to be worth it, since preliminary evidence indicates that estriol protects against breast cancer as opposed to promoting it like estradiol does. As a consequence, the higher the proportion of estriol in an estrogen supplement, the less progesterone that is required to provide protection against the potential cancer-promoting effects of estrogen. And since many women stop taking progesterone because of its side effects, a lowered dose of progesterone would be a significant plus because its side effects would also decrease.

Until recently one of the major problems with natural progesterone is that it was not orally absorbed without extensive degradation. However, a new form of progesterone called micronized progesterone solved many of these early problems. But years earlier drug companies had to work fast to come up with some form of progesterone to stem the breast cancer promoting properties of Premarin. Such drugs already existed in their inventory: progestins. Progestins had a long track record as oral conceptives. Sure they had their side-effect problems, but compared to reducing the risk of breast cancer caused by Premarin, these inherent problems could be tolerated by women.

Today women have become convinced that progestins are the same as natural progesterone. They are not. The body understands how to handle progesterone, whereas progestins are unnatural drugs that have more side effects than natural hormones. This was illustrated in the PEPI study which compared natural progesterone (but now in a micronized form to enhance absorption without degradation) versus progestins. In the PEPI trial both types of progesterone were combined with Premarin (it's too bad they didn't compare estriol to Premarin at the same time) to determine the effects on breast cancer and heart disease in women. The results indicated a much lesser degree of side effects and better disease outcome when the natural progesterone was used as opposed to the standard progestins. This is important because the side effects of progestins are so great for many women that they stopped using it, despite knowing full well that they were increasing their risk of breast cancer by taking estrogen alone.

This doesn't mean that natural progesterone is without its own side-effects, such as increased irritability and depression. This is because progesterone also increases insulin secretion, which can lead to the increased formation of "bad" eicosanoids that contribute to those side effects. Nonetheless, hormone supplementation with the natural form of the hormone will always have fewer side effects than patentable analogs. So, if you are considering hormone replacement, you should demand, not ask for, natural hormones.

But the question remains, do women need estrogen replacement therapy? After all, most of our grandmothers never took estrogen, and they survived. The answer to this paradox may be found in the diet.

About 25 percent of the female population never has the symptoms associated with menopause. This number closely matches the estimated population who have a genetically low insulin response to dietary carbohydrates. That percentage of the female population who don't produce significant amounts of insulin because of genetically low insulin levels are probably not going to be adversely affected with the drop of estrogen levels. However, the other 75 percent will be negatively affected.

Also, keep in mind that estrogen replacement may have the potential to decrease heart disease, but it doesn't eliminate it. In fact, recent research has questioned how useful estrogen replacement really is in reducing the risk of heart attacks for women who have already had one.

Finally, it should be remembered that the balance of free and bound steroid hormones in the bloodstream may be as important as the actual levels of hormones in the body. This balance of free and bound hormones will be controlled by levels of the sex hormone binding proteins. All of these factors (genetic responses to carbohydrates, risk of cardiovascular disease, and levels of sex hormone binding proteins) relate to insulin levels.

As estrogen levels decrease during menopause, insulin levels will increase for these women. It is the increase in insulin levels that can be considered the underlying cause of the chronic diseases (heart disease, breast cancer, and osteoporosis) associated with postmenopausal aging. Therefore, a logical alternative to reduce the rapid rise in insulin that occurs after menopause would be a drug that would reverse this. Such a "drug" exists. It's the Zone Diet, which was designed to lower elevated insulin levels. The same dietary control of insulin will also increase the amount of sex hormone binding proteins, which sequester the estrogen that is still being produced. This is why breast cancer is so highly associated with obesity. Obesity indicates hyperinsulinemia, which means decreases in the levels of sex binding hormones. The fewer sex binding proteins you have, the more free estrogen can interact with its receptors, thus, potentially accelerating breast cancer development.

If you are a woman faced with the decision whether or not to undertake hormonal replacement therapy, instead of trying to find the right combination of estrogen and progesterone to control insulin levels, it makes more sense to first reduce insulin levels with the Zone Diet followed by the other components of the Anti-aging Zone Lifestyle Pyramid. The Zone Diet will reduce insulin levels, moderate exercise (especially strength-training) will maintain, if not actually increase, bone mass, and reduction of cortisol by meditation will decrease cortisol-induced bone loss. Once you have made the Anti-aging Zone Lifestyle Pyramid an integral part of your life, then ask what are the smallest amounts of natural estrogen and natural progesterone required to maintain maximal health after menopause.

That is the goal of anti-aging: using the minimum amount of administered hormones to maximize quality of life by improving hormonal communication. But, just as you can't build a house on sand, you must have a firm hormonal foundation to build upon. The Anti-aging Zone Lifestyle Pyramid provides that foundation for every woman.

CHAPTER 20

TESTOSTERONE:
HORMONE OF STRENGTH,
HORMONE OF DESIRE

If there is a hormone that is considered an aphrodisiac for both males and females, it's testosterone. That's right, the same hormone that is required to develop muscle mass and strength. One hormone, many functions.

You usually think of testosterone as purely a male hormone, just as you think of estrogen as purely a female hormone. In reality, it is the balance of these hormones that determines your masculinity or feminity. Males make about 5 mg per day of testosterone. This is fifty times more than the amount of testosterone that women make on a daily basis. Women, on the other hand, make two to three times more estradiol than men. These differences in testosterone and estradiol levels in males are due to the increased production of testosterone coupled with the relative inactivity of the aromatase enzyme that converts testosterone to estradiol in males. As testesterone production falls and the activity of the aromatase enzyme increases, testosterone levels fall with a corresponding increase in estradiol levels. As a result, the ratio of testosterone to estradiol moves in an unfavorable direction for males. These aromatase enzymes are found in the fat cells, and as you will see later, the more fat you carry as a male, the more your testosterone gets converted into estradiol.

Like most endocrine hormones, the story of testosterone starts in the hypothalamus. The synthesis of testosterone starts with the secretion of gonadotropin-releasing hormone (GnRH). This is the same hormone responsible for starting the synthesis of estrogens. GnRH (as it also does in females) causes the release of both luteinizing hormone (LH) and follicle-stimulating hormone (FSH) from the pituitary gland into the circulation.

In males, LH seeks out a special group of cells (Leydig cells) in the testes, which through its second messenger (cyclic AMP), begins the synthesis of testosterone. (Similar actions of FSH via cyclic AMP are used to signal the start of estrogen synthesis in the ovaries.) Meanwhile, FSH seeks out the Sertoli cells to initiate the development of sperm (again mediated via cyclic AMP). I think you are getting the picture that without adequate generation of cyclic AMP, it's difficult being a male (see Figure 20-1 on page 222).

Once testosterone is made in the testes, it is released and then circulates bound to the sex hormone binding protein (the same one used by estrogens). If free testosterone is released from the binding protein, it can then diffuse into the target cell and bind to its receptor in the cytoplasma of the cell. Once complexed to this receptor, it is transported into the nucleus of the cell where it stimulates certain genes that promote new protein synthesis.

That's how testosterone is made and exerts its biological action, but what does it really do? Obviously, one of the primary functions of testosterone is the sexual differentiation of males from females. It is also the beginning of behavioral differentiation between the two sexes. The first stage of this differentiation begins in the womb, followed by a rapid drop in testosterone before birth. Just after birth testosterone levels increase again for a few years and then rapidly drop throughout prepuberty. Then, testosterone accelerates dramatically at puberty and slowly decreases with age. This gradual drop-off of testosterone levels as you age is known as andropause.

Aside from its effects on sexual differentiation, testosterone also has a major impact on the growth of muscle mass (it increases it) and fat content and its distribution (it makes you leaner). Basically, testosterone makes males look good. Testosterone also has powerful effects on the brain in terms of the differentiation of the hypothalamus and cortex (which depends on the ratio of testosterone to estradiol). This is why males and females think and react differently when faced with similar situations. In addition, one thing that testosterone does for both sexes is to increase development of libido. In essence testosterone is what makes men look, feel, and think differently than women, but it also makes both genders sexually attracted to each other.

The history of testosterone has been checkered. As I mentioned in the opening chapter, the era of scientifically based anti-aging began

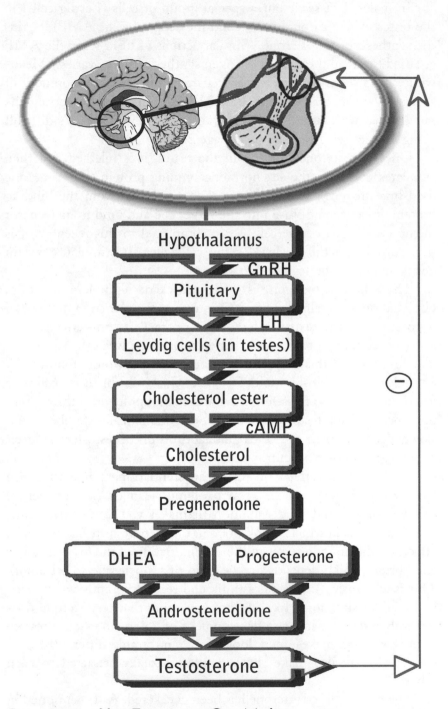

Figure 20-1   How Testosterone Gets Made

when Charles Edouard Brown-Séquard injected ground-up dog testicles into himself in 1889 and then reported his sexual rejuvenation. Although, his research was ignored (really laughed at), we now know that he was conducting the first hormonal replacement experiments by injecting himself with testosterone, the primary hormone found in the testes of any male animal species.

But the work of Brown-Séquard was not totally ignored and played a major role in steroid chemistry in the 1930s, finally leading to the chemical synthesis of testosterone independently accomplished by Leopold Ruzicka and Adolf Butenandt, who both shared the 1939 Nobel Prize in Chemistry.

The next major push of testosterone research occurred in the early 1950s. Russian sport scientists began to experiment with the use of synthetic anabolic steroids. Anabolic steroids are structurally similar to testosterone but have been chemically modified to increase the anabolic (muscle building) potential of testosterone while decreasing virilizing (i.e., masculinizing) aspects of natural testosterone. Thus, human experimentation in both male and female athletes soon led to their world dominance in strength events.

Nor, were the benefits lost upon American coaches who had to compete against these hormone-augmented Russians, especially in weight lifting. Synthetic testosterone-like hormones were soon routinely given to any athlete whose performance would be enhanced by greater muscle mass. And that included NFL football players and body-builders. Soon drug usage became widespread.

Self-experimentation became the norm with massive levels of widely different anabolic hormones used by athletes. Eventually in the 1980s there was enough concern over the problem that drug testing was instituted. By this time the mantle of anabolic steroid research had shifted from Russia to East Germany, where anabolic steroid supplementation became routine at a very early age for any elite East German athlete. The increasing use of anabolic steroids also brought new knowledge on how to avoid their detection by developing shorter-acting drugs or using masking agents. Soon, it was only the incredibly stupid athlete (or his or her coach) who was caught using anabolic steroids. Olympic Games' authorities and the NFL were patting themselves on the back for a job well done for detecting steroid use during competition. However, strength records were falling and the size of the typical NFL lineman started to accelerate as if a new genetic modification had been inserted into a select segment of the population.

As I mentioned, genetic changes are very slow, but somehow in less than a generation, the average size of an NFL lineman increased by some 60 pounds! It has been said that these changes were due to greatly improved weight-training techniques—but they used the same kind of barbell as they did 30 years ago. In fact, today the weight of every member of the offensive lines of many college teams often exceeds 300 pounds, and not all of them are good enough to go to the NFL. Something was happening out there to make strength athletes much bigger and stronger. Finally, after years of stating that anabolic steroids had only placebo-like effects, even the *New England Journal of Medicine* confirmed that testosterone replacement does indeed increase strength in athletes. Just as athletes have been saying for years.

Despite the fact that anabolic steroids (including testosterone) are now considered to be part of the same class of highly regulated drugs such as cocaine, there is a growing lobby for their potential use in hormonal replacement therapy for males.

Studies have indicated that lower levels of testosterone in males correlate with an increased risk of heart disease. Part of the reason is that testosterone is required in the production of the red blood cells needed to transfer oxygen. Low levels of testosterone are also associated with the accumulation stored body fat and increased osteoporosis in males. Yet, higher levels of testosterone can increase both psychological aggression and the production of the "bad" eicosanoid (TXA_2), which increases the likelihood of platelet aggregation and heart disease.

As you might expect, supplementation with testosterone in unskilled hands (because of its myriad functions) can be fraught with danger. As mentioned earlier, aging does decrease testosterone levels in males, although not as rapidly as estrogen levels drop in females. This leads to the concept of andropause, which is the male equivalent of menopause. The similarity of andropause to menopause is shown in Table 20-1 on page 225.

As you can see, there is a striking correlation between these two passages. In both, body fat begins to increase, there is a decrease in the psychological status (i.e., loss of short-term memory, depression, anxiety, and loss of confidence), along with an increase in cardiovascular disease, osteoporosis, and sexual cancers (prostate and breast). You can see why the golden years for both sexes are not always that golden.

One reason why these two conditions are so closely related is that both the stimulation of the ovaries to synthesize estrogen and the synthe-

TABLE 20-1

Andropause and Menopause

ANDROPAUSE	MENOPAUSE
Testosterone decreases	Estrogen decreases
Body fat increases	Body fat increases
Psychological status decreases	Psychological status decreases
Cardiovascular disease increases	Cardiovascular disease increases
Osteoporosis increases	Osteoporosis increases
Prostate cancer increases	Breast cancer increases

sis of testosterone by the testes are controlled by the levels of follicle-stimulating hormone (FSH) and luteinizing hormone (LH) released from the pituitary. As you recall, both FSH and LH require adequate levels of cyclic AMP to initiate their biological actions. Any decrease in the number of Leydig cells (the cells in which 95 percent of male testosterone is actually made) or decreasing cyclic AMP production in the Leydig cells decrease levels of testosterone in males as they age.

It is estimated that at age 50, male testosterone levels are 33 to 50 percent less than they were at age 25. And by age 80, testosterone levels may drop by more than 60 percent of what they were at age 25. However, these drops may not mirror the actual extent of testosterone reduction. The amount of free testosterone falls more dramatically than total testosterone levels (which include both free and bound testosterone). While, these decreases in testosterone levels are not as great as the fall in estrogen levels during menopause, what is important for males is the ratio of estradiol (which is formed from testosterone) to testosterone. During andropause, estradiol levels in males remains relatively constant, but because of falling testosterone, the ratio of estradiol to testosterone increases. In addition, both estrogen and testosterone use the same sex hormone binding protein to circulate in the plasma. However, testosterone has a greater affinity for the sex hormone binding protein than does estrogen. And any excess insulin will decrease overall levels of the sex hormone binding protein. As a result, as the levels of the binding protein decrease, relatively more testosterone is bound to it compared to estrogen. Therefore, the ratio of free estrogen to free testosterone increases at a faster rate. This apparently increases the risk of heart disease by changing the lipid profile. This effect is readily observed in transsexuals who wish to change from male to female. In the course of treatment, large doses of estrogens are given, resulting in a rapid deterioration of their cardiovascular risk profiles. Conversely, when testosterone is given to males with low testosterone levels, their lipid profiles improve and cardiovascular risk decreases. In addition to increased libido, it appears that testosterone is also required to work in concert with vasodilators, such as nitric oxide, for maximum erectile function.

In females, a very different testosterone picture emerges after menopause. Before menopause, only 25 percent of a female's testosterone is produced by the ovaries with 25 percent coming from the adrenal glands and 50 percent from the peripheral tissues. However, after menopause, a woman's total testosterone levels drop by as much as 50 percent. Much of the lack of sexual desire that women may experience during and after menopause may be a direct consequence of decreased testosterone production. (The same is true of men during andropause.) This is why many new forms of estrogen replacement formulations now include small amounts of testosterone to make up for the deficiency. Without sufficient levels of testosterone in both males and females, desire for sex drops dramatically.

Can you increase testosterone without hormonal supplementation? Of course you can, and this is where the Anti-aging Zone Lifestyle Pyramid comes in. From a molecular standpoint, you can see that many of the complex series of events that lead to testosterone synthesis, are mediated through cyclic AMP. Maintaining a baseline level of cyclic AMP in the target cells increases the fidelity of the various hormonal signals required to make testosterone. This cyclic AMP "booster" can be increased by the constant production of "good" eicosanoids generated by the Zone Diet, thus decreasing the likelihood of a drop-off in testosterone levels as you age.

An indirect effect of the Zone Diet on testosterone levels in males is the reduction of excess body fat. The enzyme responsible for converting testosterone to estradiol is concentrated in the fat cells. As you increase your percentage of body fat, the amount of the enzyme also increases. This was dramatically illustrated in a recent report by Allan Mazur, an Air Force physician, who followed airmen potentially exposed to Agent Orange in Vietnam for a 10-year period. Those airmen who had increased their body fat by more than 10 percentage points over this 10-year period had constantly declining levels of testosterone. For those whose body fat increased between zero and 10 percentage points, their testosterone levels remain relatively constant over this 10-year period. Finally, airmen who had lost body fat had their testosterone levels consistently increasing from year to year. These results are shown in Figure 20-2.

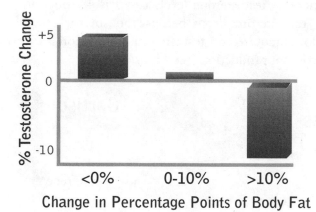

Figure 20-2   Effect of Changes in Body Fat Percentage on Testosterone Levels

Therefore, the surest way to maintain (if not actually increase) testosterone levels is by reducing excess body fat. The only way you can lose excess body fat is to lower insulin.

Another part of the Anti-aging Zone Lifestyle Pyramid that can raise testosterone levels is anaerobic exercise. Weight-training is one of the best ways to raise testosterone levels in both males and females. The building of muscle mass and strength is a coordinated effort between testosterone and growth hormone. With weight training, the levels of both hormones increase especially if relatively short rests (approximately 1 minute) are allowed between sets. Since loss of muscle mass and strength is the primary cause of functionality loss in later life, following a lifelong strength exercise program is one of the best insurance policies for a better quality of life for both males and females.

When you weight train, realize that testosterone is under circadian rhythm control. It peaks in the morning, and then falls during the day. Actually the highest levels occur between 2 A.M. and 4 A.M. and stay elevated until about 9 A.M. By 3 P.M., testosterone levels will have dropped by some 40 percent compared to the morning. This is why it's better to do strength training in the morning than at night. Maybe it is not too surprising that Bill Pearl (the only man ever to defeat Arnold

Schwarzenegger for the Mr. Universe title) always did (and still does) his training at 3 A.M. in order to make maximum use of his testosterone levels.

The final component of the Anti-aging Zone Lifestyle Pyramid that can increase testosterone levels is cortisol reduction. As cortisol levels rise, testosterone drops because one of the steroid precursors (pregnenolone) required for testosterone production is diverted toward increased cortisol production (see Figure 20-3).

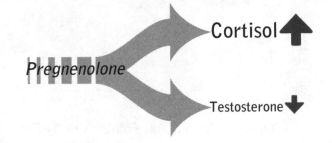

Figure 20-3   Stress Increases Cortisol Production at the Expense of Testosterone Synthesis

If there is a true antimuscularity drug, it is chronic stress. This was demonstrated in one experiment with young soldiers undergoing Army Officer Candidate Training. At the peak of training, their testosterone levels dropped by 30 percent. Within weeks after the course ended (thus, removing the psychological and physical stress), their testosterone levels returned to their pretraining levels. Thus, stress is one of the most serious threats to testosterone production. And chronic stress is a fact of life in the latter part of the twentieth century. But stress can also be created by intensive exercise, especially excessive weight training. After approximately 45 minutes of intensive weight training, testosterone levels drop and cortisol levels begin to increase. Any further weight training at that point is like spitting into the wind. Better to simply stop at that point and realize that you have done all the hormonal modulation you can do in that session by weight training. So, while testosterone is anabolic, cortisol is catabolic. The more you reduce excess cortisol, the greater the anabolic benefits of testosterone.

So if you want more sexual desire, better strength, and better cardiovascular health (if you are a male) maintaining testosterone levels will be a key. And as I have shown again and again, the Anti-aging Zone Lifestyle Pyramid is the best "drug" to achieve that goal.

CHAPTER 21

GROWTH HORMONE:
TURNING BACK THE
HANDS OF TIME?

If there is one hormone that may reverse the aging process, it is growth hormone. Of all the hormones tested in humans, this one seems to have the most anti-aging potential. Growth hormone is also unique because the body is still able to make large amounts of it as we age, though it does become increasingly more difficult to release growth hormone from the pituitary gland into the bloodstream.

The secretion of growth hormone decreases by 10 to 15 percent in each decade of life, so that in many elderly individuals it is almost non-existent in the bloodstream. Yet, nearly 10 percent of the mass of the pituitary gland is composed of growth hormone. Can the Anti-aging Zone Lifestyle Pyramid enhance the release of more growth hormone from the pituitary or do you have to take injections of growth hormone to restore youthful levels in the bloodstream? Before I answer that question, let me explain what growth hormone does and how it works.

As the name suggests, growth hormone promotes growth. It also increases lean body mass, decreases stored body fat, and increases skin thickness. All of these changes are associated with the reversal of the aging process. This was the conclusion of the landmark study in 1989 by Donald Rudman, who injected genetically engineered growth hormone into elderly men (with deficient levels of growth hormone) on a weekly basis for 6 months. At the end of the study, they had gained lean body mass, lost body fat, and observed an increase in skin thickness. It should be noted, however, that loss of excess body fat was the only true biological marker that had changed. Nonetheless, the authors of the study stated, "It was as if they had become 10 to 15 years younger."

Needless to say, since that time there has been a dramatic increase in the use of this hormone in various longevity clinics throughout the world to reverse aging. And old men are not the only ones using this hormone. World class athletes are also avid users for three reasons. First, they believe it works to increase recovery times from one bout of exercise to the next. Second, they believe it increases muscle mass formation and causes loss of excess body fat. And third, and perhaps most important, it can't be detected.

As might be expected, growth hormone secretion begins in the hypothalamus, with the secretion of growth hormone releasing hormone (GHRH). GHRH then interacts with the receptors on the surface of the pituitary gland to initiate the release of growth hormone directly into the bloodstream (see Figure 21-1 on page 231).

It may not be surprising to discover that the signal delivered by

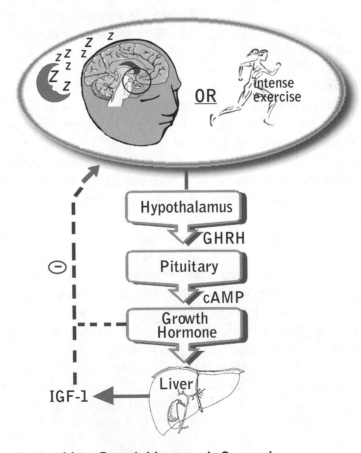

Figure 21-1   How Growth Hormone Is Secreted

GHRH to release growth hormone is mediated through cyclic AMP. And this may be one of the keys as to why growth hormone levels decrease with age. Although, the receptors for GHRH in the pituitary are fully functional as you age, if there is a less than adequate levels of cyclic AMP in the pituitary gland, growth hormone is not released into the bloodstream. On the other hand, if by brute force you flood the pituitary gland of elderly individuals with increased GHRH, growth hormone release reaches the same levels found in young adults. So the problem is not a lack of growth hormone, but the inability of GHRH to generate enough cyclic AMP to stimulate the release of growth hormone into the bloodstream. When pituitary cells are exposed to a "good" eicosanoid like PGE_1 (which increases cyclic AMP levels), increased growth hormone release is the result. Once again, "good" eicosanoids act as a backup system to boost the levels of necessary second messengers (like cyclic AMP) in case the more "sophisticated" hormonal signaling system of GHRH breaks down. And unlike GHRH, the production of "good" eicosanoids can be directly controlled by the Zone Diet.

It turns out that growth hormone is secreted in rhythmic pulses from the pituitary gland with more than 75 percent of the output occurring at night. (Remember the old wives' tale of growing in your sleep. It's true.) In fact, for most individuals the largest pulse of growth hormone is secreted during deep sleep (Stages III and IV) that occurs prior to REM sleep. The pulsatile nature of growth hormone release is a consequence of two hormones from the hypothalamus constantly fighting each other. One of these hormones is GHRH and other is somatostatin. GHRH stimulates cyclic AMP formation, somatostatin decreases cyclic AMP formation. If the balance of these two hormones becomes tilted toward increased somatostatin (i.e., decreased cyclic AMP formation), then growth hormone secretion is dramatically reduced. Another factor that can decrease growth hormone production in the pituitary are elevated levels of insulin which inhibit its synthesis.

Like many polypeptide hormones (such as insulin and glucagon), growth hormone doesn't stay around in the bloodstream very long. Its lifetime is measured in minutes with a half-life of only 5 to 6 minutes. During this short time period, growth hormone has two primary targets. The first is the fat cells and the second is the liver. Fat cells contain specific growth hormone receptors, which, when activated, stimulate the release of stored fat that contains the energy required for growth and building new muscle. The liver is where growth hormone stimulates the release of a new set of hormones called insulin-like growth factors (IGF).

All the muscle building actions of growth hormone don't come from growth hormone directly, but are mediated through the release of IGFs from the liver. Unlike growth hormone, which is stored in the pituitary gland, IGF is made on demand and immediately released into the bloodstream. Thus, there is no direct hypothalamic control of IGF levels.

As the name insulin-like growth factor implies, these hormones are very similar in structure to insulin. There are three IGFs, not surprisingly known as IGF-1, IGF-2, and IGF-3. They are all about the same size as insulin. Therefore, many of the problems that insulin has in getting to its receptors (i.e., insulin resistance) will also be encountered by IGF as they try to reach their receptors. The most important of these three IGF hormones, IGF-1, is the one responsible for stimulation of muscle mass formation. Unlike growth hormone (or insulin for that matter), IGF-1 is associated with a binding protein that can maintain very stable levels of this hormone in the bloodstream so that its half-life is about 12 to 15 hours compared to the 5- to 6-minute lifetime for growth hormone. However, once dissociated from this binding protein, IGF-1 degrades within a matter of minutes.

While IGF-1 is bound to its binding protein, it can't interact with its receptors, but this binding protein complex does provide a long-lasting circulating reservoir of IGF-1 and provides a control mechanism for its anabolic (i.e., muscle building) characteristics.

If you are using levels of IGF-1 as an indicator of growth hormone decline, you really can't tell if (a) IGF-1 is not being released from the liver because there's not enough growth hormone or (b) whether it's being degraded at a faster rate because of the lack of protective IGF-1 binding proteins. And as we have seen with so many other hormones, the levels of IGF-1 and its binding protein are under profound dietary control, in particular the levels of insulin. The higher the levels of insulin, the lower the levels of IGF-1 binding protein. Less IGF-1 binding protein means faster degradation of IGF-1 and lower overall levels of IGF-1 in the bloodstream. Another factor that controls the levels of IGF-1 in the bloodstream is calorie restriction. IGF-1 levels will generally fall with reduced calorie intake, but, if enough protein is provided, IGF-1 levels will remain constant. Thus the ratio of IGF-1 to insulin will play an important role in building muscle mass, since insulin inhibits the release of growth hormone and thus reduces IGF-1 formation. As the ratio of IGF-1 to insulin increases, muscle mass is maintained or increased. As the ratio decreases, muscle mass will be lost.

As might be expected, as the levels of growth hormone decrease with age, so do the levels of IGF-1, falling by nearly 50 percent after the age of 40. Of course, increasing IGF-1 levels (by injections of growth hormone or even injections of IGF-1 itself) is not without danger because most tumor cells have IGF-1 receptors. And growth factors, such as IGF-1 and insulin, can increase the risk of cancer. In fact, one proposed anticancer treatment involves increased production (or injection) of IGF-1 binding proteins to prevent interaction of free IGF-1 with receptors on tumor cells. But who cares about an increased chance of cancer if you can turn back the aging process? It sounds exactly like the early days of Premarin.

Presently, the only pharmacological way to increase growth hormone levels is by injections of genetically engineered growth hormone. This is why there is such excitement about a new generation of growth hormone, secretologues. These are small peptides that bypass the need for GHRH to be released from the hypothalamus, because they directly stimulate the release of growth hormone from the pituitary. More important, it appears that these peptides are orally active, which means pills, not injections. No wonder drug companies are very excited about developing these orally active growth hormone releasers, especially in light of the success of Viagra. Of course, there is still that slight problem of increased cancer risk.

But before one gets too carried away with growth hormone, some recent placebo-controlled studies have placed a slight damper on the growing enthusiasm for this hormone. Rudman's early research on growth hormone injections, which created all the excitement, consisted of open studies (non-placebo controlled), which looked at compositional changes, but not strength. One of the universal markers of aging is strength loss and the corresponding loss of muscle mass. Muscle mass is different than lean body mass. Lean body mass is the sum total of all body weight that is not body fat. It includes water, bones, tendons, and muscle mass. Usually muscle mass is about 40 percent of lean body mass, which means the other 60 percent is composed of components (like water) that have very little to do with strength. In

1997, using elderly, but still-functional males, it was shown that similar compositional changes (increase in lean body mass and loss of fat mass) seen in the Rudman study were repeated, however, there was no improvement in the strength of those males receiving growth hormone versus those who only received the placebo injections. Since there was no change in strength, the researchers concluded that muscle mass was not actually increased. The observed increases in lean body mass was primarily due to increased water retention, not increasing muscle mass. On the other hand, testosterone replacement does increase strength with weight training compared to the placebo group undergoing the same weight-training. In fact, other studies have shown that weight-training alone in the elderly can increase strength by nearly 100 percent. So, perhaps we have to wait a little longer before we crown growth hormone as the ultimate anti-aging hormone.

The thing about growth hormone injections (and this is true of virtually all hormone replacement) is that the normal release of the natural hormone is altered and reduced. This was clearly demonstrated in 1983 in a trial using trained weight lifters who were given injections of growth hormone. The control group also consisted of trained weight lifters who were given placebo injections. Both groups continued their weight-lifting programs throughout the study. These individuals were by no means deficient in growth hormone, unlike the subjects in Rudman's research. As a result of the injections, the natural secretion of growth hormone was severely depressed. Like Rudman's subjects, these trained athletes saw significant changes in their body composition, but there was no corresponding data to indicate that their strength had increased compared to other athletes in the study who had received placebo injections.

There is no question that growth hormone injections will decrease fat, because there are discrete growth hormone receptors on fat cells. An increase in muscle mass, however, requires the presence of other hormones (primarily testosterone) in addition to growth hormone (and really IGF-1). And if an individual has insulin resistance, then it is likely he or she will also have IGF-1 resistance, which makes it more difficult for IGF-1 to reach its target receptors on the muscle cells. The best way to reduce insulin resistance (and possibly IGF-1 resistance) is by reducing insulin levels. Therefore, to effectively build new muscle mass, you have to make sure that testosterone is stimulated and that IGF-1 is not impeded from reaching its target receptors. The best way to achieve both goals is to make sure that insulin levels are not elevated.

This is why the Anti-aging Zone Lifestyle Pyramid becomes the key to not only reverse the decline in growth hormone levels with age, but also to realize all the potential benefits of this hormone. The starting point is the Zone Diet, because it sets a platform to amplify the signal carried by GHRH to the pituitary by boosting the levels of its second messenger (cyclic AMP) required to initiate the release of growth hormone. Any breakdown in this cycle mediated by cyclic AMP can be overcome by "good" eicosanoids, especially those like PGE_1, which increase cyclic AMP levels. This fact was demonstrated more than 25 years ago when pituitary cells exposed to PGE_1 increased the release of growth hormone. So you can begin to see that many of the underlying factors (increased vasodilation mediated through increased production of second messengers induced by PGE_1) involved in treating erectile dysfunction and increasing testosterone production are the same ones needed to increase the release of growth hormone from the pituitary. The growth hormone is there in the pituitary as you age. You just have to boost the second messenger (cyclic AMP) to get it out.

The other part of the Anti-aging Zone Lifestyle Pyramid required to increase growth hormone levels is exercise, in particular anaerobic exercise. The stress of weight-training or other forms of anaerobic exercise (like wind sprints) sets in motion the signals to the hypothalamus that result in increased growth hormone secretion. Growth hormone doesn't come out during intense exercise, but in a 15-to-30-minute period just after the cessation of exercise. Weight-training also causes the release of testosterone that is required to work in tandem with IGF-1 to form new muscle mass.

You can increase growth hormone levels by injections of growth hormone or by following the Anti-aging Zone Lifestyle Pyramid. The Zone Diet not only increases cAMP levels formation, but simultaneously reduces insulin levels that can block growth hormone release and the action of IGF-1. Couple the Zone Diet with a consistent weight-training program to increase both growth hormone and testosterone release, and you have the ideal growth hormone enhancement program that truly turns back the hands of time.

CHAPTER 22

SEROTONIN:
YOUR MORALITY HORMONE

What separates civility from animal behavior? Unfortunately, not much. However, there is one hormone that is quickly becoming recognized as a morality hormone. Differences in concentrations of this hormone may offer us an insight on what we call civilized behavior. The hormone is serotonin.

Although, serotonin is one of possibly hundreds of neurotransmitters in your brain, it may be among the most important. Your serotonin levels influence whether or not you are depressed, prone to violence, irritable, impulsive, or gluttonous. In essence, it functions as a surrogate parent in the brain constantly telling you to just say no. It also has a significant impact on the primary pillar of aging: excess insulin.

Serotonin is a paracrine hormone that travels very short distances from one nerve cell to another. It interacts with its receptor to transmit its signals and then is taken back up by the original secreting nerve to get ready for its next job. When this system works well, the brain functions smoothly, including the hypothalamus. Remember the hypothalamus is the integration center for incoming sensory inputs. This information is delivered by various nerves, and really by the neurotransmitters moving from one nerve to another.

Much of our recent understanding about the importance of serotonin on brain function and hormonal output has come with the development of drugs that can increase its levels in the synaptic junction by preventing its re-uptake by the original secreting nerves. This results in higher levels of serotonin in the synaptic junctions between nerves, giving the brain greater opportunity to alter communication between nerves. The best known drug that inhibits the re-uptake of serotonin is Prozac.

Given the commercial success of these Prozac-like drugs (including Paxil and Zoloft) you might hypothesize that (1) we have developed a new generation of Prozac-deficient adults, (2) stress has dramatically increased in one generation, or (3) changes in our diet have radically altered the natural levels of serotonin. I believe the third is the correct interpretation, but to explain why, I need to tell you in greater detail what serotonin does.

Serotonin is also the precursor to melatonin. Both hormones are under dietary control since they ultimately come from the amino acid tryptophan as shown in Figure 22-1.

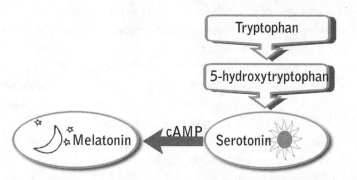

Figure 22-1   Synthesis of Serotonin and Melatonin from Tryptophan

This relation between serotonin and melatonin is best demonstrated in the pineal gland. Serotonin levels in the pineal gland are the highest during the day and fall during the night. Melatonin levels rise at night, and they fall during the day. This makes perfect sense since melatonin is synthesized from serotonin. Furthermore, the synthesis of melatonin from serotonin is mediated by increased levels of cyclic AMP, which means the Zone Diet can facilitate this dynamic balance. The rise and fall of these two hormones in the pineal gland creates the circadian rhythms that control our daily activities. As a consequence of these rhythms, the release of many endocrine hormones is also controlled by the temporal cycling of serotonin and melatonin. For example, growth hormone is released primarily at night prior to REM sleep, whereas cortisol and testosterone peak in the early morning hours prior to waking, and their levels drop throughout the day.

Serotonin's importance comes from its ability to act as a general organizer, especially concerning the limbic system of the brain that controls many so-called primitive behaviors. This is an important point because the hypothalamus is located within the limbic system. The generalized role of serotonin is reinforced by the fact that there is not just one serotonin receptor, but more than a dozen different types of serotonin receptors. Unlike most neurotransmitters, it appears that serotonin's role is not to convey information as much as to inhibit the flow of information. Serotonin acts like a policeman controlling traffic by inhibiting some of our more base instincts by controlling input into the hypothalamus. In essence, too little serotonin may mean less control over our more animal-like impulses.

This rather bold statement is reinforced by the strong association between low serotonin levels and violence and aggression. Just as the rhesus monkey makes a good model for studying aging because of its close genetic similarity to man, it also makes a good model for studying the effects of serotonin on violence. Monkeys who have the lowest levels of serotonin tend to be the most violent. On the other hand, monkeys bred for non-aggressive behaviors have much higher than normal levels of serotonin. Interestingly, dominance (we call that leadership in humans) within the monkey groups has no relation to serotonin levels. Leadership apparently requires a more complex integration of competition and restraint just as Michael Corleone demonstrated in *The Godfather* as opposed to his two brothers, Sonny (low serotonin) and Fredo (high serotonin). The same trend appears in humans. Violent criminals tend to have low levels of serotonin. Our moods as well as our behavior are also affected by serotonin. In particular, serotonin plays a major role in depression. Depression has always been part of the human condition, but it appears to be reaching epidemic levels. It is estimated that clinically defined depression costs the country nearly 50 billion dollars annually in medical treatment.

But this may only be the tip of the iceberg. A far greater problem is subclinical depression, which might be described as a milder form of the blues. Symptoms of subclinical depression can include rapid changes in weight, irritability, fatigue, sleeping longer than usual, feelings of worthlessness, lack of interest or pleasure in most activities, and decreases in mental function (like thinking, concentrating or making decisions). Upon closer inspection many of these symptoms appear in the eicosanoid status report that I developed many years ago, and are indicators of the increased production of "bad" eicosanoids. Since eicosanoids are important in the release and uptake of neurotransmitters, it would be reasonable to assume that there may be a connection between the two hormonal systems.

Knowing why low serotonin levels contributes to the symptoms of depression comes from an understanding of how this hormone works at the molecular level. Nerve impulses have to constantly make decisions about which pathway to follow. This decision-making process occurs at the synaptic junctions between nerve cells. Think of these synaptic junctions as a very complex traffic rotary. Keeping the nerve impulse going from the sending nerve (the presynaptic nerve) to the receiving nerve (the postsynaptic nerve) depends on the amount and types of neurotransmitters released from the sending nerve and the type of receptors found on the surrounding nerves. If appropriate receptors on the receiving nerve are triggered by the sufficient levels of the neurotransmitter, then the nerve impulse will be regenerated in this nerve and move forward carrying its information to the hypothalamus for the appropriate hormonal action. This is where serotonin comes in. Its role is to inhibit this information flow. If there is enough serotonin released with the other neurotransmitters, then the regeneration of the nerve impulse along the receiving nerve is halted. On the other hand, if there isn't enough serotonin, the nerve impulse goes merrily along its way. And if the nerve impulse is coming from the limbic region of the brain, where much of our animal behavior is located, the end biological action may be one consistent with symptoms associated with the blues, depression, or in extreme cases violence.

Here's where drugs like Prozac come in. They inhibit the re-uptake of serotonin by the original nerve. This is why they are known as selective serotonin re-uptake inhibitors or SSRIs. Using these drugs increases the lifetime of serotonin in the synaptic junction, and thus the greater extent it can inhibit transmission of the nerve impulse. You can also see why highly elevated serotonin levels might be so calming that you would consider an earthquake a relaxing experience, like sitting in a vibrating chair.

Is there a better way to increase serotonin levels in the synaptic junction without using these SSRI drugs? The most obvious way would be to consume more serotonin. What better way to increase levels in the brain? Unfortunately, there's a little problem with that approach. Serotonin also increases platelet aggregation. So, while you would get more serotonin in the brain, you would also greatly increase your chances of a heart attack. Some trade off for feeling less depressed.

A second option might be to supplement your diet with the precursor of serotonin, the amino acid tryptophan. Actually, this is not a bad option, except that the FDA has banned the sale of tryptophan due to a contaminated batch made by a Japanese biotechnology company several years ago. The contaminant caused a disease known as eosinophilia myalgia syndrome (EMS). Even though the manufacturing problem has been corrected and the contaminant identified, sale of tryptophan is still banned. However, there is one source of tryptophan that the FDA has not banned, and that's called food. Which foods are rich in tryptophan? Turkey and milk.

Maybe it's not a lack of serotonin that causes the problems of depression, but the inability to release it effectively. One of the problems with diagnosing depression (and therefore the treatment of it) is that there are no good markers of disease progression nor its treatment other than how you feel. However, new research indicates that such a marker may be available: the levels of "bad" eicosanoids.

It turns out that depression is highly correlated with elevated levels of "bad" eicosanoids, in particular PGE_2. As early as 1983 it was reported that levels of "bad" eicosanoids in the spinal fluid were two to three times higher in depressed patients than normal controls. These results were confirmed when it was found that saliva levels of the same eicosanoid (PGE_2) were also elevated in depressed patients. Since PGE_2 is also pro-inflammatory, it is not surprising that multiple sclerosis (which is mediated by inflammation) is also characterized by low serotonin levels. This fact explains why the Zone Diet seems to have equally beneficial effects in both depressed patients and individuals suffering from multiple sclerosis. By lowering the production of "bad" eicosanoids (such as PGE_2), while simultaneously increasing the production of "good" eicosanoids (such as PGE_1, which is not only anti-inflammatory, but also elevates mood), you are altering the hormonal environment within the central nervous system. There are two ways to increase the production of "good" eicosanoids: (1) decrease insulin production and (2) increase EPA consumption. Therefore, by simply decreasing insulin production with the Zone Diet (plus EPA) you have an exceptionally powerful (not to mention less toxic) approach to treating depression compared to taking SSRI drugs.

Unfortunately, there is much confusion about the role of diet, particularly carbohydrates in serotonin production. It is known that high-carbohydrate meals can generate a transient increase in serotonin levels, leading to the hypothesis that eating high-carbohydrate meals is the best way to treat depression. If so, Americans should be the happiest people on the face of the earth (while they have also become the fattest). Here lies the difference between acute and chronic ingestion of high-carbohydrate meals. The longer you follow a high-carbohydrate diet, the more likely it is that insulin levels will continue to rise. Excess insulin leads to the overproduction of "bad" eicosanoids (such as PGE_2) which are strongly associated with depression.

But can elevated serotonin levels actually increase insulin production? The answer comes from new research that indicates how changes in the balance of serotonin to other neurotransmitters, such as dopamine, affect insulin levels. Dopamine and serotonin act as a neurotransmitter axis. If serotonin levels increase, dopamine levels generally decrease as they have directly opposing actions. The balance of these two neurotransmitters is most important in the ventromedial nucleus (VMN) of the hypothalamus. As the serotonin-to-dopamine ratio is increased, there is a corresponding increase in insulin levels and development of insulin resistance. If you increase dopamine levels with certain drugs (such as bromocriptine), then the serotonin-to-dopamine ratio drops and insulin levels decrease in both Type 2 diabetics and overweight (i.e., hyperinsulinemic) individuals. Generating too much serotonin only accelerates the rate of aging because of the increase in insulin levels. Preliminary observations suggest that longer-term use of SSRI drugs does increase obesity which is not good news for any successful anti-aging program.

One final note about drugs that actually increase the release of serotonin as opposed to the SSRIs that only inhibit their re-uptake. Serotonin-enhancing drugs, such as fenfluramine and dexfenfluramine, were the basis of the phen/fen and redux weight loss craze a few years ago until it was realized that a significant increase in life-threatening primary pulmonary hypertension and malfunctioning heart valves were observed. This led to their immediate removal from the market. Obviously a far safer way to lose excess body fat is to reduce insulin as opposed to increasing serotonin. Of course, you can't patent the Zone Diet, but it works without side effects.

With too little serotonin, you get depression and violence. With too much serotonin, you accelerate the aging process by increasing insulin. If you want better morality and civility to complement a longer life, then maintaining serotonin within a zone will be an important key. The answer may not be increased levels of serotonin, but simply a better eicosanoid balance. The only drug that can achieve that goal is the Zone Diet.

CHAPTER 23

THYROID:
THE MYSTERY OF METABOLISM

For years obesity has been blamed on a slow metabolism caused by decreased levels of thyroid hormones. This condition is known as hypothyroidism. You don't hear much about hypothyroidism today, but is it still a problem? It must be since 36 million thyroid prescriptions were filled in 1997. This makes it the second most prescribed drug after Premarin, which had 45 million prescriptions filled in 1997.

Obviously, judging by the number of prescriptions written, thyroid hormones must do a lot of things. They do. They control the body's heat production by increasing oxygen consumption, affect metabolism (especially cholesterol metabolism), control brain maturation in neonates, affect behavior in children and adults, and control growth and development.

I say thyroid "hormones," because there are three. T4 is the primary hormone secreted from the thyroid gland, but it is converted to T3 in the peripheral tissue. T3 is the most active form, being three to eight times more active than T4. Unfortunately, T4 has a much shorter lifetime in the bloodstream. There is also a thyroid hormone called reverse T3, which is metabolically inactive but can occupy thyroid receptor sites. However, about 40 percent of T4 is converted into reverse T3 (rT3), which is metabolically inactive. So the vast bulk of your thyroid activity will be controlled by the levels of T3 in the bloodstream.

Like most endocrine hormones, our journey begins back in the hypothalamus. Depending on the type of input received about environmental conditions, the hypothalamus secretes a small peptide known as thyroid releasing hormone (TRH). The binding of TRH to its receptor in the pituitary causes the release of thyroid stimulating hormone (TSH) into the bloodstream. The TSH binds to receptors on the thyroid gland. The second messenger used by TSH to initiate its biological action in the thyroid gland is our old friend cyclic AMP. It is only through the initating action of cyclic AMP that T4 is secreted into the bloodstream to seek out its target tissues.

Because thyroid hormones are relatively water insoluble, they must be bound to appropriate binding proteins (i.e., thyroxine binding globulin or (TBG) to circulate in the bloodstream.) Like other water-insoluble hormones (such as cortisol, estrogen, progesterone, and testosterone) that travel in the bloodstream complexed to binding proteins, it is only the free thyroid hormone that can impart its biological signal. The levels of the free hormone then circulate back to the hypothalamus to complete the feedback loop by shutting down any further secretion of TRH. This completes the hypothalamus-pituitary-thyroid axis (see Figure 23-1).

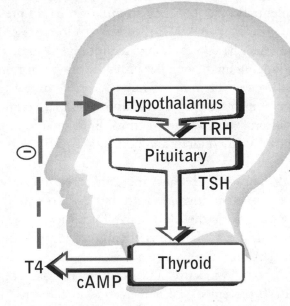

Figure 23-1   Hypothalamus-Pituitary-Thyroid Axis Controls Metabolism

Once the free thyroid hormone enters the cell, it binds to its receptor and is transported into the nucleus. Once in the nucleus, it can either up-regulate or down-regulate various genes to increase or decrease the amount of messenger RNA produced. This messenger RNA then leaves the nucleus and once back into the cytoplasma of the cells, various proteins are synthesized from it. One of those proteins is known as Na, K ATPase. This protein causes the breakdown of ATP to release energy in the form of heat, which is your primary source of increased body heat production. This might seem like a very inefficient process—giving up valuable ATP production for relatively useless heat—until you think about it.

Much of the heat energy you produce is needed simply to keep the body warm. Imagine what percentage of the total daily energy is used to keep a house warm in New England on a winter day. Compared to the amount of energy used to keep the lights on, the television warmed up, and the stove cooking, your furnace is a true energy hog. The same is true of your body. Keeping it at 98.6 degrees takes a lot of energy. Why not run the body at a lower temperature and save energy? It turns out that the enzymes in your body, which are your biochemical factories, and the brain that controls the nervous system works most efficiently at this temperature. At higher temperatures, enzyme structure falls apart (denaturation) and the brain begins to shut down. At lower temperatures, the enzyme factories are not nearly as active, and the brain shuts down. The human body runs best in a very limited temperature zone. That's the price for being warm-blooded.

The cheapest and most abundant source of energy to keep your body warm is stored body fat. You have plenty of it, and it is exceptionally rich in energy, containing more than twice the energy per gram of fat compared to protein or carbohydrate. It doesn't take a rocket scientist to realize that burning stored fat for energy to keep the body in its ideal temperature zone is a pretty smart thing to do. The cells that have the highest levels of Na, K ATPase activity are specialized fat cells known as brown adipose tissue (BAT).

One of the many tasks of thyroid hormones is to stoke those specialized BAT cells to keep burning stored fat to produce heat for the rest of your body. The reason these specialized fat cells are called brown fat is that they are rich in mitochondria, which represent the cellular factories that convert fat to heat in a series of complex biochemical reactions.

Although, keeping your brown fat cells turning out heat to keep your body warm is only one of the many functions of thyroid hormones, it is one of the best indicators of how well your thyroid hormone system is functioning. The standard exploratory test for hypothyroidism is measuring your temperature in the morning under your armpit. Should this recorded temperature be consistently low, then that is a pretty good indication that your thyroid hormones may not be fully functioning.

If the thyroid hormone's message is not getting through, there will be less heat production and thus less use of stored body fat to make new stores of ATP. Thus, having a slow metabolism (i.e. low thyroid action on the DNA in the brown fat cells) can make it difficult to lose excess body fat.

However, the discovery of thyroid hormones had little to do with slow metabolism but rather with their role in heart disease. Unlike the derision that Charles Edouard Brown-Séquard met in response to his early work with testosterone, the study of thyroid hormones followed a very different path. Much of our knowledge on the myriad functions of thyroid hormones comes from autopsy work that began in the late nineteenth century and from the strange relationship that hypothyroidism had with heart disease. Pathologists in the late nineteenth century noticed high levels of atherosclerosis when performing autopsies on patients who died of severe hypothyroidism. The appearance of atherosclerosis before the turn of the century was such a rare event, that its strong correlation with severe hypothyroidism was unusual. Invariably, there were high levels of a mucin-like substances (now known as mucopolysacchrides) associated with the atherosclerotic lesions in the arteries of these hypothyroid patients. In 1891, only two years after Brown-Séquard injected himself with ground-up animal testicles, extracts of animal thyroid were isolated. Upon injection, this extract successfully treated severe hypothyroidism (known as myxedema). Some four years later, it was shown that removal of the thyroid gland from animals that ate only a vegetarian diet (like rabbits) would produce rapid development of atherosclerosis, again suggesting a linkage between hypothyroidism and heart disease.

That observation was substantiated in 1921 in animals that had their thyroid glands removed. The usual development of atherosclerosis in these animals could be completely prevented by giving them thyroid extracts. It was about this time that the study of heart disease and its relation to thyroid hormones took a turn for the worse.

Heart disease was considered a relatively uncommon disease in the nineteenth century, even though many individuals lived to an advanced old age. Autopsies performed in the late nineteenth century are still valid today, as the eye can easily determine the presence or absence of atherosclerotic lesions. Unfortunately, autopsies have become a rare event today because of the time involved. So why did heart disease become such a potent killer in the latter half of the twentieth century? The answer is complex, but it probably has relatively little to do with the current perceived villain of heart disease: cholesterol.

The starting point for making cholesterol the poster boy for heart disease was a 1913 paper that demonstrated feeding large amounts of cholesterol to rabbits would cause the appearance of atherosclerotic lesions. This set off a frenzy lasting more than 80 years to implicate poor cholesterol as the devil incarnate of heart disease. Unfortunately, it took 50 years for investigators to discover that feeding high levels of cholesterol to rabbits also suppressed their thyroid function. In fact, it was demonstrated that feeding high levels of cholesterol to rabbits would not cause atherosclerosis if they were given thyroid hormones at the same time.

Throughout much of the early part of the twentieth century, there were numerous references suggesting that low thyroid levels are highly correlated with heart disease and that thyroid supplementation eliminated many symptoms of heart disease. It is also known that hypothyroidism increases trigylceride levels and lowers HDL cholesterol levels. Since the triglyceride/HDL cholesterol ratio is a surrogate marker for insulin, this would suggest that hypothyroidism increases insulin or that increased insulin lowers thyroid levels. In either case, the result would be the same.

The troubling part of this hypothyroid-heart disease connection is in the measurement of thyroid hormones. While many endocrine hormones decline rapidly with aging, thyroid levels in the bloodstream don't seem to drop as fast. Or is something happening outside the bloodstream that is not easily detected?

If there is any hormone system that depends on patient observation (other than eicosanoids) it is thyroid hormones. One of America's greatest physicians, Sir William Osler, stated at the turn of the century, "If you let the patient talk long enough, they will eventually make the diagnosis." In the era of managed care, that is all but impossible. Now, there is heavier reliance on blood chemistry and less on patient diagnosis. When it comes to hypothyroidism, that can be a dangerous situation.

All blood testing is by definition a snapshot of the blood. It tells you nothing of the cellular levels of the hormone nor how well the hormone is really doing its job. I illustrated this earlier in the chapter on eicosanoids when I explained that blood levels of essential fatty acids may be misleading, and that's why the use of my Eicosanoid Status Report gives a much more profound insight into what is really happening at the cellular level. Another example is insulin resistance, in which the blood levels of insulin appear normal or even elevated— but because of insulin resistance the hormone is unable to do its job. How well your thyroid hormones are functioning is best determined by your own description of your symptoms, confirmed possibly by a blood or urine test. It is estimated from blood tests that perhaps only 4 percent of the elderly population has low thyroid function. Yet, a lot more thyroid is being prescribed, which means from a functional standpoint that supplemental thyroid is giving benefits to patients with otherwise "normal" blood levels.

Standard blood tests depend on blood levels of the thyroid stimulating hormone (TSH) or the T4 hormone. Although, these are the standard tests, they may not indicate thyroid inefficiency at the cellular level. As a result, a person can have "normal" test results, but still have symptoms of low thyroid. This is why many experts recommend a 24-hour urine collection with complete chromatographic analysis of both the thyroid and adrenal hormone levels coupled with an exhaustive patient diagnosis based on symptoms. The reason that adrenal function should also be checked is because of the need for cortisol to convert T4 to T3. If adrenal output is low, then supplemental thyroid could overwhelm the limited adrenal reserve and cause additional hormonal problems.

In cases of severe hypothyroidism, known as myxedema, some very characteristic symptoms emerge. Weight gain, dry skin, brittle hair and fingernails, increased joint pains (and increases in other auto-immune disorders), decreased resistance to infection (depressed immune system), slowly healing wounds, slow and clumsy speech, depression and decreased sexual function are commonplace. On closer inspection, many of these symptoms that characterize severe hypothyroidism seem very similar to those found in Type 2 diabetics who are hyperinsulinemic by definition.

However, the best indication of your thyroid status comes from asking yourself if you have any of the following symptoms described in Table 23-1 on page 249.

As you may have noticed, many of the symptoms of low thyroid function are similar to those seen in individuals with a poor eicosanoid

TABLE 23-1

Some Common Indicators of
Low Thyroid Hormone Function

Cold intolerance
Depression
Fatigue
Sleepiness
Muscle weakness
Brittle fingernails and hair
Elevated cholesterol
Dry skin
Weight gain

balance, again suggesting a linkage between the two hormonal systems.

Therefore, if poor eicosanoid balance and hyperinsulinemia are linked to hypothyroidism, then the Zone Diet offers a significant intervention for improving thyroid efficiency. First, the Zone Diet will increase the levels of cyclic AMP, thereby enhancing the action of TSH in the formation and release of T4 from the thyroid gland. Second, it will decrease elevated levels of insulin, which appear to cause accelerated degradation of T3, the truly active form of thyroid hormones. Third, increasing T3 reduces the production of precursors of "bad" eicosanoids by decreasing the activity of the delta-5-desaturase enzyme just as glucagon and EPA do.

Another linkage between hypothyroidism and hyperinsulinemia may result from increased cortisol levels. As cortisol levels rise, thyroid production is reduced. In other words, you can create hypothyroidism by excessive cortisol production. Is this the best way to reduce cortisol? Follow the Anti-aging Zone Lifestyle Pyramid in general and the Zone Diet in particular.

To flip the coin now, let's ask if the thyroid can be too active? Yes it can, and the condition is called Graves' disease. The solution? Although, there are certain drugs and surgeries that can decrease elevated thyroid output, the usual course of action is to simply destroy the entire thyroid gland with radioactive iodine, leaving the patient with no thyroid activity (this is very severe hypothyroidism) and then placing the patient on lifetime thyroid replacement therapy.

Finally, let's come back full circle to the belief 30 years ago that obesity was a consequence of slow metabolism attributed to a low thyroid function. In other words, "It's not your fault that you're fat. You simply have a slow metabolism." In fact, one of the early pioneers in thyroid replacement therapy was Broda Barnes, who recognized the linkage between hypothyroidism and hyperinsulinemia. Not surprisingly, he was also one of the pioneers in the use of a prototype Zone Diet to correct hyperinsulinemia more than 20 years ago. He stated the following:

> It would appear that a rational and natural approach to overcoming obesity should employ a slightly modified diet containing approximately one gram of protein for each kilo (2.2 pounds) of body weight and a minimum of fifty grams of carbohydrate to avoid ketosis. Enough fat should then be added to keep the appetite satisfied and still not quite enough to satisfy the body needs, thus allowing a weight loss of one or two pounds per week.

His words mirror the basic guidelines for the Zone Diet. Consume adequate levels of low-fat protein, enough low-glycemic carbohydrates to prevent the generation of ketosis, and sufficient levels of monounsaturated fat to produce satiation. Broda Barnes developed a good treatment for both hyperinsulinemia and hypothyroidism, probably because these are two manifestations of the same eicosanoid imbalance. The only thing Broda Barnes didn't know was the role insulin plays on eicosanoid formation. Other than that, he was ahead of his time.

CHAPTER 24

DHEA AND MELATONIN:
THE HYPE BROTHERS?

There are no other hormones that have received more hype in the last few years than dihydroepiandrosterone (DHEA) and melatonin. I believe much of their reputation as anti-aging hormones comes from the fact that they are available in health food stores and can be taken in capsule form. And although much of this fad has now passed, the question remains: Do they have a role in reversing the aging process? Since DHEA comes from the adrenal gland and melatonin comes from the pineal gland, it is probably best to look at each one separately to ask what is fact and what is fad.

First, let's look at all of the supposed benefits of DHEA supplementation and compare them to improvements that I have observed with an improved eicosanoid balance as shown in Table 24-1.

TABLE 24-1

Comparison of Benefits of DHEA and Improved Eicosanoid Balance

DHEA	IMPROVED EICOSANOID BALANCE
More energy	More energy
Reduced heart disease risk	Reduced heart disease risk
Fat loss	Fat loss
Better memory	Better memory
Improved immune function	Improved immune function

As you can see from this table, all the suggested benefits of DHEA supplementation are remarkably similar to the benefits of improved eicosanoid balance. This strongly suggests a linkage between the two hormonal systems.

It is true that DHEA is the most abundant steroid hormone produced by the body and is synthesized in the range of 25 to 30 mg per day. But the second most abundant is cortisol, which is synthesized at a rate of about 10 to 20 mg produced every day under normal conditions. If stress is higher, then cortisol output is higher.

The reason why the body is producing so much DHEA is that it inhibits cortisol action by binding to its receptors. Thus, DHEA represents another feedback control mechanism to fine-tune eicosanoids by inhibiting the inhibitor (cortisol) of eicosanoid synthesis. Obviously, if DHEA production is decreased for whatever reason, there is no control rod to prevent excess cortisol from wreaking havoc on eicosanoid synthesis.

This inhibitory relationship of DHEA to cortisol is similar to the relationship between glucagon and insulin. It's not so much that hormone levels change with aging, but that their controlling partners decrease at a faster rate, so that the ratio of the paired hormones within a hormonal axis becomes uncoupled. If the ratio of insulin to glucagon increases, hyperinsulinemia results and cortisol levels also increase. If the ratio of cortisol to DHEA increases, eicosanoid synthesis is suppressed and insulin levels increase. You can never affect one hormone system without affecting another. Combine these hormonal axis disturbances with decreasing concentrations of second messenger cyclic AMP in target cells, and you have a prescription for systemwide hormonal miscommunication—and that is the basis for aging.

Like cortisol, DHEA is primarily synthesized in the adrenal cortex. Its production is activated by the same hormone (ACTH) that signals the beginning of cortisol synthesis. The action of ACTH on the adrenal glands is governed by the levels of cyclic AMP. Therefore the synthesis of DHEA in the adrenal cortex is also governed by the levels of cyclic AMP.

If adequate levels of cyclic AMP are generated in the adrenal cortex, the first step in DHEA synthesis begins with the release of cholesterol from cholesterol ester storage droplets. This free cholesterol then moves to the mitochondria where through a series of free radical reactions it is converted into pregnenolone. Pregnenolone is an interesting branch point for steroid hormones. One branch can take it toward the production of progesterone, another to DHEA, and still another toward cortisol production. These are shown in Figure 24-1.

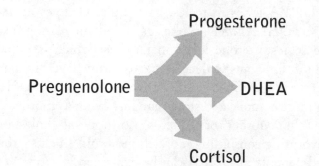

Progesterone

Pregnenolone   **DHEA**

Cortisol

Figure 24-1   Pregnenolone has Various Hormonal Outcomes

It is true that DHEA levels do drop remarkably as we age and that men with higher DHEA levels do appear to have less heart disease and lower overall mortality than age-matched males with lower levels. (However this is more likely caused by decreased insulin which would result in increased DHEA.) Impotence is also associated with lower DHEA levels. As you might remember from an earlier chapter, men with lower testosterone levels also have higher rates of heart disease. As a result, many have argued that DHEA is the mother hormone for the sex hormones testosterone and estrogen (and as we all know, sex sells) as shown by its metabolism in Figure 24-2.

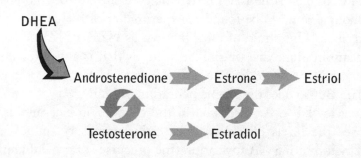

DHEA

Androstenedione ➤ Estrone ➤ Estriol

Testosterone ➤ Estradiol

Figure 24-2   DHEA Can be a "Loose Cannon" in Sex Hormone Metabolism

However, synthesis of these sex hormones is very tightly controlled, and increased DHEA doesn't necessarily mean better sex, but sex has a lot to do with how DHEA affects you. For example, there is an association of decreased DHEA levels and increased heart disease in males, but not in females. Likewise increasing insulin levels will decrease DHEA levels in males, but similar changes in insulin have no effect on DHEA levels in females. While increasing insulin levels will increase testosterone levels in females (which is not desirable), increased insulin seems to decrease testosterone levels in males (which is also not desirable). Such gender-driven differences of DHEA effects make it a more complicated story than just being a "mother" hormone. (In reality, the "Mother" of all steroid hormones is cholesterol, and no one is advocating consuming more cholesterol.) I believe that most of the touted benefits of DHEA can be explained in terms of its role as an inhibitor of the biological actions of corticosteroids, especially cortisol. As explained in an earlier chapter, cortisol levels tend to increase with age if adequate levels of glucagon are not produced. Therefore, the ratio of cortisol to DHEA is a more critical parameter in aging than simply measuring the amount of DHEA in the bloodstream. Since increased cortisol levels lead to an overall slowdown of all eicosanoid production (both "good" and "bad"), then it becomes reasonable to link decreasing DHEA production to a corresponding decrease in eicosanoid production. The lower the levels of DHEA, the greater the inhibition of all eicosanoid synthesis (due to the lack of cortisol inhibition), including the production of "good" eicosanoids. Reinforcing this connection is the fact that the synthesis of DHEA requires cyclic AMP, which can be generated by "good" eicosanoids.

An example of the role DHEA plays as an indirect modulator of eicosanoid action can be found in experiments with a certain strain of inbred mice. This strain of mice (known as NZB x NZW) develop a severe autoimmune disease similar to lupus that is always fatal. It has been shown that the addition of DHEA to their diet will prolong their life span. But so does the supplementation of high levels of the omega-3 fatty acid, EPA. As discussed in the chapter on eicosanoids, EPA improves the levels of PGE_1 (an anti-inflammatory "good" eicosanoid), by inhibiting AA formation (the precursor of pro-inflammatory "bad" eicosanoids). Likewise, restricting their calories has an even greater impact on their longevity. Finally and most telling are experiments that show direct injections of PGE_1, or analogs of PGE_1, will completely prevent the certain early mortality in these animals. Thus, if "good" eicosanoids completely protect the animals from early death, whereas DHEA only slightly prolongs their life, you can probably guess which of the two hormones is most important for anti-aging.

It is also not too surprising that many of the symptoms associated with low DHEA levels are very similar to the clinical conditions associated with Cushing's syndrome, which is caused by an overproduction of cortisol. With Cushing's syndrome, the overproduction of cortisol results in eicosanoid production grinding to a halt.

What could cause this decrease in DHEA associated with aging? One possible explanation is the inadequate production of cyclic AMP induced by "good" eicosanoids. Without adequate levels of cyclic AMP, it is impossible to maintain high levels of DHEA production. Therefore, the best way to increase DHEA production may be to maintain adequate levels of "good" eicosanoid production (with the corresponding increase in cyclic AMP levels) by following the Zone Diet. In fact, this is confirmed in experiments with rhesus monkeys on calorie-restricted diets in which levels of DHEA were increased compared to the typical age-related decrease observed in other monkeys fed a higher calorie diet. So before you reach for a bottle of DHEA at the health food store, think about the Zone Diet first.

What about melatonin, the other hype brother? The main function of melatonin has always been assumed to be the control of circadian rhythms based on light and dark cycles. Many hormones, such as cortisol, testosterone and growth hormone are strongly influenced by such rhythms. Cortisol and testosterone levels peak in the early morning and then drop off during the day, whereas growth hormone peaks during the deep sleep phase just prior to REM sleep. So if there is a drop-off in melatonin production, it might be expected that the circadian rhythms that govern these particular hormones will be thrown out of kilter.

The circadian rhythms of hormones also influence a wide variety of other physiological responses. For example, heart attacks are twice as likely to occur in the morning. Or consider that women are much more likely to go into labor between 1 A.M. and 2 A.M. as opposed to midday. Eating a large meal is more likely to cause weight gain if eaten at night as opposed to eating the same meal in the morning. Drug metabolism is also changed. Aspirin has a longer lifetime in the bloodstream if taken in the morning as compared to taking it in the evening. Obviously if you decrease melatonin levels, the circadian rhythms orchestrated through melatonin will also become uncoupled. That's what happens with age as much of the rhythm of hormonal ebb and flow is lost.

The pathway to melatonin in the pineal gland is via serotonin as shown in Figure 24-3.

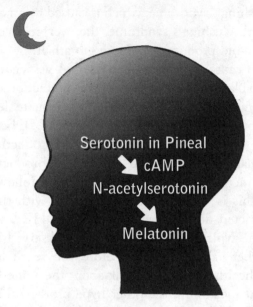

Serotonin in Pineal

cAMP

N-acetylserotonin

Melatonin

Figure 24-3   Melatonin Synthesis Requires Cyclic AMP

Serotonin levels in the pineal gland rise in response to light, whereas melatonin levels increase in the dark. The conversion of serotonin to melatonin requires cyclic AMP. Like many hormones, the levels of melatonin drop dramatically with age. By age 80, the serum levels of melatonin are only about 10 percent of what they were at age 20. It has always been thought that the primary function of melatonin was to control the biological clock located in the suprachiasmatic nuclei (located in the hypothalamus), which is governed by the cycles of light and dark. It is this biological clock that is responsible for circadian rhythms that control many of the undulating hormone levels in the body. In darkness, there is a release of the neurotransmitter norepinephrine, which acts through the second messenger cyclic AMP to cause the synthesis of melatonin from serotonin. Therefore, one reason that melatonin levels decrease with aging may be the decreased production of cyclic AMP in the pineal gland necessary for its synthesis.

Melatonin levels in the pineal gland rise during darkness and then rapidly fall upon exposure to light (in fact it only takes about one hour of exposure to light to stop melatonin synthesis). Since melatonin is very lipid soluble, once it is made, it immediately leaves the pineal cell by diffusion either into the bloodstream or into the brain.

Melatonin exerts its biological effects by *decreasing* cyclic AMP levels, and thus decreases the activity of every hormone that requires cyclic AMP as its second messenger for action. Melatonin also increases the production of somatostatin that prevents the release of growth hormone. Somatostatin also works by decreasing cyclic AMP levels. So, obviously, excess levels of melatonin don't bode well for better hormonal communication.

With this as a background, let's look at all the suggested benefits of melatonin supplementation compared to the benefits of improved eicosanoid balance. These are listed in Table 24-2.

TABLE 24-2

Comparison of Benefits of Melatonin and Improved Eicosanoid Balance

MELATONIN	IMPROVED EICOSANOID BALANCE
More energy	More energy
Better sleep	Better sleep
Reduced risk of heart disease	Reduced risk of heart disease
Immune function improvement	Immune function improvement

Like DHEA, it would appear that many of the benefits of melatonin are strikingly similar to those achieved through better eicosanoid balance. Is it possible that melatonin also has a role to play in eicosanoid synthesis? Yes, it does.

The real interest in melatonin began with observations that supplementation of this hormone could increase the maximum life span of animals. Although the extension of maximum life span (approximately 20 percent) with melatonin supplementation is not nearly as great as by calorie restriction (approximately 50 percent), it is interesting to note that calorie restriction does increase melatonin levels almost twofold in rats compared to control rats fed their normal caloric diet. Extension of maximum life span in test animals is the first test that must be passed for any anti-aging strategy. But why would an increase in life span be connected to the biological clock? Obviously, maintaining circadian rhythms are important. Earlier I discussed the potential mechanism of aging put forward by Valdimar Dilman that a clock in the hypothalamus sets aging in motion. Maybe that can be interpreted as the loss of circadian rhythm with decreasing melatonin production. Or might melatonin be involved in something else other than making sure that circadian rhythms are maintained? A second potential role of melatonin in aging began to emerge in 1993. That was the discovery that melatonin is an antioxidant with some unique properties.

As mentioned earlier, mankind has lost the ability to make some very basic antioxidants, such as vitamin C, vitamin E, and beta carotene. Yet we have conserved melatonin and various defensive antioxidant enzyme systems, such as superoxide dimutase, catalase, and gluthione peroxidase. From an evolutionary perspective, you usually only retain those genes that are most important for survival. The reason that these antioxidant enzymes and melatonin have been retained is that they represent a combined defense system against the extremely destructive hydroxyl free radical.

As I said earlier in this book, of all the free radicals, the hydroxyl free radical is the most active and therefore, the most dangerous. The antioxidant enzymes (superoxide dimutase, glutathione peroxidase, and catalase), work in concert to prevent the production of the hydroxyl free radical. However, melatonin is incredibly successful in quenching the hydroxyl free radical if it is formed. If hydroxyl free radicals are produced, they will exert their greatest damage in the brain. If there is one area of the body you want to prevent from free radical damage, it is the brain, which is nearly 50 percent fat by weight and more than one-third of that fat is polyunsaturated fat (which is exceptionally prone to free radical attack). Since the pineal gland is in the center of the brain, the synthesis and secretion of melatonin is at the ideal site to quench hydroxyl free radicals. In essence, melatonin is your free radical defense of last resort for the brain.

Eicosanoids, especially "good" eicosanoids are important because they maintain hormonal communication, and thus their protection has been the utmost priority during evolution. Because melatonin is very lipid-soluble, it can freely diffuse throughout the brain, which makes it the ideal hydroxyl free radical scavenger to minimize the oxidation of polyunsaturated fatty acids and thus maintain eicosanoid formation in the brain.

This begins to explain the remarkable similarity of the purported benefits of melatonin supplementation with those achieved through a better eicosanoid balance. They are simply two sides of the same coin. You need melatonin to protect essential fatty acids, so that they can be made into "good" eicosanoids. You need "good" eicosanoids to maintain adequate levels of cyclic AMP to convert serotonin into melatonin. The Zone Diet plays a critical role in that transformation since it has already been shown in calorie-restricted animals that melatonin levels increase. This is also indicated in rhesus monkeys undergoing calorie restriction because their body temperature drops by about a single degree. Melatonin lowers the core body temperature, thus the temperature drop observed in rhesus monkeys on calorie-restricted diets is consistent with increased melatonin production.

Maybe DHEA and melatonin aren't the hype brothers after all. They play unique roles either through inhibiting cortisol action (i.e., DHEA), which would limit eicosanoid synthesis or by protecting the essential fatty acids (i.e., melatonin) from oxidation by hydroxyl free radicals so that they can be synthesized into eicosanoids. Any decrease in the production of DHEA and melatonin with time adversely affects eicosanoid production, which has devastating consequences for accelerating the aging process. And since the synthesis of both DHEA and melatonin rely upon adequate levels of cyclic AMP, the increased production of "good" eicosanoids should reduce, if not prevent, their decline with age. While they aren't the miracle hormones reported by the popular press, they do have a significant role to play in maintaining eicosanoid balance, which is the real key to anti-aging.

CHAPTER 25

NITRIC OXIDE:
THE NEW KID ON THE BLOCK

What if there were a hormone that needed no receptor? What if this hormone could only travel incredibly short distances before it quickly self-destructs? What if this hormone were also a component of air pollution and cigarette smoke, yet could help control your cardiovascular, immune, and nervous systems? More important, what if this hormone was the key to solving erectile dysfunction?

Such a hormone was discovered in 1987. It's called nitric oxide, and it is one of the smallest molecules known. And it's a free radical to boot. Yet, this reactive free radical provides the latest clue on the power of the diet to alter hormonal response.

As I have already stated, free radicals are an enigma. You need some to survive, but too many are destructive. Earlier I talked about free radicals derived from oxygen. But since the air we breathe is nearly 80 percent nitrogen, you can also make nitrogen free radicals, such as nitric oxide. Nitric oxide bears a striking resemblance to the superoxide free radical formed from oxygen (see Figure 25-1).

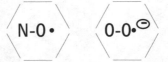

Figure 25-1   Comparison of Nitric Oxide to Superoxide Free Radicals

However, unlike oxygen free radicals, nitric oxide is relatively stable. In fact, it is possible to maintain nitric oxide in a gaseous form for more than 40 years. This relative lack of activity, especially compared to the highly reactive hydroxyl free radical (which attacks virtually every organic molecule it bumps into), makes nitric oxide an interesting carrier of information.

Nitric oxide is a proto-hormone. It evolved before the first true hormones, eicosanoids. It has no receptor, and once it is made it freely diffuses as a gas in all directions. But nitric oxide is very quickly quenched by any iron-bearing enzymes or proteins. And that is how it transmits its information.

One of those iron-bearing enzymes is called guanylate cyclase. This particular enzyme is important because it makes the second messenger called cyclic GMP. As long as nitric oxide is bound to this enzyme, it continues to produce cyclic GMP. This second messenger has many similar properties to cyclic AMP. One of those cellular responses is increased vasodilation. The drug Viagra works by preventing the degradation of cyclic GMP generated in the penis to maintain an erection for a longer period of time due to the vasodilation effects of cyclic GMP.

Eventually, nitric oxide interacts with oxygen (to form the nitro-syldioxyl radical), which removes it from the guanylate cyclase enzyme (see Figure 25-2).

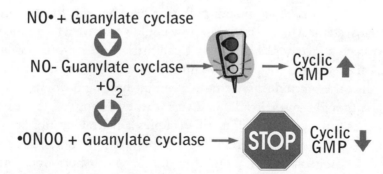

Figure 25-2   Nitric Oxide Controls Cyclic GMP Synthesis

When that happens any further cyclic GMP production immediately stops. It is a very elegant start-stop mechanism.

Even though nitric oxide is a component of air pollution and cigarette smoke, the only way your body can make it internally is by using the amino acid arginine. Arginine is the substrate for the enzyme known as nitric oxide synthease (NOS). Therefore, without a protein-adequate diet that contains enough arginine, it's impossible to have enough of the raw material to make nitric oxide. The reaction is shown in Figure 25-3 on page 262.

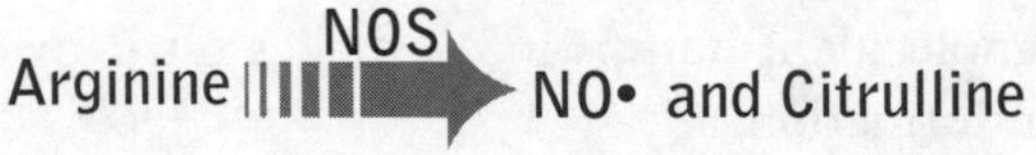

$$\text{Arginine} \xrightarrow[\hspace{1.3cm}]{\text{NOS}} \text{NO}\cdot \text{ and Citrulline}$$

Figure 25-3   Synthesis of Nitric Oxide Requires Arginine

The story of nitric oxide began some 90 years ago when researchers noted that patients fighting bacterial infections had increased amounts of nitrate in their urine. Although, this observation couldn't be explained at the time (and I will explain its significance later), it was the first indication of the importance of nitric oxide. Then about 20 years ago it was noted that something coming from endothelial cells that surround the arteries was causing them to relax. Using typical scientific word-smithing, this substance was named endothelial derived relaxing factor (EDRF). Whatever this EDRF might be, it was pretty interesting because it seemed to maintain blood flow by preventing vasoconstriction of blood vessels.

For years researchers tried to isolate EDRF and finally succeeded in 1987. And when researchers realized it was nitric oxide, there was chaos in the endocrinology community. How could a contaminant found in cigarette smoke and air pollution have benefits for the cardiovascular system? More disturbing, how could you have a hormone that didn't need a receptor? That's why I call nitric oxid a proto-hormone. It doesn't require a receptor to communicate information nor does it have any other hormonal system involved in shutting down its production. Although, nitric oxide predates the evolution of the earliest hormones (i.e., eicosanoids), it still occupies a central location in communicating biological information. So unhappy or not, researchers started finding out more about this unique proto-hormone, and as they did, even more amazing stories emerged. In fact, the 1998 Nobel Prize in Medicine was awarded to Robert Furchgott, Ferid Murad, and Louis Ignarro for their early research on this gaseous proto-hormone.

Let's start with the cardiovascular system. You need a smooth steady flow of blood to prevent clot formation. When blood begins to collect in little turbulent pools caused by transient obstructions in this normally smooth flow, some real problems begin, such as the clotting of platelets that obstruct arteries causing heart attacks or stroke.

Imagine blood flow as a collection of tiny streams, any one of which has the potential to become constricted. When that happens, the smooth flow of blood is interrupted and turbulence in the other tiny streams occurs. At the first sign of turbulence, the endothelial cells that line the bloodstream (and represent the biological barrier between the blood and the smooth muscle cells that comprise your arteries, capillaries, and veins) begin to make nitric oxide. The immediate consequence of this very localized production of nitric oxide is a transitory vasodilation or relaxation of the smooth muscle cells in that vicinity to compensate for the restriction upstream. The iron-containing hemoglobin found in the red blood cells that flow past the endothelial cells becomes a sink for this newly formed nitric oxide, so that the nitric-oxide generated vasodilation is controlled, thus preventing blood pressure from becoming too depressed.

This is also how nitroglycerine works. During an angina attack, you aren't making enough nitric oxide to control the vasoconstriction of the arteries. Once the nitroglycerine is in the bloodstream, it immediately becomes a substrate for the production of nitric oxide, which causes the necessary vasodilation to temporarily relieve the angina.

It was only with the discovery of nitric oxide that the mechanism of how nitroglycerine works was finally understood. Like aspirin, nitroglycerine had been in use for nearly a century without anyone knowing why it worked. Just as the mechanism of aspirin's action was discovered to be its effect on eicosanoids, the mode of action of nitroglycerine was the increased generation of nitric oxide.

The same underlying mechanism behind nitroglycerine's use in the treatment of angina is also used by Viagra to maintain blood flow to the genital area. Remember, that Viagra was first developed as a cardiovascular drug to promote sustained vasodilation by preventing the degradation of cyclic GMP. Thus, Viagra works not by increasing nitric oxide production, but by decreasing the degradation of cyclic GMP (generated by nitric oxide) that relaxes the blood vessels. While Viagra was a poor cardiovascular drug, it did seem to have some spectacular effects on one very limited part of the circulatory system: the arteries that feed the corpus cavernosa in the penis. Filling the corpus cavernosa with blood is required to maintain an erection—and that requires vasodilation. Since the arteries that surround the corpus cavernosa are very small, Viagra has a larger effect on those small arteries than on the much larger arteries found in the heart.

Although, Viagra alone was not strong enough to affect the cardiovascular system, if it is used in combination with nitroglycerine or other nitrates, a potentially life-threatening situation of extreme low blood pressure can result. And for a number of Viagra users, it has been deadly.

Since nitric oxide is a free radical, it should not be too surprising that like oxygen free radicals, it can also be used to kill invading organisms. Nitric oxide works by attacking the iron-containing enzymes of bacteria, and thus represents a unique inhibitor of their growth (since bacteria, especially anaerobic bacteria, depend on these enzymes for survival). It can also interact with the superoxide free radical generated by lymphocytes to form the powerful peroxynitrite anion, which is exceptionally toxic to invading bacteria (see Figure 25-4).

$$NO^{\bullet} + O_2^{\bullet\ominus} \quad \Longrightarrow \quad ONOO^{\ominus}$$

Figure 25-4   Synthesis of the Peroxynitrite Anion

Since peroxynitrite is eventually degraded to nitrate, this finally explains observations dating from the turn of the century as to why bacterial infections were often accompanied by nitrate increases in the urine of surviving animals and humans.

However, perhaps the most fascinating role nitric oxide plays may be in the central nervous system. Here nitric oxide helps guide the formation of new synaptic junctions between nerves. Nitric oxide is very lipid (fat) soluble, which means it can diffuse readily between lipid structures in all directions. This is a great advantage in the brain since it contains the highest concentration of fats of any organ in the body. It is the ideal molecule for helping to direct and reinforce new neural pathways needed for the development of short-term memory. Ironically, this is done by conveying information in the wrong direction.

This reverse information flow is achieved through two of the major excitatory neurotransmitters in the brain (glutamatic acid and aspartic acid). When a nerve is actively firing and releasing these neurotransmitters, a specific receptor on the target nerve opens channels to allow calcium ions to flow into the nerve. This influx of calcium activates the NOS enzyme that makes nitric oxide from arginine. Once generated, the nitric oxide flows back in a direction opposite to that from which the excitatory neurotransmitter was released. In doing so, it interacts with the guanylate cyclase enzyme in that nerve to make cyclic

GMP and helps reinforce the linkage between these two nerves. Nerves that aren't actively firing don't get this nitric oxide reinforcement, and their linkage begins to weaken. This is is the basis of short-term memory. As you age, long-term memory appears to be relatively unaffected, but short-term memory is compromised. One possible explanation is that your neural cells are having difficulty making adequate levels of nitric oxide to reinforce the formation of new neural pathways that are the basis of memory.

So how can you make more nitric oxide if it is so important? Eat a diet that is protein adequate and make sure the protein is rich in arginine. Turkey is one such protein source. Soybean products (like tofu or imitation soybean meat products) are another. In fact, soy protein is exceptionally rich in arginine compared to most animal products. By making turkey and soy protein products a more significant part of your diet you can boost nitric oxide production.

But can you make too much nitric oxide? Although nitric oxide is quickly quenched if there are excessive amounts of superoxide free radicals nearby, nitric oxide can be converted into the exceptionally toxic peroxynitrite anion normally used to kill invading bacteria. This often occurs during a stroke. This increase of peroxynitrite anion is one reason for neural death that takes place during a stroke. Having a stroke (either major or mini) means that local oxygen transfer is constricted, and superoxide production begins to dramatically increase. Under these conditions, peroxynitrite formation increases with devastating consequences (i.e., death) for local nerves.

So the newest kid on the block really predates all hormones. As important as nitric oxide is, like eicosanoids, it is totally controlled by the diet. In fact, nitric oxide can stimulate the enzymes (especially cyclo-oxygenase) that make eicosanoids. These two hormonal systems are in close communication. Therefore, the way to orchestrate their actions to reverse aging is to eat a Zone Diet rich in arginine-containing proteins. Not a difficult price to pay if you want better cardiovascular, immunological and brain function (not to mention better sex).

PART V

WHAT ELSE SHOULD YOU KNOW?

CHAPTER 26

ANTI-AGING SUPPLEMENTS:
BEYOND THE ANTI-AGING ZONE
LIFESTYLE PYRAMID

So far I have discussed how the Anti-aging Zone Lifestyle Pyramid is the primary key to reverse aging by reducing each of the four pillars of aging (excess insulin, excess blood glucose, excess free radicals, and excess cortisol). You can't put any of those components into a two-piece hard-shell capsule and take them once a day. Yet, that is exactly what millions of Americans are trying to do. In 1997, for the first time in history, sales of nutritional supplements were greater than the sales of all cardiovascular drugs combined. America is going on a self-medication kick that is unprecedented.

Do supplements have a place in reversing the aging process? Yes they do, but only if they are used after you have established a proper hormonal foundation through the consistent application of the Anti-aging Zone Pyramid.

What types of supplements am I talking about? They include hormone replacement either by prescription or over-the-counter sales. They also include vitamins and minerals that have utility in hormone synthesis. And finally they include herbs that have hormonal effects.

Let's start with the most powerful supplements, hormones, especially the hormones that require a prescription. There is a good reason for this: they're exceptionally powerful drugs.

Estrogen and Progesterone

As you may remember, the most widely used hormone supplement for estrogen replacement is Premarin. Considering the availability of natural estrogens, the continued use of Premarin, which contains of more than 50 percent of estrogens that are foreign in the human body, strikes me as one of the most ridiculous things in modern medicine. This is compounded by the fact that Premarin doesn't contain estriol, which appears to generate many of the benefits of estrogen replacement with far fewer side effects, such as the increased incidence of breast cancer. In fact, it may turn out that estriol is actually protects against breast cancer.

Finding supplies of natural estrogens is easy because many compounding pharmacies (these are pharmacies that actually custom-make drugs as opposed to simply distributing drugs from the pharmaceutical companies) will make individualized prescriptions. More difficult is finding a physician who knows how to fine-tune the balance of estrogen to your unique biochemistry. It will take about 2 to 3 months of experimentation to find the right balance of natural estrogens for your biochemistry. This means constantly paying attention to how your body is reacting to them and then discussing these symptoms with your physician who can alter the balance (if required) of natural estrogens. Always keep in the mind the bimodal effect of estrogen. At low levels, it can reduce insulin resistance, but at higher levels it can increase insulin resistance and therefore insulin output. If your goal is anti-aging, then using the lowest possible amount of natural estrogen is a must.

Estrogens, however, are rarely given without the simultaneous intake of progesterone, not only to reduce the likelihood of breast cancer but also increase the building of bone density. Like estrogen, the widespread availability of natural progesterone makes it difficult to understand the continued prescription of artificial analogs of progesterone (i.e., progestins). If you think finding the right amount and type of natural estrogen is difficult, you increase the complexity to a much greater degree when you add progesterone to your hormonal mix. Remember, that progesterone can also increase insulin resistance. If you are using natural progesterone (and that should be a no-brainer), then you have two methods of application. The first is micronized progesterone in pill form. The PEPI trial demonstrated the superiority of this form of natural progesterone relative to progestins. The other form is transdermal delivery using various creams or gels. Many women do wonderfully well on natural estrogen (especially estriol) but have a very difficult time once they include progesterone into the mix. For these individuals, the transdermal route allows a method of reducing progesterone dosage to a lower level before any side effects from too much progesterone (even natural progesterone) arise.

As you can quickly see, the key to determining the right balance of estrogen and progesterone requires listening to your body and then communicating that information to a knowledgeable physician (who also takes the time to listen) so that you can both work as a team to develop the appropriate dosage. In the era of managed care, that seems almost like Fantasy Land. But such physicians do exist. Your job is to find one.

Thyroid and Cortisol

The second most prescribed hormone replacement in the country is for the thyroid. Once again, how you feel and how well you communicate with a knowledgable physician will be of far greater utility than any blood test.

For years the primary source of thyroid hormone replacement was extracted from animal glands, and therefore contained a mixture of both T4 and T3 (the most active form of thyroid hormone). Drug companies, however, have spent a lot of money (primarily in marketing) to convince physicians that a synthetic version containing only T4 is the only appropriate thyroid replacement. That's fine as long as you are converting T4 into T3. Unfortunately, in many individuals that transformation of T4 to T3 is highly compromised, thus giving only T4 may not be sufficient.

However, as with estrogen, the picture is more complex. Thyroid replacement increases metabolism and that puts a greater stress on the adrenal glands to secrete enough cortisol to prevent a runaway metabolic engine. In addition, you need sufficient levels of cortisol to convert T4 into the more active form of T3. If your adrenal output is compromised, then without adequate supplementation of cortisol, thyroid replacement can have dangerous consequences in terms of cardiovascular complications.

It is very likely that some patients will need both thyroid and cortisol replacement simultaneously. Isn't that contradictory if excess cortisol is one of the pillars of aging? No, because lack of cortisol (especially in the face of increased metabolism) will also increase the rate of aging because it lowers the ability to respond to stress. Although, the relative outputs of thyroid and cortisol are best determined by a 24-hour urine collection (to average out the different outputs of cortisol caused by circadian rhythms), in the final analysis how you feel will determine the amounts and ratio of thyroid and cortisol (if required). Again it comes back to listening to your body, recording the information, and finding a knowledgable physician to work with you to fine-tune your hormonal supplementation program.

Growth Hormone

No hormone replacement therapy has raised more excitement than growth hormone. As mentioned earlier, it is a powerful hormone that appears to reverse many of the signs of aging. Unfortunately, it must be given by injection. The actual goal of growth hormone injections is to raise IGF-1 levels (since it is the anabolic mediator of growth hormone) to a concentration consistent with the levels found in early adulthood. This is not quite as straighforward as it appears because of the complicating factor caused by insulin. First, excess insulin makes it more difficult to release growth hormone from the pituitary (very few people are totally growth hormone deficient). Second, excess insulin can create not only insulin resistance, but also IGF-1 resistance making it increasingly more difficult for IGF-1 to reach the target tissue. Third, excess insulin can decrease levels of IGF-1 binding protein. The less IGF-1 binding protein you have in the bloodstream, the more rapidly IGF-1 is degraded and the less IGF-1 you have to interact with target cells. This is why I believe that the ratio of IGF-1 to insulin is more important than the absolute levels of IGF-1. The higher the ratio, the better the results you will obtain with growth hormone injections.

Preliminary communication with physicians using growth hormone replacement therapy indicates that free IGF-1 levels are initially increased, but after about a year, the levels decrease by about 50 percent. One course of action would be simply to increase the amounts of growth hormone being injected. However, growth hormone has its own array of side effects, including the development of insulin resistance and thus an increase in insulin levels. And that is the last thing you want to have happen if anti-aging is your goal.

Unless you are controlling insulin by the Zone Diet, I believe many of the benefits of growth hormone replacement therapy will be minimized on a long-term basis. Conversely, the more that insulin is controlled by the Zone Diet, the lower the dose of growth hormone needed to realize its full potential benefit as an anti-aging supplement.

Like all hormonal supplementation, the right amount of growth hormone injections (which is always the least, consistent with physiological results) will be counterbalanced by the ability of the individuals to control their own insulin levels. If you aren't controlling insulin, then you may be spitting into the wind if you are taking growth hormone injections.

Testosterone

Testosterone replacement is just around the corner. It increases libido in both males and females, and it appears to decrease the likelihood of heart attacks and osteroporosis in males. Unfortunately for females, testosterone (over and beyond the amount to increase libido) also increases the likelihood of heart attacks. Like growth hormone, testosterone requires injections or implants; like growth hormone, unless you are controlling insulin, testosterone injections may be self-defeating on a long-term basis. As you remember, testosterone is the substrate to make estrogens. The more insulin you produce, the greater the accumulation of stored body fat. It is that stored body fat that contains the enzyme that converts testosterone into estrogen. It is not just testosterone levels that count, but the ratio of testosterone to estrogen that should be maximized in males. The only way to reduce estrogen formation is to reduce excess body fat. That can only be achieved by lowering insulin. And that requires the Zone Diet.

All of the above hormone replacement therapies require a prescription and hopefully a knowledgable physician to constantly monitor your progress. Make no mistake about it, each of these are life-long hormonal supplementation programs. We are only now learning about their long-term effects from controlled clinical trials. Unfortunately, we also have a whole new group of hormones that only require a trip to the local health food store and a friendly sales clerk behind the counter to give you their "extensive" anti-aging advice, especially on hormonal modulation.

DHEA and Melatonin

The over-the-counter sales of DHEA and melatonin represent the largest uncontrolled human experiment in the history of hormonal replacement and no one seems to care. Since there is no physician to act as an intermediary between you and these hormones, you're on your own. If you are going to experiment with your body (and nothing is wrong with that if you are willing to accept the consequences), then there is one basic guideline: never take any more of an over-the-counter hormone than your body normally makes. For DHEA that is about 25 mg per day. But that 25 mg is produced over a 24-hour period. If you want to play endocrinologist at home, then plan to take that 25 mg divided into various doses taken five times a day with most of it (about 10 mg) coming early in the morning and decreasing amounts throughout the day to simulate the natural release of DHEA from the adrenal gland. That's pretty hard work, but if want to play the game, then play it right.

Melatonin, on the other hand, is only secreted at night throughout the sleep cycle. Taking a single dose will radically increase melatonin blood levels, but because the half-life of melatonin is short, it is very hard to maintain a consistent level throughout the night. Waking up every few hours to take your next dose doesn't make a lot of sense. The best approach is to find sustained release tablets that slowly release melatonin during sleep. (Here is an obvious pointer—don't take melatonin during the day.)

The next question is how much to take? Melatonin appears to be very safe, even though it is banned from over-the-counter sale in England, Canada, and France—and you need a physician's prescription to obtain it. If you are not working with a physician to monitor your blood levels (and if you are going to a health food store to buy melatonin then you probably aren't), plan to take no more than 1 mg of sustained release melatonin right at bedtime.

DHEA and melatonin aren't the only supplements you can buy at a health food store to alter hormones. You can also buy precursors to hormones. These are almost as good (or as dangerous) as the real thing. Three in particular come to mind.

The first is pregnenolone. This is the steroid hormone that is the precursor to DHEA. But if you remember, it is also the precursor to progesterone (not a good idea if you are a male) and cortisol (which may not be a good idea for either sex). Which of these three pathways pregnenolone will lead to is anyone's guess (of course, you could always ask the sales clerk behind the counter). It's the hormonal version of Wheel of Fortune at the health food store.

Androstenedione is another potential powder keg. Androstenedione is the immediate precursor to testosterone. There is a good reason why testosterone is a prescription drug—it's potentially dangerous. Taking androstenedione is playing Russian roulette unless you are monitoring your blood levels of testosterone to make sure you are not taking an overdose of androstenedione.

The third is 5-hydroxytryptophan, which is the immediate precursor to serotonin. The FDA in its wisdom banned the sales of tryptophan (which is stupid, because it's safe), but allows the sale of 5-hydroxytryptophan (which is stupid, because the last thing you want floating in the bloodstream is excess serotonin). Excess serotonin in the bloodstream can increase platelet aggregation, giving rise to a heart attack (not a good thing in any anti-aging program). In addition, long-term buildup of serotonin in the central nervous system increases the production of excess insulin by decreasing dopamine levels. If you go to a health food store, stick with things that are less dangerous, like vitamins and minerals.

Vitamins and Minerals

In my book, *Zone Perfect Meals in Minutes,* I outlined the most important vitamin and mineral supplements for the Zone Diet. Needless to say they are also the most important for reversing the aging process (see Table 26-1 on page 276).

Of all the supplements, the most important is fish oil, since it's rich in EPA, which will reduce AA formation and therefore help you make more "good" eicosanoids. Right behind supplemental fish oil is natural vitamin E (because it has more isomers than synthetic vitamin E). I feel that the data is overwhelming that the RDA set for vitamin E by the U.S. government is woefully inadequate in light of the clinically proven benefits of higher levels of this vitamin.

I don't care what diet (including the Zone Diet) you are following, it is virtually impossible to get adequate levels of these two nutrients. Therefore, you have to take supplements, assuming they are suitable for human consumption. Natural vitamin E definitely meets that requirement since it has been molecularly distilled to remove all the nasty things (like herbicides and pesticides) that you find in the raw material (crude soybean oil distillate) used to make vitamin E. Unfor-

TABLE 26-1

Ranking of Nutritional Supplements

TYPE	DAILY AMOUNT
Essential (if molecular distilled)	
Fish oil	3 grams (about 500 mg of EPA)
Natural Vitamin E	100–400 IU
Important	
Vitamin C	500–1000 mg
Magnesium	250–400 mg
Cheap insurance	
B3	20 mg
B6	5–10 mg
Folic acid	500–1000 μg
Beta carotene	5,000 IU
Calcium	500–1,000 mg
Chrominum	200 μg
Selenium	200 μg
Zinc	15 mg
Exotic, but expensive	
CoQ10	5–10 mg
Lycopene	3–5mg
Lutein	3–5 mg
Polyphenols	5–10 mg

tunately, all crude fish oil is contaminated with PCBs. Just like vitamin E, you want to make sure that this contaminant is removed. Only if a fish oil is molecularly distilled, can you be assured that PCBs have been removed. If not, it's buyer beware. Molecularly distilled fish oil is available, but you have to look very hard to find it.

The next group of supplements (vitamin C and magnesium) are important, although if you are eating a lot of fruits and vegetables (as you do on the Zone Diet), you should be getting adequate amounts. You need water-soluble vitamin C to work in concert with water-insoluble vitamin E to effectively remove free radicals from the body. Magnesium is the critical mineral required for effective eicosanoid synthesis. In my opinion, there is no more important mineral for cardiovascular health than magnesium.

Next come the vitamins and minerals that I term "cheap insurance policies." If you are following the Zone Diet, they are probably there in more than adequate levels, but their supplementation is easy and relatively inexpensive.

Let's look at the vitamins first. Vitamins B_3 and B_6 are required for efficient eicosanoid synthesis. Folic acid reduces any excess buildup of pro-inflammatory homocysteine, thereby reducing the likelihood of heart attacks. (If you are a vegetarian, I would also strongly recommend taking B_{12} supplements). Beta carotene is a useful (and cheap) antioxidant once you have adequate levels of vitamin E and vitamin C in your system.

Calcium is useful in preventing osteoporosis (although 40 percent of bone mass is composed of magnesium). Selenium is important not only as part of the antioxidant enzyme gluthathione peroxidase but also for the enzyme that converts T4 to T3. Zinc is important not only in eicosanoid synthesis but also in the transcription of new messenger RNA synthesis signaled by steroid and thyroid hormones. Finally, in this category is chromium, which is important in lowering insulin levels by acting as a potentiator of insulin action through interaction with the glucose tolerance factor.

The last category are the exotic, but expensive supplements. These are new antioxidants that have shown significant promise in reducing free radical formation. They are expensive, but they can fill in your anti-oxidant defenses.

Notice that the levels of the vitamins and minerals I am recommending are often considerably less than those commonly touted for anti-aging benefits. That is because I assume that you are already following the Anti-aging Zone Lifestyle Pyramid, which includes the Zone Diet. If you aren't, be prepared to spend most of the day taking a lot more "magic pills" from the health food store and seeing very little benefit on your Anti-aging Zone Report Card. I try to remind people to never let the tail wag the dog. Vitamins and minerals are useful supplements, but without the Anti-aging Zone Lifestyle Pyramid as your base, they will be relatively worthless in your effort to reverse aging.

Herbs

Finally, there are herbs. Herbs are drugs, just in a more diluted form. Sixty years ago, virtually all drugs came from botanical sources.

After all, plants have been engaged in chemical warfare for billions of years. Just find the most successful warriors in that struggle, isolate their active ingredients (usually an alkaloid), purify them, and presto you have a drug. Even today, about 25 percent of all prescription pharmaceuticals still come from botanical sources because the active ingredients are too complex to be synthesized.

Herbs are relatively nontoxic due to a significant improvement in standardization procedures. Herbs are also unique because often the partially purified crude herb is more functional than any one of the isolated ingredients. However, keep in mind that herbs are drugs, so always consult your physician if you are taking any prescription medications.

In Table 26-2 are some of the herbs that have potential for anti-aging because of their effects on hormonal systems.

TABLE 26-2

Herbs That Affect Hormones Important in Anti-aging

HERB	HORMONAL MODE OF ACTION
Coleus forshohii	Increases cyclic AMP
Garlic	Inhibits platelet aggregation
Ginger	Inhibition of eicosanoids
Ginkgo	Inhibits platelet activating factor
Ginseng	Stimulation of ACTH production
Glycyrrhizin	Enhances cortisol action
Guar gum	Reduces insulin secretion
Gugulipid	Reduces triglycerides
Genistein	Mimics estrogen

Probably the most interesting of these herbs is coleus forshohii because of its active ingredient, forskolin. This compound enhances cyclic AMP production by activating the enzyme (adenylate cyclase) that makes cyclic AMP. This is the same second messenger that is produced by "good" eicosanoids. A good dosage of this herb might be 50 mg twice a day of a standardized 18 percent forskolin content.

Garlic is another herb that has considerable scientific support. The primary ingredient in garlic that inhibits platelet aggregation is the compound ajoene. Unfortunately, ajoene is relatively unstable and the highest concentrations are found in raw and cooked garlic; lower con-centrations are found in the garlic pills sold in health food stores. Many of the benefits attributed to garlic (antiviral properties, reduc-tion of blood pressure, inhibition of cancer, anti-inflammatory action, and reduction of platelet aggregation) are related to its altering of eico-sanoid-based responses. The less processed garlic is, the more of its oxygen-sensitive compounds (like ajoene) that are available. Since raw garlic can have some toxicity, cooked garlic is probably the best source, with two to three cloves per day a recommended dosage—plus it tastes pretty good. Garlic's antibacterial benefits come from another ingredi-ent known as allicin, which is more stable for processing. If you want to take pills to get the benefits of allicin, then plan to take about 1,000 mg per day.

Ginger also appears to have a mode of action similar to cortisol (inhibition of synthesis of both prostaglandins and leukotrienes), only it is less powerful. The volatile oil extracted from ginger contains a number of sesquiterpenes that appear to be the active ingredients. Ginger extracts are only now appearing in health food stores, and about 100 mg per day is a good dose. Alternatively, like garlic, just add fresh ginger (about 1 to 2 grams per day) to your foods.

Ginkgo biloba extracts contain certain terpene molecules known as ginkgolides that work together to inhibit platelet activating factor (PAF). PAF is a powerful agent that promotes the clumping of plate-lets, especially in the cerebral circulation. Used for improving mental function, it maintains blood flow, thus supplying adequate amounts of oxygen for optimal brain function. Controlled studies have indicated some potential for this herb to treat Alzheimer's disease. A good dos-age would be 120 mg per day, but spread that throughout the day to maintain consistent blood levels of the ginkgolides.

Ginseng appears to stimulate the release of ACTH from the pitu-itary gland. ACTH stimulates the adrenal glands to make more corti-sol, but also more endorphins (your body's natural opiates). This would make sense for its reported benefits in treating fatigue and adapting to stress (i.e., adaptogen) if a person has low adrenal output. The active ingredients appear to be a number of triterpenoid saponins known as ginsenosides. (However, Siberian ginseng has different com-pounds known as eleutherosides.) Due to the stimulation of ACTH, it is best to use ginseng on an intermittent basis, and then give the body a 2- to 3-week recovery period before using it again. Unfortunately, strict standardization is not in place for this herb. If you want to try ginseng, you may have to experiment with several brands to find one that works, but still give yourself a 2- to 3-week rest every 6 weeks.

Glycyrrhizin is derived from licorice and it seems to work through the same mechanism as ginseng. If you have adrenal insufficiency, then glycyrrhizin may be of use. Since it is more standardized than ginseng, excess glycyrrhizin will have the same effects as excess cortisol production. Furthermore, it should only be used on a short-term basis for no more than 6 weeks, followed by 2 to 3 weeks of nonuse to ensure that natural cortisol production doesn't atrophy; 25 mg per day is probably a good dose. It should be taken in uneven doses throughout the day with the largest dose in the morning (to mimic cortisol output), a lower dose at noon, and the lowest dose in the early evening.

Guar gum is a soluble fiber, rich in beta glucan. Other types of soluble fibers include pectin, oat and barley fiber, and other gums, such as locust bean and acacia. Although not an herb per se, these soluble fibers play an important role in reducing the entry rate of any dietary carbohydrate into the bloodstream, thereby reducing insulin secretion. Insoluble fibers have little, if any, effect on reducing insulin secretion. Since reducing excess insulin levels is one key component of any anti-aging strategy, taking soluble fiber supplements makes good sense. A good dose would be 5 grams of soluble fiber about 30 minutes prior to every meal. This would provide 15 grams of soluble fiber per day.

Gugulipid is derived from the myrrh tree. The active ingredient is a compound known as guggulsterone. The key for gugulipid is that it can raise HDL cholesterol while lowering triglycerides, one of the key tests you want to pass on your Anti-aging Report Card. A good dose would be 500 mg of gugulipid taken three times a day.

Genistein is a phytoestrogen derived from the soybean. Since the receptor for estrogen is relatively nonspecific, a lot of different molecules can occupy it and potentially activate it. The phytoestrogens from soy have a much lower activity (approximately 0.5 percent) than natural estrogens with estrogen receptors. However, Asian women who eat a lot of soy products have nearly one thousand times the levels of these phytoestrogens in their blood than their Western counterparts do. This is one of the reasons hypothesized why Asian women seem to have less postmenopausal problems than Americans, especially osteoporosis, even though they consume virtually deficiency-like levels of calcium (about 300 mg/day).

The herbs listed above are by no means meant to be an exhaustive list. However, these herbs can be very useful adjuncts to the Anti-aging Zone Lifestyle Pyramid, just like hormonal replacement and the use of vitamins and minerals.

While these are all useful items, here are some things to avoid in the health food or grocery store. The first to beware of is excess consumption of gamma linolenic acid (GLA). Not because it isn't useful, but because it is so powerful due to its effects on eicosanoid synthesis. Most items in health food stores can't hurt you too much. GLA can if you're not paying very close attention to your Eicosanoid Status Report. Since most people won't, rather than taking a capsule with far too much GLA (45 to 240 mg per capsule), stick with a serving of oatmeal that contains one to two mg. Even that amount may be too much for some people, so be forwarned! If you want to use borage, black currant, or evening primrose oil capsules, find a knowledgable physician to work with. However, if you think finding a physician who understands hormonal replacement is tough, then it is even more difficult to find one who understands the impact of GLA on eicosanoid modulation. To use GLA without working with a physician who understands its powerful hormonal modulating actions is like lighting a cigarette with a stick of dynamite. You can do it, just be very, very careful.

Another thing to avoid is any product that contains extracts of Mexican yams. As you recall, Russell Marker revolutionized steroid chemistry using extracts of Mexican yams for his starting material. While you can convert those starting materials in a laboratory into steroid hormone precursors, it is impossible to do so in your body.

And the health food store is not the only place to use caution. There's danger lurking in your grocery store. Any product that contains trans-fatty acids will disrupt essential fatty acid metabolism, and thereby cause eicosanoid imbalances. If you see the phrase, "partially hydrogenated vegetable oils" run in the other direction. Virtually every fast food restaurant uses partially hydrogenated vegetable oils to cook French fries.

Likewise, beware of food additives that should have never become part of the food supply. Two in particular are aspartame and olestra. Aspartame is a methyl ester of a dipeptide containing aspartic acid. When aspartame breaks in the heat or upon prolonged storage, methanol (wood alcohol) is formed. Not a very pleasant thing to ingest if you are trying to reverse aging. Unfortunately, when you ingest aspartame, the same methanol is formed in your body. That fact that aspartic acid is an excitatory neurotransmitter that in excess can cause nerve death, this is another good reason to avoid this food additive.

Another loser in the food additive wars is olestra. This fake fat prevents the uptake of carotenoid-based antioxidants. The jury will be out for the next 20 years on whether inhibition of carotenoid uptake will increase cancer risk. If you would like to join this ongoing human experiment as an unpaid guinea pig, then try to consume as many products as possible that contain this fake fat.

What I have tried to do in this chapter is to give a balanced overview to supplements complementary to the Anti-aging Zone Lifestyle Pyramid. Many of these make great sense to add to your baseline age-reversal program. Others may detract from it. The best way to tell is to listen to your body and pay close attention to the dialog that it is continually trying to carry on with you.

CHAPTER 27

THE SKIN ZONE:
BEAUTY IS SKIN DEEP

What is the good of a successful anti-aging program if no one can tell the difference? For better or worse, the appearance of your skin is usually seen as one of the first indications of not only your age, but also your general health. During youth, it is elastic, ruddy, and smooth. As you age, it begins to take on the appearance of flaky leather covered with age spots and pallor. Are these simply cosmetic concerns or does the condition of your skin give you an insight as to the rate of aging inside your body? More important, what can be done to reverse aging in the skin that makes hormonal sense?

To answer these questions, let's begin with the skin itself. It is the largest organ in your body accounting for about 15 percent of the total dry weight of the body. More important, it is the primary defense between you and an otherwise hostile environment. And unlike most organs, it is constantly growing. Skin cells (i.e., fibroblasts) are constantly being made to renew the outer layers of the skin, which are constantly lost to the environment. But as you age, the rate of new skin cell synthesis can drop by nearly 50 percent.

The skin is composed of two parts. The first part is called the epidermis, which is composed primarily of an upper layer (i.e., stratum corneum) made up of dead skin cells that have a unique lipid composition. Unlike most membranes that are composed primarily of phospholipids, skin lipids in the epidermis are primarily ceramides, wax esters, and cholesterol esters. These dead cells are also surrounded by keratin (a structural protein) that prevents the dead cells from flaking off. The stratum corneum provides an extremely hydrophobic barrier to the outside world. In addition, this same barrier prevents loss of internal moisture from the skin to the outside. This layer of dead skin cells acts as a protective barrier, but they are constantly sloughed off at the surface of the skin by wear and tear. The lower level of the epidermis consists of skin cells that move upward to replace those in the stratum corneum that are being lost. This entire process from the synthesis of a new skin cell to it becoming part of the stratum corenum takes between 15 to 30 days.

The epidermis also contains a number of cells called melanocytes. These are responsible for the release of melanin, the compound responsible for tanning and protection of the skin against UV radiation. As melanocytes decrease with age, your protection against UV radiation also decreases. This leads to the appearance of age-spots that are accumulations of cross-linked proteins and fats catalyzed by UV radiation, due to the absence of sufficient melanin. Likewise, the graying of hair is also caused by a decrease in the number of melanocytes within the hair follicles. Melanocyte-stimulating hormone (MSH) controls the number of these melanocytes. The release of MSH from the pituitary gland requires cyclic AMP. Thus, the appearance of age-spots and the graying of your hair are highly visible indications that cyclic AMP levels are probably running low in your pituitary, and therefore other pituitary hormones requiring cyclic AMP (such as growth hormone and ACTH) are having a more difficult time being released into the bloodstream.

Below the epidermis is the dermis, where living cells are processed on a continual basis. Unlike the epidermis, the dermis is rich in capillaries that bring fresh nutrients and oxygen necessary for the continued growth of new skin cells. With age the number of these capillaries decrease giving rise to the appearance of pale skin, coupled with decreased nutrient flow and waste removal, as well as decreased temperature regulation to control excess body heat. Lack of temperature regulation is compounded by the decreased number of sweat glands, making it more difficult to dissipate heat from the body.

However, much of skin aging involves structural changes in the dermis, in particular the structural proteins (collagen and elastin) that maintain its flexibility. Wrinkled skin is a combination of reduced collagen synthesis coupled with free radical-induced cross-linking of collagen fibers. This also occurs in the elastin fibers generating a lack of elasticity in the skin. Much of the free radical damage is due to decreased levels of melanocytes and a corresponding lack of melanin secretion to protect against sun-induced free radical damage. Each of these effects can be positively affected by the Zone Diet.

But before I go into how this is accomplished, let me give you some history of the relationship of the skin to diet and eicosanoids.

The fact that some fats are essential was discovered 70 years ago in rat studies in which certain fats (polyunsaturated fats) were withheld from the diet. Within a very short period of time, significant deterioration of the skin took place, almost as if the skin was undergoing accelerated aging. Adding these polyunsaturated fats back to the diet, restored the skin within a short period of time. Soon these fats became known as vitamin F. That terminology is no longer used as we now recognize these essential fats to be both omega-6 and omega-3 fatty acids. Why they are important to skin aging is a combination of their structural properties and their effect on eicosanoids.

From a structure perspective, even though the stratum corenum is composed of dead cells, their ability to form a tight junction is critical for keeping the skin from losing water. The first sign of essential fatty acid deficiency is the breakdown of this barrier resulting in dry, flaking skin. It turns out that only omega-6 essential fatty acids can restore this structural function. However, that doesn't mean that omega-3 essential fatty acids are not important because they are critical in generating more "good" eicosanoids and fewer "bad" ones—this is important in stimulating the synthesis of new structural proteins.

As I stated earlier, the real structure of the skin is maintained by elastin and collagen in the dermis. With increasing age, the synthesis of these structural proteins decreases. However, the synthesis of both these structural proteins can be restimulated by "good" eicosanoids. Another structural protein that is also stimulated by "good" eicosanoids is keratin, the protein component of the hair and fingernails. It is also the protein component of the stratum corneum necessary to maintain the integrity of this barrier to the outside world. Each of these three structural proteins is affected by improved eicosanoid balance generated by the Zone Diet. The increase in keratin synthesis is the easiest to spot visually, especially in terms of your fingernails and hair texture which are largely composed of keratin. That's why these parameters are part of your Eicosanoid Status Report. If you are using the Zone Diet and observing significant increases in fingernail growth and strength, then you can be sure that other internal structural proteins (collagen and elastin) in the skin are also being stimulated.

Perhaps the best examples of collagen stimulation by "good" eicosanoids are the molecular events that occur during the ripening of the cervix at birth. Here you can actually see massive amounts of new collagen synthesis before your very eyes, all induced by eicosanoids. That same type of collagen synthesis can take place on a smaller scale in the skin as long as the micro-environment in the skin is making more "good" eicosanoids. This is how the drug Retin-A removes wrinkles from the skin. Actually it is stimulating the microproduction of collagen that fills in the wrinkles. Retin-A is a nonspecific eicosanoid stimulator. It stimulates the "good" eicosanoids that cause collagen synthesis. Unfortunately, it also stimulates the "bad" eicosanoids that generate pro-inflammatory compounds that make your face look like a lobster. Thus the ideal skin "drug" would increase "good" eicosanoids while simultaneously decreasing the production of "bad" eicosanoids. The Zone Diet is such a "drug."

The reduction of the "bad" eicosanoids also has profound effects on inflammatory skin conditions. Decreasing the levels of arachidonic acid (AA) in the skin through the Zone Diet also decreases the likelihood of producing "bad" eicosanoids (primarily hydroxy essential fatty acids). "Bad" eicosanoids are also implicated in the development of skin cancer. In addition, serious skin disorders, including psoriasis and eczema, are both caused by an overproduction of "bad" eicosanoids (in particular, excessive amounts of leukotrienes). So, whether your goal is the prevention of sunburn, psoriasis, or skin cancer, the Zone Diet becomes one of your greatest allies.

However, the most important benefit of the Zone Diet for the skin is the increase in blood flow. "Good" eicosanoids are powerful vasodilators that increase blood flow. If a person has a shallow skin tone, it usually indicates that blood flow is probably constricted, not only in the skin, but also in the cardiovascular system as well. On the other hand, the ruddy vibrant skin complexion one usually associates with good health is purely a consequence of improved blood flow and improved nutrient delivery to the skin that is essential for new structural protein synthesis, especially the hair.

The increase in blood flow to the skin is the primary mechanism behind the use of Rogaine, a drug to promote hair growth. Rogaine (like Viagra) was a failed cardiovascular drug. However, one of its side effects was increased hair growth mediated through its vasodilation action. The same benefits can be generated by the Zone Diet as "good" eicosanoids are not only excellent vasodilators, but they also stimulate the synthesis of keratin, the structural protein of hair that Rogaine can't affect.

The old saying that beauty is skin deep is correct. You can control the appearance of the skin by altering its hormonal environment using the Zone Diet. However, aging skin is also a signpost of an aging body. The skin is truly the window to your internal world, which provides a clue to the speed at which you are aging. And the Zone Diet provides the "drug" to alter that rate of skin aging.

CHAPTER 28

EMOTIONS:
THE MIND-BODY-DIET
CONNECTION

Are emotions powerful? You bet they are! Are hormones powerful? You know by now that the answer is yes. Then is it possible that emotions are ultimately controlled by hormones? If so, is it possible to use the Zone Diet to modulate emotions?

Emotions are stored in the limbic system of the brain. Recall from an earlier chapter that the limbic system consists of the hypothalamus and the hippocampus. The hippocampus stores dry, unemotional facts for recall, and the hypothalamus acts as the commander-in-chief of your hormonal armies. However, within the limbic system lies the amygdala, which does most of the processing of emotional memories. The integration of incoming stimuli are filtered through the hippocampus, amygdala, and neocortex to decide whether or not an appropriate hormonal response needs to be generated by the hypothalamus. So, it is really in the limbic system that the "mind-body" connection exists, and hormones initiated by the hypothalamus via the pituitary dictate how your body will respond to the mind. Another way of putting it: emotions are pretty complex.

One of the best examples of this is the hormone β-endorphin, your natural opiate that makes you feel good. The parent compound of β-endorphorin is β-lipotropin, which is secreted simultaneously with ACTH from the pituitary gland in response to stress. If you remember, the key event that controls the secretion of ACTH is adequate levels of cyclic AMP. Likewise, it is the key for release of the parent compound of β-endorphorin. The β-endorphin (which has morphinelike characteristics) is then cleaved from β-lipotropin. (see Figure 28-1 on page 289).

Once β-endorphin binds to its receptor, it *decreases* cyclic AMP

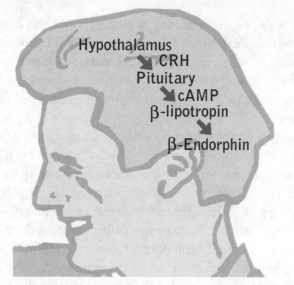

Figure 28-1   Beta Endorphin Synthesis Requires Cyclic AMP

levels essentially "numbing" the cell by shutting it down temporarily. So your "feel good" hormones work by reducing information flow, just as serotonin does.

I believe these hormonal responses, as illustrated with β-endorphin, are the basis of the mind-body connection. First of all, there is no distinction between the brain and emotion, if we define emotion as how hormones (like natural opiates, such as β-endorphorins) cause pleasure by altering information flow. Or, how other hormones (like an overproduction of "bad" eicosanoids) can lead to depression. Once you begin to define emotions in terms of hormonal communication, you now have a starting point to develop strategies to improve emotional control. The fidelity of this emotional information will be controlled to a great extent by your eicosanoid balance. The "mind-body" connection really becomes the "mind-body-diet" connection. A hormonally correct diet becomes your primary tool to improve emotional control. Conversely, a hormonally incorrect diet is your passport to emotional chaos.

One of the major breakthroughs of twentieth century science was understanding the duality of matter. Sometimes matter behaves as if it were matter, at other times as if it were energy. In fact, matter and energy are interconvertible. That same duality can be applied to emotions and hormones. Emotions can't be isolated, but hormones can.

One is the realm of the spiritual, the other is on the cutting edge of medical research. Since both transmit complex information, they can be considered different forms of information constantly converting back and forth. Like energy that can never be destroyed (although it can be interconverted), information is also immortal. It transcends both time and space.

Controlling energy is now possible to a degree never before imagined. A nuclear reactor is simply a controlled nuclear bomb. And what controls a nuclear reactor? Control rods. Take out the control rods, and ground zero is not too far away. The control rods for biological information are slightly different because they consist of hormonal feedback loops constantly communicating within their appropriate hormonal axis. No one hormone ever acts by itself, and most have a myriad of interactions that we are just beginning to understand. But as I have explained in the earlier chapters of this book, increased production of "good" eicosanoids represent a cyclic AMP booster system to maintain information fidelity to virtually all of these hormonal feedback loops. Essentially, eicosanoids are the control rods for biological information flow, and thus their modulation will have a dramatic impact on emotions.

This leads to a very exciting possibility. Since eicosanoids are controlled by the Zone Diet, it should be possible to use the Zone Diet to manipulate emotions. Often the reverse is true, that emotions manipulate the diet. If you are depressed or stressed, you reach for comfort food that is usually carbohydrate-rich. Although, there will be a temporary increase in blood glucose levels to the brain, there is a price to be paid for this acute influx of carbohydrates—increased secretion of insulin. Increased insulin suppresses the normal hormonal action of glucagon, thus forcing your body to increase cortisol production (i.e., more stress) to maintain adequate blood glucose levels. Elevated insulin also enhances the increased production of "bad" eicosanoids, which generates more depression. You might solve the emotional problem temporarily with your comfort food, but in the process you have set in motion a cascade of hormonal events that will continue to uncouple the tight feedback loops of hormonal communication—a sure-fire prescription for accelerated aging and further emotional trauma. On the other hand, improved control of insulin and the corresponding improvement of eicosanoid balance will lead to better emotional health.

There is no better example of this than looking at a young child whose emotional control is not as sophisticated as that of an adult. Give them a carbohydrate-rich meal and initially they respond positively. But within an hour or two, they become surly and uncooperative. On the other hand, feed them a balanced Zone meal and for the next 4 to 6 hours, they are a pleasure to be with. The "drug" of choice is yours, as is the emotional outcome. Use the right "drug," and emotional life is good. Use the wrong "drug," and emotional life can be very unpleasant.

This is not to say that the Anti-aging Zone Lifestyle Pyramid in general, and the Zone Diet in particular, can totally control emotions, but it can significantly influence them. The integration of emotions is mediated through the hypothalamus, just as the hypothalamus is responsible for integrating biological inputs into appropriate hormonal responses. The information contained in emotions is more complex than are the direct hormonal responses, which affect physiological systems, but their action is probably mediated by many of the same second messengers used by the endocrine hormonal systems. The most likely second messenger candidate is cyclic AMP, whose levels can be enhanced by "good" eicosanoids. Therefore, without adequate levels of "good" eicosanoids constantly driving integration of emotional inputs, the resulting hormonal communication becomes garbled and incoherent. In other words, you become an emotional mess.

An example of this linkage between hormones and behavior can be found in the relationship of hormones to stress and depression. From the earlier chapter on cortisol, you know that increased chronic stress translates into higher cortisol levels, which can accelerate aging by the inhibition of "good" eicosanoid synthesis. This same inhibition on eicosanoid formation has a dramatic impact on the immune system. Therefore, it should not be too surprising that in stressful situations, such as the death of a loved one or caring for someone with a chronic disease like Alzhemier's, that the efficiency of the immune system (levels of natural killer cells, lymphocyte production, and antibody formation) is depressed. In addition, increased cortisol levels cause increased involution of the thymus and the loss of tissue mass in the spleen and peripheral lymph nodes, thus creating still another hit to the immune system.

On the opposite extreme, laughter is associated with decreased cortisol production and increases in natural killer cells and activated T-cells. This is why Norman Cousins wrote his book on laughter as the best medicine against cancer. It makes perfect hormonal sense, especially if combined with the Anti-aging Zone Lifestyle Pyramid.

Depression is yet another disease that has a profound effect on the immune system. It was recognized by the Roman physician Galen that depressed women were more prone to breast cancer than their more cheerful counterparts. Perhaps such a revelation is not so surprising, since depressed patients have much higher levels of "bad" eicosanoids than do normal individuals, and one consequence of an overproduction of "bad" eicosanoids is the depression of the immune system. This also explains why depressed patients have decreased levels of natural killer cells, lymphocytes, and T-helper cells, just as patients under chronic stress have elevated cortisol levels.

The brain and the immune system are linked together in an intricate balance of the endocrine, nervous and immune systems as shown in Figure 28-2.

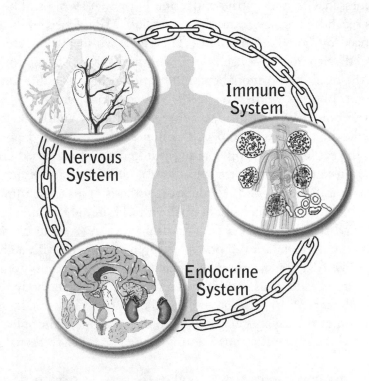

Figure 28-2   Nervous, Immune and Endocrine Systems
               are All Linked Together

This is why you find receptors for neuropeptides in the strangest places outside the brain, such as lymphocytes, macrophages, and granulocytes. These cells are the key players in your immune system, which is ultimately controlled by eicosanoids. If the language of emotions is mediated via hormones, neuropeptides, and cytokines, then the grammar of emotion may be mediated by eicosanoids.

What good is successful anti-aging if you aren't improving your emotional health simultaneously? To a great extent emotional health depends upon looking inside yourself and then making appropriate lifestyle changes. The Anti-aging Zone Lifestyle Pyramid should be your primary tool to make that change. Other people or institutions can only take you so far. At some point you have to take the baton yourself and finish the race. Otherwise you deserve the emotional state you are in.

CHAPTER 29

THE FUTURE OF MEDICINE

As we approach the twenty-first century, we stand on the threshold of a brave new world of hormonal modulation. It has taken us a little more than a century from Charles-Edouard Brown-Séquard's announcement that he reversed aging by using injections of ground-up animal testicles to this day when our knowledge of endocrinology is growing exponentially. Hormones have been around for millions of years, but now we are finally beginning to understand them—and more important how to control them. I believe, that controlling hormone levels and improving their communication within the body will become the central focus of health care in the future. I also believe, they are the key to reversing the aging process. And that is the real goal everyone desires.

To reverse the aging process, you don't have to wait for some new drug from the pharmaceutical industry. You already have the opportunity to begin your personal anti-aging program today using the Anti-aging Zone Lifestyle Pyramid. The core of that pyramid is the Zone Diet, which offers the only proven drug to reverse aging because it represents calorie restriction without deprivation or hunger. In my earlier books, *The Zone, Mastering the Zone, Zone Perfect Meals in Minutes,* and *Zone Food Blocks,* I have tried to give you "how-to" basics for turning your kitchen into a food pharmacy for twenty-first century medicine. In this book, I have tried to outline some of the fundamental interactions of hormones that can be controlled by that food pharmacy. In that pharmacy, hormonal responses generated by your diet will either accelerate the aging process or reverse it.

Medicine in America is changing rapidly, but not because of managed care. Managed care is simply a fancy name for cost-cutting. The

real change in medicine is being driven by the consumer. Self-medication is the new mantra. As I stated earlier, for the first time in history,
sales of vitamins and minerals are now greater than all cardiovascular
drugs combined. The consumer is now looking to the local health food
store for salvation. I feel the reason for this new consumer activism is
threefold.

First, consumers have better access to information. The Internet
allows everyone to play doctor or at least think they can. Unfortunately, some of the advice on the Internet is simply dead wrong. Second, consumers are tired of being treated as second-class citizens
because of by the new realities of managed care. They figure they can
do better by going to the local health food store. But the third, and
most important, reason is that consumers are scared. What they fear
is not disease, but aging. They are going to try every magic pill in the
health food store to prevent aging because they have seen the realties
of aging in their parents, and they don't like what they see. This fear
is only increased as they drive by growing numbers of nursing homes
catering to people who are living longer, but without functionality.
They see themselves in the same nursing homes in the not too distant
future. Driven by this fear of aging, they often rely upon an untrained
sales clerk behind the health food counter for their anti-aging advice.
Talk about the blind leading the blind.

Yet, this same fear of aging has the potential to be channeled into
a new beginning for twenty-first century medicine. One reason is that
the consumer is becoming proactive. And any anti-aging program requires you to be pro-active on a lifetime basis. Anti-aging is like pregnancy. You can't be half pregnant—either you are or you aren't.
Likewise either you are reversing aging or accelerating it. And if you
want to be proactive about reversing aging, you have to follow the
Zone Diet.

The Zone Diet goes back to the foundations of medicine some
2,500 years ago when Hippocrates said, "Let food be your medicine,
and let medicine be your food." He was talking about the hormonal
effects of food on the body. It has taken us 25 centuries to finally
realize that. And the most powerful way to alter hormonal response is
by the Zone Diet, since it is a calorie-restricted diet designed to maintain hormones within discrete zones throughout the day.

Herbert Benson, a cardiologist at Harvard and a leading proponent of stress reduction, has stated that basically all medicine can be viewed as a three-legged stool (see Figure 29-1 on page 296).

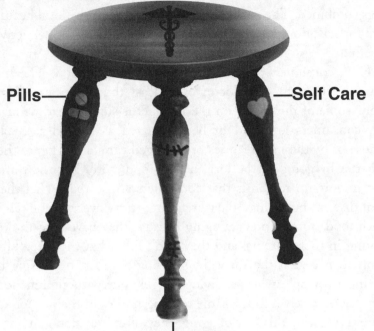

Pills—   **—Self Care**

Interventions

Figure 29-1   Three-legged Stool of Medicine

You need all three legs for stability. The first leg of the stool is pills. These can be either pharmaceuticals, vitamins, minerals, or herbs. Anything you can put into a two-piece capsule or a syringe. There will always be place for these. The second leg of the stool is intervention. This could be surgery, chiropractic manipulation, or acupuncture. There will always be a need for these interventions. Finally, and most important, is the third leg, which is self-care. This leg is composed of the Anti-aging Zone Lifestyle Pyramid. Of all the legs of this three-legged stool, the self-care leg will be the most important in the next century because it has the greatest potential to control your hormones and, therefore, your rate of aging.

On the other hand, the longer we ignore the importance of the self-care component of medicine, the more we are writing a prescription for a national health care disaster. Currently, the American health care system is like the Titanic heading for an iceberg. That iceberg is the epidemic of hyperinsulinemia (the primary pillar of aging) that currently engulfs our country. This epidemic of hyperinsulinemia was unleashed 15 years ago with the government decision to defeat obesity by making the adoption of a low-fat, high-carbohydrate diet by every American a national priority. As we have seen, the result of our war on obesity has been an abject failure because no one had thought of the hormonal consequences of these dietary recommendations.

As the baby boomers in America turn 50, the likelihood of chronic diseases (such as heart disease, cancer, diabetes, and autoimmune diseases) associated with aging will begin to rise exponentially due to the immutable law of mortality doubling times. You have to increase the mortality doubling time to reverse aging. The only way to increase it is to alter the fundamental mechanisms of aging. That change can be made by calorie restriction and primarily by reducing the excessive amounts of carbohydrates in our current diet. But, who in the medical establishment is going to step forward to admit they made a massive mistake by telling Americans to eat more carbohydrates? Instead of going to the core of our national crisis (the diet they recommended), our leadership is simply rearranging the deck chairs on this Titanic-like vessel as our health system heads on a direct collision course with this hyperinsulinemic iceberg. The end result will not be a pleasant sight.

Frankly, I don't think that anyone honestly believes that Americans are healthier now than they were 15 years ago before the new mantra of eating carbohydrates until the cows come home was implanted in our national psyche. And with hyperinsulinemia growing in our country, it is unlikely that Americans will be any healthier in the future (take a look at the children of today) unless a drastic reevaluation of the dietary advice being given to Americans is made. While I have little faith in the establishment to make such a change, I do count on the new proactive stance of Americans to take matters into their own hands. The Anti-aging Zone Lifestyle Pyramid shows how to do something about aging today. I hope this book has given you the hormonal reasons to do so.

The only proven way to reverse aging is by calorie restriction. There is no controversy about that. Calorie restriction is one of the few areas of consensus in anti-aging research. The "drug" to achieve the guaranteed anti-aging benefits of calorie restriction can only be found in your kitchen, not in a health food store or in a pharmacy.

If you want to change your future, your "drug" of choice will be food. What I have tried to demonstrate is that calorie restriction can be achieved using the Zone Diet without deprivation or hunger, that it works, and that your entire hormonal landscape will be positively affected by it.

Also, as we approach the new millennium, spirituality is in the air. New-Age thinking is trying to understand the role of man and his relationship to the world. This has spawned much in terms of trying to understand the "mind-body" connection. A significant part of the problem is in our definitions. Rather than trying to go back in time to try to find ancient writings (whose definitions are even more obscure), I believe we should go forward and use our new understanding of hormones to better define this connection. We should really talk about the "mind-body-diet" connection, as all three are intimately interconnected through the language of hormones.

Food is more than simply an anti-aging drug, because of the effect that it has on emotions. If you want a longer life with better physical health, food is your passport. If you want better emotional relationships, food is your passport. If you want better oneness with the world around you, food is your passport. Passport to what? To controlling eicosanoids, which ultimately control the "mind-body-diet" connection that is your portal to a better quality of life. Although, the Zone Diet is the centerpiece of your anti-aging program, you also need to follow the Anti-aging Zone Lifestyle Pyramid on a lifetime basis to achieve the maximum benefits of a longer life with better quality.

What I have tried to do in this book is to come full circle. It's not living longer that should be your first goal, it's living better. It's enjoying life and trying to achieve balance and harmony. It's living in a Zone, in which hormonal communication within your body moves with frightening precision. Inside that Zone, life is good. Outside that Zone, life is much more difficult than it has to be. The choice is yours. You have the "drug" to enter the Zone. The question is, will you?

APPENDIX

RESOURCES

The message of this book is that the Zone Diet is the key to anti-aging. To speed up that process, I strongly recommend that you read the first 20 pages of my book, *Zone Perfect Meals in Minutes*. This is the ultimate beginner's primer for the Zone Diet. After you have read that book, then read *Mastering the Zone* for additional hints on how to quickly and easily integrate the Zone Diet with the foods you already eat. Only then would I recommend reading *The Zone* as it deals with eicosanoids on the same technical level as this book deals with hormones.

I am the first to admit this book is complex and that it may take several readings before all the scientific concepts sink in. Furthermore, the knowledge of hormones is constantly changing. For the most current information on hormones and aging (along with helpful hints and new Zone recipes) contact my web site at www.drsears.com. In addition, this web site has several discussion groups devoted to specialized Zone topics.

If you don't have a computer, call 1-800-352-6195 for more information.

If you are a physician and want to know more about practical aspects of applied endocrinology, I strongly recommend that you contact the Broda Barnes Research Foundation at (203) 261-2101 for information on upcoming medical seminars. Likewise, if you are an individual with questions relative to thyroid and adrenal dysfunction, I also strongly urge you to contact the Barnes Foundation for information, especially with regard to a 24-hour urine analysis that I believe is critical for making any judgments before embarking on any type of hormonal supplementation.

GLOSSARY

Adenosine Triphosphate (ATP): This is the primary fuel used by cells to generate the biochemical reactions essential for life.

Adrenals: The glands located on the top of the kidneys that are responsible for the production of stress-related hormones, such as cortisol, DHEA, and adrenaline.

Adrenocortiotrophic Hormone (ACTH): The hormone released from the pituitary that interacts with receptors on the adrenal gland to begin the process of cortisol and DHEA production. ACTH uses the second messenger cyclic AMP to signal target cells in the adrenal glands.

Advanced Glycosylation Endproduct (AGE): The polymerized end products of protein cross-linked with glucose. AGE's tend to adhere to capillaries and arteries increasing the risk of heart disease, blindness, and kidney failure. AGE's are best estimated by the levels of glycosylated hemoglobin in the bloodstream.

Aerobic Capacity: The body's ability to process oxygen. It is a combination of lung capacity, the size of the capillaries, the pumping action of the heart, and transfer of oxygen from red blood cells to target tissues.

Aerobic Exercise: Exercise with a low enough intensity to facilitate adequate oxygen transfer to the muscle cells so that no buildup of lactic acid is observed. This type of exercise is useful for reducing insulin levels and lowering blood glucose.

Aging: The general deterioration of the body with increasing age.

Amino Acids: These are the building blocks of protein. There are eight essential amino acids the body cannot make and, therefore, must be included in the foods you eat.

Amygdala: The portion of the limbic system in the brain that processes emotions.

Anaerobic Exercise: Exercise at an intensity that exceeds the ability to supply oxygen to the muscle cells leading to the buildup of lactic acid. Anaerobic exercise stimulates the synthesis of both growth hormone and testosterone.

Anabolic Steroids: Synthetic analogs of testosterone that maintain the anabolic (i.e., muscle-building effects) while reducing the virilization effects of testosterone.

Anti-aging Zone Lifestyle Pyramid: The combination of the Zone Diet, moderate exercise, and meditation that interact to reduce the four pillars of aging (excess insulin, excess blood glucose, excess free radicals, and excess cortisol). Of the three components of the Anti-aging Zone Lifestyle Pyramid, the Zone Diet is by far the most important.

Arachidonic Acid: An essential fatty acid that is the immediate precursor to "bad" eicosanoids found in fatty red meats, egg yolks, and organ meats.

Autocrine Hormones: Hormones that act upon the secreting cell. They are used to sample the immediate environment surrounding the cell. Eicosanoids are the best-known example of autocrine hormones.

Binding Proteins: Proteins that bind to water-insoluble hormones, such as sex hormones, cortisol, and thyroid; or certain water-soluble proteins, such as insulin-like growth factor to maintain stable circulating levels of the hormone in the bloodstream.

Biological Marker of Aging: Any physiological marker that appears to be universal in an aging population.

Biological Response Modifier: Any molecule that can modify the biological response of cells to changes in its external environment.

Blood Glucose: The primary source of energy for the brain. Elevated blood glucose levels cause diabetes and accelerate aging.

Calorie Restriction: The reduction of calories that maintains adequate levels of protein and essential fats while also supplying adequate amounts of micronutrients (vitamins and minerals).

Corticotropin-Releasing Hormone (CRH): The hormone released from the hypothalamus that interacts with the pituitary to produce ACTH. This hormone uses cyclic AMP for its second messenger.

Cortisol: The hormone released from the adrenal glands in response to stress or low blood glucose. It's primary mode of action in times of stress is to shut down eicosanoid synthesis. Its synthesis in the adrenal gland requires the second messenger, cyclic AMP.

Cyclic AMP: A second messenger that begins the biological response initiated by a hormone. Cyclic AMP is derived from ATP. Many endocrine hormones use cyclic AMP as their second messenger.

Cyclic GMP: A second messenger that begins the biological response initiated by a hormone. Cyclic GMP is the second messenger induced by nitric oxide.

Dehydroepiandrosterone (DHEA): A steroid hormone produced in the adrenal glands. Its primary function is to inhibit the binding of cortisol.

Diabetes: A condition in which blood glucose is not well controlled. Type 1 diabetics make no insulin, whereas Type 2 diabetics are characterized by the overproduction of insulin, but the inability of the target cells to respond to the insulin.

Dopamine: A neurotransmitter that works in an axis with serotonin.

Eicosanoid: A hormone derived from a 20-carbon atom, polyunsaturated fat. Eicosanoids are made by every cell in the body. As autocrine hormones, they are constantly produced by the cell to sample the external environment. "Good" eicosanoids generate cyclic AMP.

Endocrine Hormones: Hormones that are secreted from a discrete gland and then travel through the bloodstream to target tissues.

Endocrinology: The study of hormones. A more inclusive definition would be the study of biological communications.

Endocytosis: The process by which extracelluar molecules (including hormones) enter a cell.

Endothelial Cells: The cells that line the vascular system. They act as a barrier between the bloodstream and target cells that hormones must pass through in order to reach their receptors and exert their biological action.

β-Endorphin: A hormone derived from the pituitary that induces opiate-like responses to decrease pain. The release of its precursor hormone (β-lipotropin) requires cyclic AMP.

Essential Fatty Acids: These are fats the body cannot make and therefore must be part of the diet. Essential fatty acids are also the building blocks of eicosanoids. There are two groups, omega-3 and omega-6 fatty acids, each gives rise to a different group of eicosanoids.

Estrogens: A group of three steroid hormones that convey female characteristics and control fertilization. The production of estrogen is stimulated by follicle-stimulating hormone (FSH), which uses cyclic AMP as its second messenger.

Exocytosis: The process by which intracellular chemicals (including hormones) are released.

Follicle-Stimulating Hormone (FSH): The hormone released from the pituitary that stimulates estrogen production in females, and sperm production in males. FSH uses cyclic AMP as its second messenger.

Free Radical: Any molecule that contains an unpaired electron. Free radicals are unstable and will extract electrons from other biological molecules, which generates more free radicals.

Functionality: The ability to live in an unassisted fashion.

Gland: A discrete organ responsible for the secretion of hormones. There are nine separate glands in the body. Three are in the brain (hypothalamus, pineal, and pituitary), three are in the throat area (thyroid, thymus, and parathyroid), two are in to midsection (pancreas and adrenals), and one is in the gonad area (testes for males and ovaries for females).

Glucagon: The hormone from the pancreas that causes the release of stored carbohydrate in the liver to restore blood glucose levels. Glucagon uses the second messenger cyclic AMP to exert its biological action.

Glucose: The only simple carbohydrate that circulates in the bloodstream. Glucose is the primary fuel used by the brain. It can also be stored in the liver and muscles in a polymer form known as glycogen.

Glucose Tolerance: The ability of muscle cells and the liver to remove glucose from the bloodstream. As you age, glucose tolerance decreases.

Glycemic Index: A measure of the rate at which a carbohydrate will enter the bloodstream as glucose. Some simple sugars, like table sugar, will enter the bloodstream slower than many complex carbohydrates, such as bread, rice, and potatoes. The faster a carbohydrate enters the bloodstream, the higher its glycemic index. The higher the glycemic index of a carbohydrate, the greater the increase in insulin levels. Fruits and vegetables tend to have a low glycemic index, whereas breads, pasta, grains, and starches tend to have a high glycemic index.

Glycogen: The storage form of glucose. Only glycogen from the liver can be used to restore blood glucose levels.

Glycosylated Hemoglobin: A measure of the long-term control of blood glucose determined by the amount of carbohydrate-modified hemoglobin in the red blood cells. The higher the amount of glycosylated hemoglobin, the worse the control of blood glucose levels.

Growth Hormone: The hormone released from the pituitary that interacts with fat cells to release fatty acids and also the liver to produce insulin-like growth factors.

Growth Hormone-Releasing Hormone (GHRH): The hormone released from the hypothalamus that causes the release of growth hormone from the pituitary. GHRH uses cyclic AMP as its second messenger.

High Density Lipoprotein (HDL): The "good" cholesterol that helps remove cholesterol from cells. If insulin levels go up, then HDL levels go down. The lower your HDL level, the more likely you are to suffer cardiovascular complications.

Hippocampus: The portion of the limbic system in the brain that integrates incoming nerve impulses to the hypothalamus, and is also the memory center for the brain.

Hormones: Biological compounds that communicate information at a distance. Hormones require specific receptors to begin their biological action and use second messengers to initiate the cellular process that uses that information.

Hormone Releasing Factors: Hormones released from the hypothalamus that directly affect the pituitary and initiate the release of other hormones into the bloodstream. Many hormone releasing factors use cyclic AMP as their second messengers.

Hyperinsulinemia: The excess production of insulin. This is usually a consequence of insulin resistance in which the cells do not respond to insulin to reduce blood glucose levels.

Hypothalamus: The portion of the brain's limbic system that integrates incoming information and either increases or decreases the release of certain hormones that instruct the pituitary gland to release hormones.

Insulin: The hormone that drives incoming nutrients into cells for storage. Excess insulin is the primary pillar of aging.

Insulin-like Growth Factor (IGF): The hormone released from the liver in response to growth hormone. IGF-1 is the hormone responsible for building muscle.

Insulin Resistance: A condition in which the cells no longer respond well to insulin. As a result, the body secretes more insulin into the bloodstream in an effort to reduce blood glucose levels.

Interstitial Space: The space between the endothelial cells and target cells, such as the liver or the smooth muscle cells that line the vascular bed.

Lean Body Mass: The total body weight minus the fat mass. Lean body mass consists of water, bones, collagen, and muscle.

Life Expectancy: The average age at which 50 percent of newborn children survive.

Limbic System: The part of the brain that is concerned with more primitive impulses and maintaining biological homeostasis.

Longevity: The percentage of the maximum life span that an organism will reach before it dies.

Luteinizing Hormone (LH): The hormone released from the pituitary gland that stimulates the production of testosterone in males and the production of progesterone in females. This hormone uses cyclic AMP as its second messenger.

Macronutrient: Any food that contains calories and, therefore, can generate hormonal responses. Protein, carbohydrate, and fat are macronutrients.

Maximum Life Span: The longest period of life that an animal can expect to reach.

Melatonin: The hormone made in the pineal gland that controls circadian rhythms. It is also a powerful antioxidant for hydroxyl free radicals.

Micronutrient: Vitamins and minerals that have no caloric value and little direct impact on hormonal response.

Mortality Doubling Time: The amount of time required for the death rate to double after reaching adulthood.

Nitric Oxide: A protohormone that generates cyclic GMP. Nitric oxide is a free radical.

Omega-3 Fatty Acids: A special type of polyunsaturated essential fatty acids found primarily in cold-water fish and purified fish oils. This type of fat is exceptionally beneficial to your cardiovascular system because of its effect on promoting the formation of "good" eicosanoids.

Omega-6 Fatty Acids: The type of ployunsaturated essential fatty acids found in protein and most seed oils. This type of fat can generate both "good" and "bad" eicosanoids.

Percentage Body Fat: This describes the percentage of your total weight that is composed of fat. The higher your percentage of body fat, the greater the likelihood of chronic disease, such as heart disease, cancer, or diabetes.

Pineal: The gland located within the brain that synthesizes melatonin.

Pituitary: The gland from which a number of hormones are released into the bloodstream. These hormones include growth hormone, ACTH, β-lipocortin (the precursor to β-endorphorin), FSH, LH, and TSH.

Progesterone: A hormone produced in response to luteinizing hormone (LH) released from the pituitary gland. It is required to flush out the uterus if an egg is not fertilized. It is also useful for the stimulating the growth of new bone mass.

Progestins: Synthetic analogs of progesterone that have some of the properties of natural progesterone.

Receptor: A molecule that recognizes a unique hormone. Once that hormone is bound to the receptor, the information carried by the hormone can now exert its biological action.

Second Messenger: Molecules that are synthesized in response to hormones binding to their receptors. Second messengers initiate the biological action of the hormone.

Serotonin: A neurotransmitter important in filtering out information. If its levels are low, it can be the underlying cause of depression and violence.

Telomer: A small segment at the end of nuclear DNA that becomes shorter with every replication of the DNA. DNA will no longer replicate beyond a certain point of telomere reduction.

Testosterone: The hormone that promotes the building of muscle mass in males and libido in both sexes.

Thymus: The gland responsible for the production of certain white cells known as T-lymphocytes that are important for immune function. The thymus is very sensitive to excess cortisol.

Thyroid: The gland in the throat that synthesizes thyroid hormones that affect metabolism.

Thyroid-Releasing Hormone (TRH): The hormone released from the hypothalamus that instructs the pituitary to release TSH.

Thyroid-Stimulating Hormone (TSH): The hormone released from the pituitary that causes the thyroid gland to produce T4 hormone. TSH uses the second messenger cyclic AMP to initiate the synthesis of T4.

Triglycerides (TG): The form of fat found in various lipoproteins in the bloodstream. High levels of triglycerides are usually indicative of high levels of insulin. The ratio of TG/HDL is a powerful indicator of insulin levels and is strongly predictive of future cardiovascular events.

Type 2 Diabetes: A diabetic condition characterized by the overproduction of insulin (hyperinsulinemia), increased AGE production, and decreased longevity.

T3: The active form of T4 synthesized in the peripheral tissue.

T4: The thyroid hormone that is released from the thyroid gland in response to TSH, which generates cyclic AMP.

Ventromedial Nucleus (VMN): The part of the hypothalamus sensitive to excess glucose.

Zone Diet: A calorie-restricted diet that provides adequate protein, moderate levels of carbohydrates along with essential fats, and micronutrients spread throughout the day in three meals and two snacks that approximately maintains the protein-to-carbohydrate ratio being maintained the same at each meal or snack.

A Week in the Anti-aging Zone

Below are some very easy-to-prepare Zone meals for both the typical female and typical male. Once you look at these meals, you will realize it's easy to stay in the Zone on lifetime basis. As large as these meals may appear to be, always make sure to include a late afternoon snack and late evening snack. Furthermore, these Zone meals and snacks are representative of calorie-restricted diets that are the only proven "drug" to reverse aging. Hundreds of other Zone meals can be found in *Mastering the Zone* and *Zone Perfect Meals in Minutes*.

Bon appétit.

A Week in the Zone for The Typical Female

BREAKFAST DAY 1

SOY PATTIES AND FRUIT

2 soy patties
1 oz. low-fat cheese
Fruit salad of
    $^2/_3$ cup mandarin oranges and
    $^3/_4$ cup blueberries sprinkled with
    3 teaspoons slivered almonds

Broil soy patties according to package directions. Add cheese slices and continue to broil until cheese melts.

LUNCH DAY 1

CHEF SALAD

1 large tossed salad containing 1 cup lettuce, $^1/_4$ cup chickpeas, 1 cup
    chopped mushrooms and $^2/_3$ cup sliced celery

1 tablespoon olive oil and vinegar dressing
3 oz. deli-style turkey breast
1 oz. reduced fat cheese
1 pear

DINNER DAY 1

BROILED FISH

4 ½ oz. fish fillet of your choice
1 teaspoon olive oil
Lemon or ginger slices
2 tomatoes, split, sprinkled with Parmesan cheese and broiled
1 cup cooked green beans
½ cup grapes

Brush fish with olive oil. Place lemon slices on top. Broil 10 minutes per inch of thickness. Do not turn.

BREAKFAST DAY 2

YOGURT AND FRUIT

1 cup plain, low-fat yogurt mixed with
½ cup cubed pineapple and
3 teaspoons slivered almonds
1 oz. Canadian bacon or 3 turkey bacon strips, served on the side

Mixed together and enjoy.

LUNCH DAY 2

PITA PIZZA

1 mini pita pocket, cut in half pizza-style
1 oz. reduced fat mozzarella cheese
2 oz. Canadian bacon, extra lean or 2 oz. lean chicken breast or 3 oz. lean
    ground beef
Green pepper and onion, chopped, enough to top pizza

1 large tossed salad containing 3 cups shredded lettuce, ½ raw green
   pepper, ½ raw cucumber and 1 raw tomato
1 tablespoon olive oil and vinegar dressing

Spray a nonstick pan with vegetable spray, cook bacon for 1 minute,
turning once. In same pan sauté vegetables to desired degree of tenderness. Put bacon, then vegetables on pita rounds. Sprinkle each with
cheese. Broil until cheese melts.

DINNER DAY 2

VEGETARIAN STIR-FRY

1 cup vegetable protein crumbles or
   4 oz. firm tofu
1 oz. reduced-fat shredded cheese
1 teaspoon olive oil
1 cup chopped onion
1 ½ cups broccoli florets
1 ½ cups sliced mushrooms
1 plum

If tofu is used, drain and crumble. Sauté tofu or vegetable crumbles
in a nonstick pan. Add onions, broccoli, and mushrooms. Stir-fry on
medium heat. Stir in cheese and heat until the cheese is melted.

BREAKFAST DAY 3

SCRAMBLED EGGS AND BACON

4 egg whites or ½ cup egg substitute
Sprinkling of low-fat mozzarella cheese
1 teaspoon olive oil
1 oz. lean Canadian bacon or 3 turkey bacon strips
1 cup grapes
⅔ cup cubed honeydew melon

Spray a nonstick pan with vegetable spray. Beat egg whites with olive
oil and a little milk if desired. Fold in cheese. Scramble.

LUNCH DAY 3

TUNA SALAD

3 oz. albacore tuna packed in water mixed with
    1 tablespoon olive oil and vinegar dressing
Chopped celery
1 side salad
½ cantaloupe stuffed with ½ cup boysenberries

DINNER DAY 3

FOILED FISH

4 ½ oz. fish fillet of your choice (flounder is suggested)
Sprinkling of Parmesan cheese
Freshly ground pepper, to taste
Squirt of lemon juice
Chopped onion, to taste
1 side salad
1 tablespoon olive oil and vinegar dressing
2 cups cooked green beans
½ apple

Tear off a good-sized piece of foil. Spray the center lightly with vegetable spray. Put fish in the center of the foil. Top with onion, pepper, lemon juice and cheese. Fold foil over fish, leaving space around the fish. Carefully turn up and seal the ends and the middle so that juices don't leak out. Bake in a 425° oven for 18 minutes. When done, carefully open foil to prevent steam burns.

BREAKFAST DAY 4

FRUIT SALAD

¾ cup low-fat cottage cheese
1 cup pineapple

⅓ cup mandarin oranges
3 macadamia nuts, crushed

Mix together and enjoy.

LUNCH DAY 4

VEGETARIAN BURGER

1 soy burger patty
1 oz. reduced-fat cheese
Lettuce and tomato slice
Dill pickle wedge, optional
1 teaspoon reduced-fat mayonnaise
1 side salad
2 teaspoons olive oil and vinegar dressing
1 cup unsweetened applesauce, sprinkled with cinnamon

Spray nonstick pan with vegetable spray. Cook soy burgers 5 to 8 minutes on each side. Note: Check package instructions. Cooking directions vary from product to product.

DINNER DAY 4

BARBECUED CHICKEN

3 oz. chicken breast, no skin
Lemon slices
Onion slices
1 to 2 teaspoons barbecue sauce
1 cup cooked green beans sauteed in garlic with
   3 teaspoons slivered almonds
1 apple

Preheat oven to 450°. Cover chicken breast with slices of onion and lemon. Bake for 15 minutes. Reduce heat to 350°. Baste with barbecue sauce. Cook for 10 to 15 minutes or until done.

BREAKFAST DAY 5

OLD-FASHIONED OATMEAL

²/₃ cup slow-cooking oatmeal
¹/₃ cup applesauce
Nutmeg
Cinnamon
1 scoop protein powder (7 grams of protein powder)
3 teaspoons almonds, slivered
2 oz. lean Canadian bacon or 6 turkey bacon strips

Cook oatmeal according to package directions. Sprinkle with cinnamon and nutmeg. Mix in slivered almonds, applesauce, and protein powder into hot, cooked oatmeal.

LUNCH DAY 5

VEGETARIAN CHILI

1 cup vegetable protein crumbles
1 teaspoon olive oil
Onions, chopped, to taste
Garlic, to taste
Pepper, to taste
Mushrooms, to taste, chopped
1 cup chopped, stewed tomatoes with liquid
¹/₄ cup kidney beans, drained and rinsed
Chili powder, to taste
Pepper, to taste
1 oz. reduced-fat cheese

Sauté the crumbles in the oil with the chopped onion, garlic, pepper, and mushrooms. Add tomatoes, kidney beans, chili powder. Simmer until beans are tender. Top with shredded cheese.

DINNER DAY 5

SHRIMP SCAMPI

4 ¹/₂ oz. shelled shrimp
³/₄ cup chopped onion

1 chopped green pepper
1 teaspoon olive oil
Garlic to taste
$\frac{1}{4}$ to $\frac{1}{2}$ cup dry white wine (optional)
1 to 2 teaspoons lemon juice
Lemon wedges
1 cup cooked asparagus
$\frac{1}{2}$ apple

In a nonstick pan, sauté garlic, onion, and green pepper, until tender in olive oil. Add shrimp, white wine and lemon juice. Cook for 5 minutes stirring often until shrimp is pink. Garnish with lemon wedges.

BREAKFAST DAY 6

HUEVOS RANCHEROS

4 large egg whites or $\frac{1}{2}$ cup egg substitute
1 oz. shredded lowfat Monterey Jack cheese
1 teaspoon olive oil
Chopped onion
1 chopped green pepper
1 chopped tomato
Chili powder, optional
1 orange

Beat egg whites and olive oil with a little milk if desired. Mix in vegetables, cheese, and chili powder to taste. Spray a nonstick pan with vegetable spray. Scramble eggs.

LUNCH DAY 6

GRILLED CHICKEN SALAD

1 salad containing 1 cup lettuce, 1 cup broccoli, $\frac{1}{2}$ cup chopped green pepper, $\frac{1}{2}$ sliced tomato
1 tablespoon olive oil and vinegar dressing (sprinkled with garlic powder)

Lemon juice
3 oz. grilled chicken
Grated Parmesan cheese
Dash Worcestershire Sauce
1 pear

Prepare salad. Drizzle salad dressing over the salad. Squeeze the lemon over the salad. Season with Worcestershire Sauce and grind pepper over all. Toss until well combined. Place chicken on top.

DINNER DAY 6

BROILED SALMON

4 ½ oz. salmon fillet
Rosemary, to taste
Tarragon, to taste
Dill, to taste
1 teaspoon olive oil
Lemon, optional
2 cups cooked zucchini
2 tomatoes, split, sprinkled with Parmesan cheese and broiled
½ apple

Rub the fillet with the herbs and then brush with oil. Broil for 10 minutes per inch of thickness, turning and basting once. Garnish with lemon, if desired.

BREAKFAST DAY 7

VEGETABLE OMELETTE

1 large whole egg plus
    4 large egg whites or
    ½ cup egg substitute
1 teaspoon olive oil
1 cup cooked asparagus tips
Diced tomato, onion, and mushrooms

²/₃ cup mandarin oranges
(Note: If you don't like asparagus, substitute another vegetable or add
   another block of fruit.)

Cook asparagus tips and sauté vegetables. Beat eggs, adding 1 tablespoon of milk if desired. Stir in sautéed chopped vegetables. Spray
nonstick pan with vegetable spray. Cook eggs on medium low heat
until eggs are almost set. Lift edge of omelette with spatula to let
liquid drain to the bottom. Place asparagus tips on top of omelette and
fold over. Continue cooking, turning when necessary until done.

LUNCH DAY 7

STUFFED TOMATO

2 tomatoes
3 oz. albacore tuna packed in water
1 tablespoon light mayonnaise
Chopped celery and onion to taste
1 apple

Drain tuna. Mix mayonnaise, celery, and onion. Stuff in the tomato.

DINNER DAY 7

BEEF KABOBS

3 oz. lean beef, cut into cubes
Kabob vegetables, such as onions, green peppers, mushrooms, and cherry
   tomatoes
Marinade
1 spinach salad consisting of 3 cups raw spinach ½ onion, ½ cup raw
   mushrooms, and 1 tomato
1 tablespoon olive oil and vinegar dressing
1 nectarine

Marinate the meat in your favorite marinade for several hours or overnight. If you have no favorite, try combining olive oil, low-sodium soy

sauce, red wine vinegar, lemon juice, Worcestershire sauce, dry mustard, and pepper. Thread meat and vegetables on skewers. Brush with marinade. Broil 3 inches from source of heat (or cook on the barbecue grill) 18 minutes for rare and 25 minutes for well done. Turn once during cooking time and baste with marinade once or twice.

A Week in the Zone for The Typical Male

BREAKFAST DAY 1

SOY PATTIES AND FRUIT

2 soy patties
2 oz. low-fat cheese
Fruit salad of
   1 cup mandarin oranges and
   ³/₄ cup blueberries sprinkled with
   4 teaspoons slivered almonds

Broil soy patties according to package directions. Add cheese slices and continue to broil until cheese melts.

LUNCH DAY 1

CHEF SALAD

1 large tossed salad containing 1 cup lettuce, ¼ cup chickpeas, 1 cup
   chopped mushrooms and ²/₃ cup sliced celery
4 teapoons olive oil and vinegar dressing
3 oz. deli-style turkey breast
1 ½ oz. deli-style ham
1 oz. reduced fat cheese
1 pear
½ orange

DINNER DAY 1

BROILED FISH

6 oz. fish fillet of your choice
1 ⅓ teaspoons olive oil
Lemon or ginger slices
2 tomatoes, split, sprinkled with Parmesan cheese, and broiled
2 cups cooked green beans
½ cup grapes

Brush fish with olive oil. Place lemon slices on top. Broil 10 minutes per inch thickness. Do not turn.

BREAKFAST DAY 2

YOGURT AND FRUIT

1 cup plain, low-fat yogurt mixed with
    ½ cup cubed pineapple
½ cup blueberries and
4 teaspoons slivered almonds
2 oz. Canadian bacon or 6 turkey bacon strips served on the side.

LUNCH DAY 2

PITA PIZZA

1 mini pita pocket, cut in half pizza-style
1 oz. reduced fat mozzarella cheese
3 oz. Canadian bacon, extra lean or 3 oz. lean chicken breast or 4 ½ oz. lean ground beef
Green pepper and onion, chopped, enough to top pizza
1 large tossed salad consisting of 3 cups shredded lettuce, ½ raw green pepper, ½ raw cucumber and 1 raw tomato
4 teaspoons olive oil and vinegar dressing
1 peach

Spray nonstick pan lightly with vegetable spray, cook bacon for 1 minute, turning once. In same pan sauté vegetables to desired degree of tenderness. Put bacon, then vegetables on pita rounds. Sprinkle each with cheese. Broil until cheese melts.

DINNER DAY 2

VEGETARIAN STIR-FRY

1 ¼ cups vegetable protein crumbles or
    6 oz. firm tofu
1 oz. reduced-fat shredded cheese
1 ⅓ teaspoons olive oil
1 cup chopped onion
1 ½ cups broccoli florets
1 ½ cups sliced mushrooms
¼ cup chickpeas
2 plums

If tofu is used, drain and crumble. Sauté tofu or vegetable crumbles in olive oil in a nonstick pan. Add onions, broccoli, chickpeas, and mushrooms. Stirfry on medium heat. Stir in cheese and heat until the cheese is melted.

BREAKFAST DAY 3

SCRAMBLED EGGS AND BACON

4 egg whites or ½ cup egg substitute
1 oz. low-fat mozzarella cheese
1 ⅓ teaspoons olive oil
1 oz. lean Canadian bacon or 3 turkey bacon strips
1 cup grapes
1 ⅓ cups cubed honeydew melon

Spray a nonstick pan with vegetable spray. Beat egg whites with olive oil and a little milk if desired. Fold in cheese. Scramble.

LUNCH DAY 3

TUNA SALAD

4 oz. albacore tuna packed in water mixed with
   4 teaspoons olive oil and vinegar dressing
Chopped celery
1 side salad
½ cantaloupe stuffed with 1 cup boysenberries

DINNER DAY 3

FOILED FISH

6 oz. fish fillet of your choice (flounder is suggested)
Sprinkling of Parmesan cheese
Freshly ground pepper, to taste
Squirt of lemon juice
Chopped onion, to taste
1 side salad
4 teaspoons olive oil and vinegar dressing
2 cups cooked green beans
1 apple

Tear off a good-sized piece of foil. Spray the center lightly with vegetable spray. Put fish in the center of the foil. Top with onion, pepper, lemon juice, and cheese. Fold foil over fish, leaving space around the fish. Carefully turn and seal the ends and the middle so that juices don't leak out. Bake in a 425° oven for 18 minutes. When done, carefully open foil to prevent steam burns.

BREAKFAST DAY 4

FRUIT SALAD

1 cup low-fat cottage cheese
1 cup pineapple

⅔ cup mandarin oranges
4 macadamia nuts, crushed

Mix together and enjoy.

LUNCH DAY 4

VEGETARIAN BURGER

1 ½ soy burger patties
1 oz. reduced-fat cheese
Lettuce and tomato slice
Dill pickle wedge, optional
1 teaspoon reduced-fat mayonnaise
1 side salad
1 tablespoon olive oil and vinegar dressing
1 cup unsweetened applesauce, sprinkled with cinnamon
1 small breadstick

Spray nonstick pan with vegetable spray. Cook soy burgers 5 to 8 minutes on each side. Note: Check package instructions. Cooking directions vary from product to product.

DINNER DAY 4

BARBECUED CHICKEN

4 oz. chicken breast, no skin
Lemon slices
Onion slices
1 to 2 teaspoons barbecue sauce
2 cups cooked green beans sautéed in garlic with
    4 teaspoons slivered almonds
1 apple

Preheat oven to 450°. Cover chicken breast with slices of onion and lemon. Bake for 15 minutes. Reduce heat to 350°. Baste with barbecue sauce. Cook for 10 to 15 minutes or until done.

BREAKFAST DAY 5

OLD-FASHIONED OATMEAL

1 cup slow-cooking oatmeal
⅓ cup applesauce
Nutmeg
Cinnamon
1 scoop protein powder (7 grams of protein powder)
4 teaspoons almonds, slivered
2 oz. lean Canadian bacon or 6 turkey bacon strips
¼ cup lowfat cottage cheese

Cook oatmeal according to package directions. Sprinkle with cinnamon and nutmeg. Mix in slivered almonds, applesauce, and protein powder into hot, cooked oatmeal.

LUNCH DAY 5

VEGETARIAN CHILI

1 ¼ cup vegetable protein crumbles
4 teaspoons olive oil
Onions, chopped, to taste
Garlic, to taste
Pepper, to taste
Mushrooms, to taste, chopped
1 cup chopped, stewed tomatoes with liquid
½ cup kidney beans, drained and rinsed
Chili powder, to taste
Pepper, to taste
1 oz. reduced-fat cheese

Sauté the crumbles in the oil with the chopped onion, garlic, pepper, and mushrooms. Add tomatoes, kidney beans, chili powder. Simmer until beans are tender. Top with shredded cheese.

DINNER DAY 5

SHRIMP SCAMPI

6 oz. shelled shrimp
¾ cup chopped onion
1 chopped green pepper
1 ⅓ teaspoons olive oil
Garlic to taste
¼ to ½ cup dry white wine (optional)
1 to 2 teaspoons lemon juice
Lemon wedges
1 cup cooked asparagus
½ apple

In a nonstick pan, sauté garlic, onion, and green pepper until tender in olive oil. Add shrimp, white wine, and lemon juice. Cook for 5 minutes stirring often until shrimp is pink. Garnish with lemon wedges.

BREAKFAST DAY 6

HUEVOS RANCHEROS

6 large egg whites or ¾ cup egg substitute
1 oz. shredded lowfat Monterey jack cheese
¼ cup black beans or chickpeas
1 ⅓ teaspoons olive oil
Chopped onion
1 chopped green pepper
1 chopped tomato
Chili powder, optional
1 orange

Beat egg whites and olive oil with a little milk if desired. Mix in vegetables, cheese, and chili powder to taste. Spray a nonstick pan with vegetable spray. Scramble eggs.

LUNCH DAY 6

GRILLED CHICKEN SALAD

1 salad containing 1 cup lettuce, 1 cup broccoli, ½ cup chopped green
    pepper, ½ sliced tomato
4 teaspoons olive oil and vinegar dressing (sprinkled with garlic powder)
Lemon juice
4 oz. grilled chicken
Grated Parmesan cheese
Dash Worcestershire Sauce
1 pear
1 small breadstick or ½ mini pita pocket

Prepare salad. Drizzle salad dressing over the salad. Squeeze the lemon
over the salad. Season with Worcestershire Sauce and grind pepper
over all. Toss until well combined. Place chicken on top.

DINNER DAY 6

BROILED SALMON

6 oz. salmon fillet
Rosemary, to taste
Tarragon, to taste
Dill, to taste
1 ⅓ teaspoons olive oil
Lemon, optional
2 cups cooked zucchini
2 tomatoes, split, sprinkled with Parmesan cheese and broiled
1 apple

Rub the fillet with the herbs and then brush with oil. Broil for 10
minutes per inch of thickness, turning and basting once. Garnish with
lemon if desired.

BREAKFAST DAY 7

VEGETABLE OMELETTE

1 large whole egg plus
   4 large egg whites or
   ½ cup egg substitute
1 teaspoon olive oil
2 cups cooked asparagus tips
Diced tomato, onion and mushrooms
⅔ cup mandarin oranges
3 strips turkey bacon or 1 oz. lean Canadian bacon
(Note: If you don't like asparagus, substitute another vegetable or add
   another block of fruit.)

Cook asparagus tips and sauté vegetables. Beat eggs, adding 1 table-spoon of milk if desired. Stir in sautéed chopped vegetables. Spray nonstick pan with vegetable spray. Cook eggs on medium low heat until eggs are almost set. Lift edge of omelette with spatula to let liquid drain to the bottom. Place asparagus tips on top of omelette and fold over. Continue cooking, turning when necessary until done.

LUNCH DAY 7

STUFFED TOMATO

2 tomatoes
4 oz. albacore tuna packed in water
4 teaspoons light mayonnaise
Chopped celery and onion to taste
1 apple
½ cup grapes

Drain tuna. Mix mayonnaise, celery, and onion. Stuff into tomato.

DINNER DAY 7

BEEF KABOBS

4 oz. lean beef, cut into cubes
Kabob vegetables, such as onions, green peppers, mushrooms, and cherry
   tomatoes

Marinade
1 spinach salad consisting of 3 cups raw spinach, ½ onion, ½ cup raw
     mushrooms, ¼ cup chickpeas, and 1 tomato
4 teaspoons olive oil and vinegar dressing
1 nectarine

Marinate the meat in your favorite marinade for several hours or overnight. If you have no favorite, try combining olive oil, low-sodium soy
sauce, red wine vinegar, lemon juice, Worcestershire Sauce, dry mustard, and pepper. Thread meat and vegetables on skewers. Brush with
marinade. Broil 3 inches from source of heat (or cook on the barbecue
grill) 18 minutes for rare and 25 minutes for well done. Turn once
during cooking time and baste with marinade once or twice.

Zone Meal Tips

Making Zone meals is not exactly rocket science. In fact, it's pretty simple. Just remember that each Zone meal must contain protein, carbohydrate and fat, and you must select the same total number of items from each group to make a Zone meal. If you are the typical female, make sure that each meal has three (3) choices from each group (i.e., 3 proteins, 3 carbohydrates, and 3 fats). For example, if you select skinless, chicken breast from the protein group, simply triple the measurement. The actual portion size would be 3 ounces (3 × 1 oz.). Do the same for the carbohydrate and fat portions. Or you may mix items within each group as long as the total number of items selected equals three (3). For your carbohydrate portion you might select 2 cups of asparagus (2 portions) and ½ cup of blueberries (1 portion) for a total of three (3). If you are a typical male, have each meal containing four items from each group. Hundreds of Zone meals can be found in *Mastering the Zone* and *Zone Perfect Meals in Minutes*.

Here are some basic Zone rules to remember:

1. Always eat within 1 hour after waking
2. Never let more than 5 hours go by without eating a Zone meal or snack whether you are hungry or not.
3. Have some protein at every meal and snack.
4. Eat more fruits and vegetables, and ease off on the bread, pasta, grains, and starches.
5. Make sure you always eat your late afternoon and late evening Zone snacks.
6. Drink at least 64 oz. of liquid (water is the best choice) every day.
7. If you make a mistake, don't worry about it. Just make your next meal a Zone meal.
8. Eat a Zone snack 30 minutes before exercise.

Protein Choices

MEAT AND POULTRY (low in saturated fat)
    Beef (range fed or game), 1 oz.
    Chicken breast, skinless, 1 oz.
    Chicken breast, deli-style, 1½ oz.
    Turkey breast, skinless, 1 oz.
    Turkey breast, deli-style, 1½ oz.
    Turkey, ground, 1½ oz.
    Turkey bacon, 3 strips
    Lean Canadian bacon, 1 oz.
FISH AND SEAFOOD
    Bass (freshwater) 1 oz.
    Bass (sea), 1½ oz.
    Bluefish, 1½ oz.
    Calamari, 1½ oz
    Catfish, 1½ oz.
    Cod, 1½ oz.
    Clams, 1½ oz.
    Crabmeat, 1½ oz.
    Haddock, 1½ oz.
    Halibut, 1½ oz
    Lobster, 1½ oz.
    Mackerel,* 1½ oz.
    Salmon,* 1½ oz.
    Sardine,* 1 oz.
    Scallops, 1½ oz.
    Snapper, 1½ oz.
    Swordfish, 1½ oz.
    Shrimp, 1½ oz.
    Trout, 1½ oz.
    Tuna (steak), 1½ oz.
    Tuna, canned in water, 1 oz.
    (*rich in EPA)
EGGS
    Egg whites, 2
    Egg substitute, ¼ cup
PROTEIN-RICH DAIRY
    Cottage cheese, low fat, ¼ cup
    Lowfat cheese, 1 oz.

VEGETARIAN
  Protein powder (7 grams)
  Soy burgers, ½ patty
  Soy hot dog, 1 link
  Soy sausage links, 2 links
  Soy sausages, 1 patty
  Tofu, firm or extra firm, 2 oz.

Carbohydrate Choices

COOKED VEGETABLES
  Artichoke, 1 medium
  Artichoke hearts, 1½ cups
  Asparagus (12 spears), 1 cup
  Beans, green or wax, 1 cup
  Beans, black, ¼ cup
  Bok choy, 3 cups
  Broccoli, 3 cups
  Brussels sprouts, 1½ cups
  Cabbage, 3 cups
  Cauliflower, 3½ cups
  Chickpeas, ¼ cup
  Collard greens, 1 cup
  Eggplant, 1½ cups
  Kale, 2 cups
  Kidney beans, ¼ cup
  Leeks, 1 cup
  Lentils, ¼ cup
  Mushrooms (boiled), 2 cups
  Onions, chopped (boiled), ½ cup
  Okra, sliced, 1 cup
  Sauerkraut, 1 cup
  Spinach, 1 cup
  Swiss chard, 1 cup
  Turnip, mashed, 1½ cups
  Turnip greens, 4 cups
  Yellow squash, 1 cup
  Zucchini, 2 cups

RAW VEGETABLES

    Alfalfa sprouts, 10 cups
    Bean sprouts, 3 cups
    Bamboo shoots, 4 cups
    Cabbage, shredded, 4 cups
    Cauliflower pieces, 3½ cups
    Celery, sliced, 2½ cups
    Cucumber, sliced, 4 cups
    Endive, chopped, 10 cups
    Escarole, chopped, 10 cups
    Green or red peppers, 2½ cups
    Green pepper, chopped, 2 cups
    Hummus, ¼ cup (also contains fat)
    Lettuce, iceberg, 2 heads
    Lettuce, romaine chopped, 4 cups
    Mushrooms, chopped, 3 cups
    Onion, chopped, 1 cup
    Radishes, sliced, 4 cups
    Salsa, ½ cup
    Snow peas, 1½ cups
    Spinach, 10 cups
    Spinach salad (3 cups raw spinach, ½ raw onion, ½ cup raw
       mushrooms, and 1 raw tomato)
    Tomato, 2
    Tomato, chopped, 1 cup
    Tossed salad (3 cups shredded lettuce, ½ raw green pepper,
       ½ raw cucumber, and 1 raw tomato)
    Water chestnuts, ⅓ cup

FRUITS (Fresh, frozen or canned light)

    Apple, ½ cup
    Applesauce, ⅓ cup
    Apricots, 3
    Blackberries, ¾ cup
    Blueberries, ½ cup
    Boysenberries, ½ cup
    Cantaloupe, ¼ melon
    Cantaloupe, cubed ¾ cup
    Cherries, 8
    Fruit cocktail, ⅓ cup

Grapes, ½ cup
Grapefruit, ½
Honeydew melon, cubed, ⅔ cup
Kiwi, 1
Lemon,1
Lime, 1
Nectarine, ½
Orange, ½
Orange, mandarin, canned, ⅓ cup
Peach, 1
Peaches, canned, ½ cup
Pear, ½
Pineapple, cubed, ½ cup
Plum, 1
Raspberries, 1 cup
Strawberries, 1 cup
Tangerine, 1
Watermelon, ¾ cup

GRAINS

Barley (dry), ½ tablespoon
Oatmeal (slow cooking)** ⅓ cup (cooked)
Oatmeal (slow cooking)** ½ oz. (dry)

(**contains GLA)

Fat Choices

3 almonds
1 macadamia nut
3 olives
6 peanuts
1 tablespoon of gucamole
1 tablespoon of avocado
1 teaspoon of slivered almonds
⅓ teaspoon of olive oil
1 teaspoon of olive oil and vinegar dressing (⅓ teaspoon of olive oil to every ⅔ teaspoon of vinegar).

Zone Snacks

The Zone Diet is based on eating 3 meals plus 2 snacks per day. Making Zone Snacks is even easier than making Zone meals because they are smaller. Just like Zone meals, pick one item from each column. Of course, increase the size of any Zone snack, and you have a Zone meal within seconds. Many more Zone snacks can be found in *Mastering the Zone* and *Zone Perfect Meals in Minutes*.

Protein Choices:

¼ cup of 1% cottage cheese
1 oz. of low-fat mozzarella or other low-fat cheese
1½ oz. of low-fat sliced deli meats (turkey, chicken, ham, etc.)
1 oz. of tuna fish (water packed)

Carbohydrate Choices:

½ apple
3 apricots
⅔ cup of cubed honeydew melon
1 kiwi
¾ cup of cubed cantaloupe
1 tangerine
⅓ cup fruit cocktail
½ pear
1 cup raspberries
¼ cantaloupe
½ orange
½ cup of grapes
8 cherries
½ nectarine
1 peach

1 plum
½ canned peaches
½ cup pineapple
1 cup strawberries
½ cup blueberries
½ grapefruit

Fat Choices:

3 almonds
3 olives
1 tablespoon of gucamole
1 teaspoon of slivered almonds
1 macadamia nut
6 peanuts
1 tablespoon of avocado
⅓ teaspon of olive oil

Here are some representative Zone snacks:

Cottage Cheese and Fruit

¼ cup 1% cottage cheese
½ orange
3 almonds

Cheese and Fruit

1 oz. low-fat mozzarella string cheese
½ cup blueberries
1 teaspoon of slivered almonds

Sliced Turkey and Hummus Wrap

1 oz. of sliced turkey
¼ cup of hummus

Wine and Cheese

4 oz. of wine
1 oz. of cheese

The Fast-food Zone

Fast-food restaurants can be useful in a pinch when you need a quick Zone meal. These foods tend to be very rich in carbohydrates and fat (a deadly combination), but at least there are a few choices that are not too bad. (Nonetheless, they tend to be a little high in saturated fat, so always ask for no mayo.)

ARBY'S

Light roasted turkey deluxe
Light roast beef deluxe

BURGER KING

BK Boiler (without mayo)

DAIRY QUEEN

Grilled chicken fillet (nonbreaded) sandwich

HARDEE'S

Grilled chicken sandwich

JACK-IN-THE-BOX

Chicken fajita pita

McDONALDS

McGrilled chicken classic sandwich

TACO BELL

Chicken soft taco
Chicken fajita

WENDY'S

Chili
Grilled chicken sandwich

Zone Meals for the Business Traveler

If you are a businessperson, it is difficult to eat on the road. If you want to maintain peak mental acuity throughout the day, then food is your drug of choice. Just remember to always ask for extra vegetables in place of rice or potatoes, and never consume more protein at a meal that you can fit on the palm of your hand (and the same thickness). Of course, stay away from the rolls. If you have a glass of wine or a cocktail for dinner, then just cut back on some of your carbohydrate. Here are some good Zone choices that you can find at any hotel or restaurant.

BREAKFAST

Three-egg omelette (ideally a six egg-white omelette) plus oatmeal (don't eat the toast or the potatoes).
Breakfast buffet with scrambled eggs and fruit.

LUNCH

Grilled chicken Caesar salad. Have fruit for dessert.

DINNER

Fish or chicken with extra vegetables and no starches. Have fresh fruit for dessert.

References

Chapter 1—THE QUEST: LONGER LIFE OR BETTER LIFE

Austad, S. N. *Why We Age*. John Wiley & Sons, New York, NY (1997)

Hayflick, L. *How and Why We Age*. Ballantine Books, New York, NY (1994)

Moore, T. J. *Lifespan*. Simon & Schuster, New York, NY (1993)

Sears, B. *The Zone*. ReganBooks, New York, NY (1995)

———. *Mastering the Zone*. ReganBooks, New York, NY (1997)

———. *Zone Perfect Meals in Minutes*. ReganBooks, New York, NY (1997)

———. *Zone Food Blocks*. ReganBooks, New York, NY (1998)

Chapter 2—"WHY ARE WE LIVING LONGER?"

Austad, S. N. *Why We Age*. John Wiley & Sons, New York, NY (1997)

Browner, W. S., J. Westenhouse, and J. A. Tice. "What if Americans ate less fat." *JAMA* 265: 3285–3291 (1991)

Crawford, M., and D. Marsh. *The Driving Force*. Harper & Row, NY (1989)

Eaton B., M. Shostak, and M. Konner. *The Paleolithic Prescription*. Harper & Row, New York, NY (1988)

Finch, C. E. *Longevity, Senescence, and the Genome*. University of Chicago Press, Chicago, IL (1990)

Gooch, M., and D. Stennett. "Molecular basis of Alzheimer's disease." *Am J. of Health-System Pharmacists* 53: 1545–1547 (1996)

Hayflick, L. *How and Why We Age*. Ballantine Books, New York, NY (1994).

Lamberts, S. W. J., A. W. van den Beld, and A. J. van der Lely. "Endocrinology of aging." *Science* 278: 419–424 (1997)

Lamb, M. J. *Biology of Aging*. John Wiley & Sons, New York, NY (1977)

Lazarou J., B. H. Pomeranz, and P. N. Corey. "Incidence of adverse drug reactions in hospitalized patients." *JAMA* 279: 1200–1205 (1998)

McKeown, T. *The Role of Medicine*. Princeton University Press, Princeton, NJ (1979)

McNeill, W. H. *Plagues and Peoples*. Doubleday, New York, NY (1977)

Montagu, J. D. "Length of life in the ancient world: Controlled study." *J Royal Soc Med* 87: 25–26 (1994)

Moore, T. J. *Lifespan.* Simon & Schuster, New York, NY (1993)

Olshansky, S. J., B. A. Caranes, and C. K. Cassel. "In search of Methusalah: Estimating the upper limits to human longevity." *Science* 250: 634–640 (1990)

Pearl, R. *The Rate of Living.* Alfred Knopf. New York, NY (1928)

Preston, S. H. *Mortality Patterns in National Populations.* Academic Press, New York, NY (1976)

Roses, A. D., W. J. Strittmatter, M. A. Pericak-Vance, E. H. Corden, A. M. Saunders, and D. F. Schmechel. "Clinical application of apoplipoprotein E genotyping to Alzheimer's disease." *Lancet* 343: 1564–1565 (1994)

Roy, A. K., and Chatterjee, eds. *Molecular Basis of Ageing.* Academic Press, Orlando, FL (1984)

Saunders, A. M., W. J. Strittmatter, D. Schmechel, P. H. George-hyslop, M. A. Pericak-Vance, S. A. Joo, B. T. Rosi, J. F. Gusella, D. R. Crapper-MacLachlan, and M. J. Alberts. "Association of apolipoprotein E allele ε4 with late-onset familial and sporadic Alzheimer's disease." *Neurology* 43: 1467–1472 (1993)

Schachter F., L. Faure-Delanef, F. Gueno, H. Rouger, P. Froguel, L. Lesueue-Ginot, and D. Cohen. "Genetic associations with human longevity at the apo E and ACE loci." *Nature Genetics* 6: 29–32 (1994)

Seshardri, S., D. Drachman, and C. Lippy. "Apoprotein E-ε4 allele and lifetime risk of Alzheimer's disease." *Arch Neurology* 52: 1074–1079 (1995)

Takata, H., T. Ishii, M. Suzuki, S. Sekiguchi, and H. Iri. "Influence of major histocompatibility complex region genes on human longevity among Okinawan-Japanese centenarians and nonagenarians." *Lancet* ii: 824–826 (1992)

Wilson, P. W. F., R. H. Myers, M. G. Larson, J. M. Ordovas, P. A. Wolf, and E. J. Schaefer. "Apolipoprotein E alleles, dyslipidemia, and coronary heart disease." *JAMA* 272: 1666–1671 (1994)

Chapter 3—THE BIOLOGICAL MARKERS OF AGING

The Duke Longitudinal Studies of Normal Aging 1955–1980: An Overview of History, Design, and Findings. Springer Publishing Co., New York, NY (1985)

Evans, W., and I. H. Rosenberg. *Biomarkers.* Simon & Schuster, New York, NY (1991)

Hayflick, L. *How and Why We Age.* Ballatine Books, New York, NY (1994)

Older and Wiser: The Baltimore Longitudinal Study of Aging. NIH publication no 89-2797. U.S. Printing Office, Washington, DC (1989)

Timiras, P. S., ed. *Physiological Basis of Aging and Geriatrics,* 2nd ed. CRC Press, Boca Raton, FL (1994)

Timiras, P. S., W. B. Quay, and A. Vernakdakis, eds. *Hormones and Aging*. CRC Press, Boca Raton, FL (1995)

Chapter 4—HORMONES: THE SHORT COURSE

De Groot, L. J., M. Besser, H. G. Burger, J. L. Jameson, D. L. Loriaux, J. C. Marshall, W. D. Odell, J. T. Potts, and A. H. Rubenstein, eds. *Endocrinology*, 3rd ed. W. B. Saunders Co., Philadelphia, PA (1995)

Felig, P., J. D. Baxter, and L. A. Frohman. *Endocrinology and Metabolism*, 3rd ed. McGraw-Hill, New York, NY (1995)

Norman, A. W., and G. Litwack. *Hormones*, 2nd ed. Academic Press, New York, NY (1997)

Timiras, P. S., W. B. Quay, and A. Vernakdakis, eds. *Hormones and Aging*. CRC Press, Boca Raton, FL (1995)

Wilson, J. D., and D. W. Foster, eds. *Williams Textbook of Endocrinology*, 8th ed. W. B. Saunders Co., Philadelphia, PA (1992)

Chapter 5—MECHANISMS OF AGING: THE FOUR PILLARS OF AGING

Albanell, J., F. Lonardo, V. Rusch, M. Engelhardt, J. Langenfeld, W. Han, D. Klimstra, E. Venkatraman, M. A. S. Moore, and E. Dmitrovsky. "High telomerase activity in primary lung cancers: Association with increased cell proliferation rates and advanced pathologic stage." *J Nat Cancer Inst* 89: 1609–1615 (1997)

Austad, S. N. *Why We Age*. John Wiley & Sons, New York, NY (1997)

Banks, D. A., and M. Fossel. "Telomeres, cancer, and aging." *JAMA* 278: 1345–1348 (1997)

Baynes, J. W., and V. M. Monnier, eds. *The Maillard Reaction in Aging, Diabetes, and Nutrition*. Alan R. Liss, New York (1989)

Bernardis, L. L., and P. J. Davis. "Aging and the hypothalamus." *Physiol Behavior* 59: 523–536 (1996)

Bodnar, A. G., M. Ouellette, M. Frolkis, S. E. Holt, C-P. Chiu, G. B. Morin, C. B. Harley, J. W. Shay, S. Lichsteiner, and W. E. Wright. "Extension of life-span by introduction of telomerase in normal human cells." *Science* 349–352 (1998)

Cerami, A. "Hypothesis: Glucose as mediator of aging." *J Am Gerontol Soc* 33: 626–634 (1985)

Cerami, A., H. Vlassara, and M. Browlee. "Glucose and aging." *Sci Am* 256: 90–96 (1987)

Dilman, V. M. "Age-associated elevation of hypothalamic threshold to feedback control, and its role in development, aging and disease." *Lancet* ii 1211–1219 (1971)

———. "Hypothalamic mechanisms of aging and of specific age pathology." *Exp Gerontol* 14: 287–300 (1979)

Dilman, V. M., and V. N. Anisimov. "Effect of treatment with phenformin, diphenlhydantoin or L-dopa on life span and tumor incidence in C3H/Sn mice." *Gerontol* 26: 241–246 (1980)

Fraga, C. G., M. K. Shigenaga, J-W. Park, P. Degan, and B. N. Ames. "Oxidative damage to DNA during aging: 8-hydroxy-2'-dexoxyguanosine in rat organ DNA and urine." *Proc Natl Acad Sci USA* 87:4533–4537 (1990)

Harman, D. "Aging: A theory based on free radical and radiation biology." *J Gerontol* 11: 298–309 (1956)

Hayflick, L. "The limited in vitro lifetime of human diploid cell strains." *Exp Cell Res* 37: 614–636 (1965)

———. "The cell biology of human aging." *Sci Am* 242: 58–66 (1980)

———. *How and Why We Age.* Ballantine Books, New York, NY (1994)

Hoos, A., H. H. Hepp, T. Ahlert, G. Bastert, and D. Wallweiner. "Telomerase activity correlates with tumor aggressiveness and reflects therapy effect in breast cancer." *Int J Cancer* 79: 8–12 (1998)

Jarrett, R. J., and J. J. Kern. "Glucose tolerance, age, and circulating insulin." *Lancet* i 806–809 (1967)

Klingehutz, A. J. "Telomerase activation and cancer." *J Mol Med* 75: 45–49 (1997)

Kristal, B. S., and B. P. Yu. "An emerging hypothesis: Synergistic induction of aging by free radicals and Maillard reaction." *J Gerontol Biol Sci* 47: B107–B114 (1992)

Lamberts, S. W. J., A. W. van den Beld, and A. J. van der Lely. "The endocrinology of aging." *Science* 278: 419–424 (1997)

McLay, R. N., S. M. Freeman, R. E. Harlan, C. F. Ide, A. J. Kastin, and J. E. Zadina. "Aging in the hippocampus: Interrelated actions of neurotrophins and glucocorticoids." *Neurosci Behav Rev* 21: 615–629 (1997)

Mobbs, C. V. "Genetic influences on glucose neurotoxicity, aging, and diabetes: A possible role for glucose hysteresis." *Genetica* 91: 239–253 (1993)

Moller, D. E., and J. S. Flier. "Insulin resistance—mechanisms syndromes, and implications." *New Engl J Med* 325: 938–947 (1991)

Nakahara, H., T. Kanno, Y. Inai, K. Utsumi, M. Hiramatsu, A. Mori, and L. Packer. "Mitochrondrial dysfunction in the senescence accelerated mouse (SAM). *Free Radical Biol and Med* 24: 85–92 (1998)

Olovnikov, A. M. "Telomeres, telomerase, and aging: Origin of the theory." *Exp Gerontol* 31: 443–448 (1996)

Olshansky, S. J., B. A. Carnes, and C. Cassel. "In search of Methusaleh: Estimating the upper limits to human longevity." *Science* 250: 634–639 (1990)

Oomura, Y., and H. Yoshimatsu. "Neural network of glucose monitoring system." *K Autonom Nervous System* 10: 359–372 (1984)

Parr, T. "Insulin exposure controls the rate of mammalian aging." *Mech Ageing and Develop* 88: 75–82 (1996)

———. "Insulin exposure and aging theory." *Gerontology* 43: 182–200 (1997)

Ross, R. "The pathogensis of atherosclerosis: A perspective for the 1990s." *Nature* 362: 801–809 (1993)

Sapolsky, R. M., L. C. Krey, and B. S. McEwen. "The neuroendocrinology of stress and aging: The glucocorticoid cascade hypothesis." *Endocrine Rev* 7: 284–301 (1986)

Smith, M. A., S. Taneda, P. L. Richey, S. Miyata, S-D. Yan, D. Stern, L. M. Sayre, V. M. Monnier, and G. Perry. "Advanced Maillard reaction end products are associated with Alzheimer disease pathology." *Proc Natl Acad Sci USA* 91: 5710–5714 (1994)

Strehler, B. L. "Genetic instability as the primary cause of human aging." *Exp Gerontol* 21: 283–319 (1986)

Yen, T-C., Y-S. Chen, K-L. King, S-H. Yeh, and Y-H. Wei. "Liver mitrochrondria respiratory functions decline with age." *Biochem Biophys Res Comm* 165: 994–1003 (1989)

Yu, B. P., ed. *Free Radicals in Aging*. CRC Press, Boca Raton, FL (1993)

Chapter 6—GUARANTEED ANTI-AGING: CALORIE RESTRICTION

Austad, S. N. *Why We Age*. John Wiley & Sons, New York, NY (1997)

Bodkin NL, Ortmeyer HK, and Hansen BC. "Long-term dietary restriction in older-aged rhesus monkeys: Effects on insulin resistance." *J Gerontol Biol Sci Med Sci* 50: B142–B147 (1995)

Cefalu, W. T, J. D. Wagner, Z. Q. Wang, A. D. Bell-Farrow, J. Collins, D. Haskell, R. Bechtold, and T. Morgan. "A study of caloric restriction and cardiovascular aging in cynomolgus monkeys: A potential model for aging research." *J Gerontol Biol Sci Med Sci* 52: B98–B102 (1997)

Cerami, A. "Hypothesis: Glucose as mediator of aging." *J Am Gerontol Soc* 33: 626–634 (1985)

Dilman V. M., and V. N. Ansimov. "Effect of treatment with phenformin, diphenylhdydantoin or L-dopa on life span and tumor incidence in C3H/SN mice." *Gerontol* 26: 241–246 (1980)

Duffy P. H., R. J. Reuers, J. A. Leakey, K. Nakamura, A. Turturro, and R. W. Hart. "Effect of chronic caloric restriction on physiological variables related to energy metabolism in male Fischer 344 rat." *Mech Ageing Dey* 48: 117–133 (1989)

Fernades G., P. Friend, E. J. Yunis, and R. A. Good. "Influence of dietary restriction on immunologic function and renal disease in (NZB×NZW) F_1 mice." *Proc Natl Acad Sci USA* 75: 1500–1504 (1978)

Hayflick, L. *How and Why We Age.* Ballantine Books. New York, NY (1994)

Hansen, B. C., and N. L. Bodkin. "Primary prevention of diabetes mellitus by prevention of obesity in monkeys." *Diabetes* 42: 1809–1814 (1993)

Hensen, B. C., H. K. Ortmeyer, and N. L. Bodkin. "Prevention of obesity in middle-aged monkeys: Food intake during body weight clamp." *Obesity Res* 3: 199S–204S (1995)

Holehan, A. M. and B. J. Merry. "The experimental manipulation of ageing by diet." *Biol Rev* 61: 329–368 (1986)

Ingram, D. K., M. A. Lane, R. G. Cutler, and G. S. Roth. "Longitudinal study of aging in monkeys: Effects of diet retriction." *Neurobiology of Aging* 14: 687–688 (1993)

Iwasaki K., C. A. Gleiser, E. J. Masoro, C. A. McMahan, E.-J. Seo, and B. P. Yu. "The influence of dietary protein source on longevity and age-related disease processes of Fischer rats." *J Gerontol Biol Sci* 43: B5–B12 (1988)

Kalant, N., J. Stewart, and R. Kaplan. "Effect of diet restriction on glucose metabolism and insulin responsiveness in aging rats." *Mech. Ageing and Develop.* 46: 89–104 (1988)

Kagawa, Y. "Impact of westernization on the nutrition of Japanese: Changes in physique, cancer, longevity, and centenarians." *Prev Med* 7: 205–217 (1978)

Kemnitz, J. W., E. B. Roecker, R. Weindruch, D. F. Elson, S. T. Baum, and R. N. Bergman. "Dietary restriction increases insulin sensitivity and lowers blood glucose in rhesus monkeys." *Am J. Physiol.* 266: E540–E547 (1994)

Kemnitz, J. W., R. Weindruch, E. B. Roecker, K. Crawford, P. L. Kaufman, and W. B. Ershler. "Dietary restriction of adult male rhesus monkey: Design, methodology, and preliminary findings from the first year of study." *J Gerontology* 48: B17–B26 (1993)

Kim, J. W., and B. P. Yu. "Characterization of age-related malondialdehyde oxidation. The effect of modulation by food restriction." *Mech Ageing Dev* 50: 277–287 (1989)

Kim, M. J., E. B. Roecher, and R. Weindruch. "Influences of aging and dietary restriction on red blood cell density profiles and antioxidant enzyme activities in rhesus monkey." *Exp Gerontol* 28: 515–527 (1993)

Laganiere, S., and B. P. Yu. "Anti-lipoperoxidation action of food restriction." *Biochem Biophys Res Comm* 45: 1185–1189 (1987)

———. "Effect of chronic food restriction in aging rats: Liver cytosolic antioxidants and related enzymes." *Mech Ageing Dev* 48: 221–226 (1989)

Lane, M. A., S. S. Ball, D. K. Ingram, R. G. Culter, J. Engel, V. Read, and G. S. Roth. "Diet restriction in rhesus monkeys lowers fasting and glucose-stimulated glucoregulatory end points." *Am J Physiol* 268: E941–E948 (1993)

Lane, M. A., A. Z. Reznick, E. M. Tilmont, A. Lanir, S. S. Ball, V. Read, D. K. Ingram, R. G. Culter, and G. S. Roth. "Aging and food restriction alter some indices of bone metabolism in male rhesus monkeys." *J Nutr* 125: 1600–1610 (1995)

Lane, M. A., D. J. Baer, W. V. Rumpler, R. Weindruch, D. K. Ingram, E. M. Tilmont, R. G. Cutler, and G. S. Roth. "Calorie restriction lowers body temperature in rhesus monkeys, consistent with a postulated anti-aging mechanism in rodents." *Proc Natl Acad Sci USA* 93: 4159–4164 (1996)

Lane, M. A., D. K. Ingram, S. S. Ball, and G. S. Roth. "Dehydroepiandrosterone sulfate: A biomarker of primate aging slowed by calorie restriction." *J Clin Endocrinol Metab* 82: 2093–2096 (1997)

Lee, D. W., and B. P. Yu. "Modulation of free radicals and superoxide dimutase by age and dietary restriction." *Aging* 2: 357–362 (1991)

Maestroni, G. J. M., A. Conti, and W. Pierpaoli. "Role of pineal gland in immunity: Circadian synthesis and release of melatonin modulates the antibody response and antagonizes the immuno-suppressive effect of cortisterone." *J Neuroimmunol* 13: 19–30 (1986)

Manson, J. E., W. C. Willet, M. J. Stampfer, G. A. Colditz, D. J. Hunter, C. H. Hennekens, and F. E. Speizer. "Body weight and mortality among women." *New Engl J Med* 333: 667–687 (1995)

Masoro, E. J., B. P. Yu, and H. A. Bertrand. "Action of food restriction in delaying the aging process." *Proc Natl Acad Sci USA* 79: 4239–4241 (1982)

Masoro, E. J., M. S. Katz, and C. A. McMahan. "Evidence for the glycation hypothesis of aging from the food-restricted rodent model." *J Gerontol* 44:B20–B22 (1989)

Masoro, E. J. "Assessment of nutritional components in prolongation of life and health by diet." *Proc. Soc. Exp. Biol. Med.* 193: 31–34 (1990)

Masoro, E. J., R. J. M. McCarter, M. S. Katz, and McMahan. "Dietary restriction alters characteristics of glucose fuel use." *J Gerontol Biol Sci* B202–b208 (1992)

———. "Retardation of aging process by food restriction: An experimental tool." *Am J Clin Nutr* 55:1250S–1252 (1992)

————. "Antiaging action of caloric restriction: Endocrine and metabolic aspects." *Obesity Res* 3: 241S–247S (1995)

McCarter, R. J. and L. Palmer. "Energy metabolism and aging: A lifelong study of Fischer 344 rats." *Am J Physiol* 263: E448–E452 (1992)

McCarter, R., E. J. Masoro, and B. P. Yu. "Does food restriction retard aging by reducing the metabolic rate?" *Am J Physiol* 248: E486–E490 (1985)

McCay, C. M., M. F. Crowell, and L. A. Maynard. "The Effect of retarded growth upon the length of life span upon the ultimate body size." *J Nutr* 10: 63–79 (1935)

Means, L. W., J. L. Higgins, and T. J. Fernandez. "Mid-life onset of dietary restriction extends life and prolongs cognitive functioning." *Physiol Behav* 54: 503–508 (1993)

Meites, J. "Aging: Hypothalmic catecholamines, neuroendocrine-immune interactions, and dietary restriction." *Proc Soc Exp Biol Med* 195: 304–311 (1990)

Melov, S., D. Hinerfeld, L. Esposito, and D. C. Wallace. "Multi-organ characterization of mitochondrial genomic rearrangements in ad libitum and caloric restricted mice show striking somatic mitochondrial DNA rearrangements with age." *Nucleic Acids Res* 25: 974–982 (1997)

Merry, B. J., and A. M. Holehan. "Effects of diet on aging," in *Physiological Basis of Aging and Geriatrics,* 2nd ed., P. S. Timiras, ed. CRC Press, Boca Raton, FL, pp. 285–310 (1994)

Monnier, V. M. "Minireview: Nonenzymatic glycosylation, the Maillard reaction and the aging process." *J Gerontol Biol Sci* 45: B105–B111 (1990)

Nelson, J. F., K. Karelus, M. D. Bergman, and L. S. Felicio. "Neuroendocrine involvement in aging; evidence from studies of reproductive aging and caloric restriction." *Neurobiol of Aging* 16: 837–843 (1995)

Parr, T. "Insulin exposure controls the rate of mammalian aging." *Mech Ageing and Develop* 88: 75–82 (1996)

————. "Insulin exposure and aging theory." *Gerontology* 43: 182–200 (1997)

Ramsey, J. J., E. B. Roecker, R. Weindruch, and J. W. Kemnitz. "Energy expenditure of adult male rhesus monkeys during the first 30 mo of dietary restriction." *Am J Physiol* 272: E901–E907 (1997)

Reaven, G. M., and E. P. Reaven. "Prevention of age-related hypertriglyceridemia by caloric restriction and exercise training in the rat." *Metab* 30: 982–986 (1981)

Sohal, R. S., and B. H. Sohal. "Hydrogen peroxide release by mitochrondria increases during aging." *Mech Ageing Dev* 57: 187–202 (1991)

Sohal, R. S. "Hydrogen peroxide production by mitochrondria may be a biomarker of aging." *Mech Ageing Dev* 60: 189–198 (1991)

Sohal, R. S., H. H. Ku, S. Agarwal, M. J. Forster, and H. Lal. "Oxidative damage, mitochrondial oxidant generation and antioxidant defenses during aging
and in response to food restriction in the mouse." *Mech Ageing Dev* 74: 121–
133 (1994)

Sohal, R. S., and R. Weindruch. "Oxidative stress, caloric restriction, and aging."
Science 273: 59–63 (1996)

Sonntag, W. E., J. E. Lenham, and R. L. Ingram. "Effects of aging and dietary
restriction on tissue protein synthesis: Relationship to plasma insulin-like
growth factor 1." *J Gerontol* 47: B159–B163 (1992)

Trounce, I., E. Byrne, and S. Marzuki. "Decline in skeletal muscle mitochrondrial respiratory chain function: Possible factor in ageing." *Lancet* i 637–639
(1989)

Venkatraman, J. T., and G. Fernades. "Mechanisms of delayed autoimmune disease in B/W mice by Omega-3 lipids and food restriction," in *Nutrition and
Immunology*, R. K. Chandra, ed. ARTS, St. John's Newfoundland,
pp. 309–323 (1992)

Walford, R. L. Maximum Lifespan. W. W. Norton, New York, NY (1983)

———. The 120-Year Diet. Simon & Shuster, New York, NY (1986)

Walford, R. L., S. B. Harris, and M. W. Gunion. "The calorically restricted low-
fat nutrient dense diet in Biosphere 2 significantly lowers blood glucose, total
leukocyte count, cholesterol and blood pressure in humans." *Proc Natl Acad
Sci USA* 89: 11533–11537 (1992)

Walford, R. L., and L. Walford. *The Anti-Aging Plan.* Four Walls Eight Windows, New York, NY (1994)

Ward, W. F. "Food restriction enhances the proteolytic capacity of the aging
liver." *J Gerontol* 43: B121–B124 (1988)

Weed, J. L., M. A. Lane, G. S. Roth, D. L. Speer, and D. K. Ingram. "Activity
measures in rhesus monkeys on long-term calorie restriction." *Physiol Behav*
62: 97–103 (1997)

Weindruch, R. and R. L. Walford. *The retardation of aging and disease by dietary
restriction.* Charles C. Thomas, Springfield, IL (1988)

Weindruch, R. "Caloric restriction and aging." *Sci Am* 274: 46–52 (1996)

Wolff, S. P., Z. A. Bascal, and J. V. Hunt. "Autooxidative glycosylation: Free
radicals and glycation," in Baynes, J. W., and V. M. Monnier, eds., *The Maillard Reaction in Aging, Diabetes, and Nutrition,* pp. 259–273 (1989)

Yu, B. P. "Food restriction research: Past and present status." *Rev Biol Res in
Aging* 4: 349–371 (1990)

Yu, B. P., D. W. Lee, C. G. Marler, and J.-H. Choi. "Mechanism of food restriction: protection of cellular homeostasis." *Proc Soc Exp Bio Med* 193: 13–15 (1990)

———. "How diet influences the aging process of the rat." *Proc Soc Exp Biol Med* 205: 97–105 (1994)

Chapter 7—THE ZONE DIET: CALORIE RESTRICTION WITHOUT HUNGER OR DEPRIVATION

Eaton, B., M. Shostak, and M. Konner. *The Paleolithic Prescription.* Harper & Row, New York, NY (1988)

Jenkins, D. J. A., T. M. S. Wolever, and R. H. Taylor. "Glycemic index of foods: A physiological basis for carbohydrate exchange." *Am. J. Clin. Nutr.* 34: 362–366 (1981)

Jenkins, D. J. A., T. M. S. Wolever, S. Vukson, F. Brighenti, S. C. Cunnane, A. V. Rao, A. L. Jenkins, G. Buckley, and W. Singer. "Nibbling versus gorging: Metabolic advantages of increased meal frequency." *N Engl J Med* 321: 929–934 (1989)

Sears, B. *The Zone.* ReganBooks, New York, NY (1995)

———. *Mastering the Zone.* ReganBooks, New York, NY (1997)

———. *Zone Perfect Meals in Minutes.* ReganBooks, New York, NY (1997)

———. *Zone Food Blocks.* ReganBooks, New York, NY (1998)

Westphal, S. A., M. C. Gannon, and F. Q. Nutrall. "Metabolic response to glucose ingested with various amounts of protein." *Am J Clin Nutr* 62: 267–272 (1990)

Wolever, T. M. S. "Relationship between dietary fiber content and composition in foods and the glycemic index." *Am J Clin Nutr* 51: 72–75 (1990)

Wolever, T. M. S., D. J. A. Jenkins, A. A. Jenkins, and R. G. Josse. "The glycemic index: Methodology and chemical implications." *Am J Clin Nutr* 54: 846–854 (1991)

Wolever, T. M. S., D. J. A. Jenkins, G. R. Collier, R. Lee, G. S. Wong, and R. G. Josse. "Metabolic response to test meals containing different carbohydrate foods: Relationship between rate of digestion and plasma insulin response." *Nutr Res* 8: 573–581 (1988)

Young, V. R. "Protein and amino acid requirements in humans." *Scand J Nutr* 36: 47–56 (1992)

Young, V. R., D. M. Bier, and P. L. Pellert. "A theoretical basis for increasing current estimates of the amino acid requirements in adult men with experimental support." *Am J Clin Nutr* 50: 80–92 (1989)

Chapter 8—TYPE 2 DIABETES: CANARIES IN THE COAL MINE OF AGING

American Diabetes Association. "Economic consequences of diabetes mellitus in the U.S. in 1997." (1997)

———. "Diabetes: 1996 Vital Statistics." (1996)

Chen, Y. D., A. M. Coulston, Z. Ming-Yue, C. B. Hollenbeck, and G. M. Reaven. "Why do low-fat high-carbohydrate diets accentuate postprandial lipemia in patients with NIDDM?" *Diabetes Care* 18: 10–16 (1995)

Garg, A., S. M. Grudy, and R. H. Unger. "Comparison of effects of high and low carbohydrate diets on plasma lipoproteins and insulin sensitivity in patients with mild NIDDM." *Diabetes* 41: 1278–1285 (1992)

Garg, A., J. P. Bantle, R. R. Henry, A. M. Coulston, K. A. Griven, S. K. Raatz, L. Brinkley, I. Chen, S. M. Grundy, B. A. Huet, and G. M. Reaven. "Effects of varying carbohydrate content of diet in patients with non-insulin-dependent diabetes mellitus." *JAMA* 271: 1421–1428 (1994)

Golay, A., A. F. Allaz, Y. Mored, N. de Tonnac, S. Tankova, and G. Reaven. "Similar weight loss with low- or high-carbohydrate diets." *Am J Clin Nutr* 63: 174–178 (1996)

Kemnitz, J. W., E. B. Roecker, R. Weindruch, D. F. Elson, S. T. Baum, and R. N. Bergman. "Dietary restriction increases insulin sensitivity and lower blood glucose in rhesus monkeys." *Am J Physiol* 266: E540–E547 (1994)

van Liew, J. B., F. B. David, P. J. Davis, B. Noble, and Bernardis. "Calorie restriction decreases microalbuminuria associated with aging in barrier raised Fischer 344 rats." *Am J Physiol* 263: F554–F561 (1992)

Markovic, T. P., A. C. Fleury, L. V. Campbell, L. A. Simons, S. Balasubramanian, D. J. Chisholm, and A. B. Jenkins. "Beneficial effect on average lipid levels from energy restriction and fat loss in obese individuals with or without Type 2 diabetes." *Diabetes Care* 21: 695–700 (1998)

Markovic, T. P., A. B. Jenkins, L. V. Campbell, S. M. Furler, E. W. Kragen, and D. J. Chisholm. "The determinants of glycemic responses to diet restriction and weight loss in obesity and NIDDM." *Diabetes Care* 21: 687–694 (1998)

Parillo, M., A. A. Rivellese, A. V. Ciardullo, B. Capaldo, A. Giacco, S. Genovese, and G. Riccardi. "A high-monounsaturated-fat/low carbohydrate diet improves peripheral insulin sensitivity in non-insulin dependent diabetic patients." *Metab* 41: 1373–1378 (1992)

Rasmussen, O. W., C. Thomsen, K. W. Hansen, M. Vesterlund, E. Winther, and K. Hermansen. "Effects on blood pressure, glucose, and lipid levels of a high-monounsaturated fat diet compared with a high-carbohydrate diet in non-insulin dependent subjects." *Diabetes Care* 16: 1565–1571 (1993)

Robin, R. J., W. M. Altman, and D. N. Mendelson. "Health care expenditures for people with diabetes mellitus." *J Clin Endocrinol Metab* 78: 809A–809F (1992)

Chapter 9—EXERCISE: ANOTHER DRUG TO ALTER HORMONES

Ainsworth, B. E., W. L. Haskel, A. S. Leon, D. R. Jacobs, H. J. Montoye, J. F. Sallis, and R. S. Paffenbarger. "Compendium of physical activities: Classification of energy costs of human physical effort." *Med Sci Sports Exercise* 25: 71–80 (1993)

Alessio, H. M. "Exercise-induced oxidative stress." *Med Sci Sports Exercise* 25: 218–224 (1993)

Bernstein, L., B. E. Henderson, R. Hanisch, J. Sullivan-Halley, and R. K. Ross. "Physical exercise and reduced risk of breast cancer in young women." *J Natl Cancer Inst* 86: 1403–1408 (1994)

Blair, S. N., H. W. Kohl, R. S. Paffenbarger, D. G. Clark, K. H. Cooper, and L. W. Gibbons. "Physical fitness and all-cause mortality: A prospective study of healthy men and women." *JAMA* 262: 2395–2401 (1989)

Blair, S. N., H. W. Kohl, N. F. Gordon, and R. S. Paffenbarger. "How much physical activity is good for health?" *Ann Rev Pub Health* 13: 99–126 (1992)

Brown, R. L. *The 10-Minute LEAP.* Regan Books, New York, NY (1998)

Cooper, K. H. *Antioxidant Revolution.* Thomas Nelson, Nashville, TN (1994)

Cumming, D. C. "Hormones and athletic performance," in *Endocrinology and Metabolism,* 3rd edition, P. Felig, J. D. Baxter, and L. A. Frohman, eds. McGraw-Hill, New York, NY (1995)

D'Avanzo, B., O. Nanni, C. La Vecchia, S. Franceshchi, E. Negri, A. Giacosa, E. Conti, M. Montella, R. Talamini, and A. Cecarli. "Physical activity and breast cancer risk." *Cancer Epidemiol Biomarkers Prev* 5: 155–160 (1996)

Felig, P., and J. Wahren. "Fuel homeostasis in exercise." *N Engl J Med* 293: 1078–1984 (1975)

Fiatarone, M. A., E. C. Marks, N. D. Ryan, C. N. Meredith, L. A. Lipsitz, and W. J. Evans. "High-intensity strength training in nonagenarians: Effects on skeletal muscle." *JAMA* 263: 3029–3034 (1990)

Folsom, A. R., D. R. Jacobs, L. E. Wagenknecht, S. P. Winkart, C. Yunis, J. E. Hilner, P. J. Savage, D. E. Smith, and J. M. Flack, "Increase in fasting insulin and glucose over seven years with increasing weight and inactivity of young adults." *Am J Epidem* 144: 235–246 (1996)

Frontera, W. R., C. Meredith, K. O'Reilly, H. Knuttgen, and W. Evans.

"Strength conditioning in older men: Skeletal muscle hypertrophy and improved function." *J Appl Physiol* 64: 1038–1044 (1988)

Galbo, H, J. J. Holst, and N. J. Christensen. "Glucagon and plasma catecholamine response to graded and prolonged exercise in man." *J Appl Physiol* 38: 70–76 (1975)

————. "The effect of different diets of insulin on the hormonal response to prolonged exercise." *Acta Physiol Scand* 107: 19–32 (1979)

Goldbourt, U. "Physical activity, long-term CHD mortality and longevity: A review of studies over the last 30 years," in *Nutrition and Fitness: Metabolic and Behavioral Aspects to Health and Disease,* A. P. Simopoulos, and K. N. Pavlou, eds. 82: 229–239 (1997)

Hein, H. O., P. Saudicani, and F. Gyntelberg. "Physical fitness or physical activity as a predictor of ischaemic heart disease: A 17-year follow-up in the Copenhagen Male Study." *J Int Med* 232: 471–479 (1992)

Helmrich, S. P., D. R. Ragland, R. W. Leung, and R. S. Paffenbarger. "Physical activity and reduced occurrence of non-insulin dependent diabetes mellitus." *N Engl J Med* 325: 147–152 (1991)

Holloszy, J. O., J. Schultz, J. Kusnierkiewicz, J. M. Hagberg, and A. A. Ehsani. "Effects of exercise on glucose tolerance and insulin resistance." *Acta Med Scand* 711: 55–65 (1996)

Kraemer, W. J. "Influence of the endocrine system on resistance training adaptations." *National Strength and Conditioning Association Journal* 14: 47–53 (1992)

Lee, I.-M., J. E. Manson, C. H. Hennekens, and R. S. Paffenbarger. "Chronic disease in former college students. Body weight and mortality: A 27-year follow-up of middle-aged men." *JAMA* 270: 2823–2828 (1990)

Lee, I.-M., and R. S. Paffenbarger. "Change in body weight and longevity." *JAMA* 268: 2045–2049 (1992)

Lee, I.-M., C.-C. Hsieh, and R. S. Paffenbarger. "Chronic disease in former college students: Exercise intensity and longevity in men." *JAMA* 273: 1179–1184 (1995)

Leon, A. S., J. Connett, D. R. Jacobs, and R. Rauramaa. "Leisure-time physical activity levels and risk of coronary heart disease and death: The Multiple Risk Factor Intervention Trial." *JAMA* 258: 2388–2395 (1987)

Laron, Z., and Regal, A. D., eds. *Hormones and Sports.* Raven Press, New York, NY (1989)

Manson, J. E., E. B. Rimm, M. J. Stampfer, G. A. Colditz, W. C. Willett, A. S. Krolewski, B. Rosner, C. H. Hennekens, and F. E. Speizer. "Physical activity and incidence of non-insulin dependent diabetes mellitus in women." *Lancet* 338: 774–778 (1991)

Manson, J. E., G. A. Colditz, M. J. Stampfer. "Parity, ponderosity, and the paradox of a weight-preoccupied society." *JAMA* 271: 1788–1790 (1994)

Mayer-Davis, E. J., R. D'Agostino, A. J. Darter, S. M. Haffner, M. J. Rewers, M. Saad, and R. N. Bergman. "Intensity and amount of physical activity in relation to insulin sensitivity." *JAMA* 279: 669–674 (1998)

Meydani, M., and W. J. Evans. "Free radicals, exercise, and aging," in B. P. Yu, ed., *Free Radicals in Aging*, pp. 183–204. CRC Press, Boca Raton, FL (1993)

Paffenbarger, R. S., and W. E. Hale. "Work activity and coronary heart mortality." *N Engl J Med* 292: 1109–1114 (1970)

Paffenbarger, R. S., and E. Olsen. *Lifefit*. Human Kinetics, Champaign, IL (1996)

Paffenbarger, R. S., R. T. Hyde, and A. L. Wing. "Physical activity and incidence of cancer in diverse populations: A preliminary report." *Am J Clin Nutr* 45: 312–317 (1987)

Paffenbarger, R. S., A. L. Wing, and R. T. Hyde. "Physical activity as an index of heart attack risk in college alumni." *Am J Epidemiology* 108: 161–175 (1978)

Paffenbarger, R. S., R. T. Hyde, A. L. Wing, and C.-C. Hsieh. "Physical activity, all-cause mortality, and longevity of college alumni." *New Engl J Med* 314: 605–614 (1986)

Papadakis, M. A., D. Grady, D. Black, M. J. Tierney, G. A. W. Gooding, M. Schambelan, and C. Grunfeld. "Growth hormone replacement in healthy older men improves body composition but not functional ability." *Ann Intern Med* 124: 708–716 (1996)

Rauramaa, R., J. T. Salonen, K. Seppanen, R. Salonen, J. M. Venalainen, M. Ihanaien, and V. Rissanen. "Inhibition of platelet aggregability by moderate-intensity physical exercise: A randomized clinical trial in overweight men." *Circulation* 74: 939–944 (1986)

Rogozkin, V. A., *Metabolism and Anabolic Androgenic Steroids*. CRC Press, Boca Raton, FL (1991)

Thune, I., T. Brenn, E. Lund, and M. Garrd. "Physical activity and the risk of breast cancer." *New Engl J Med* 336: 1269–1275 (1997)

Viru, A. *Hormones in Muscular Activity:* Vol. I. *Hormonal Ensemble in Exercise.* CRC Press, Boca Raton, FL (1983)

———. *Hormones in Muscular Activity:* Vol. II. *Adaptive Effects of Hormones in Exercise.* CRC Press, Boca Raton, FL (1983)

———. *Adaptation in Sports Training.* CRC Press, Boca Raton, FL (1995)

Weltman, A., J. Y. Weltman, R. Schurrer, W. S. Evans, J. D. Veldhuis, and

A. D. Rogal. "Endurance training amplifies the pulsatile release of growth hormone: Effects of training intensity." *J Appl Physiol* 72: 2188–2196 (1992)

Willett, W. C., J. E. Manson, M. J. Stampfer, G. A. Colditz, B. Rosher, F. E. Speizer and C. H. Hennekens. "Weight, weight change, and coronary heart disease in women: Risk within the 'normal' weight range." *JAMA* 273: 461–465 (1995)

Wood, P. D., and W. L. Haskel. "The effect of exercise on plasma high-density lipoproteins." *Lipids* 14: 417–427 (1979)

Wood, P. D., M. L. Stefanick, P. T. Williams, and W. T. Haskell. "The effects on plasma lipoproteins of a prudent weight-reducing diet, with or without exercise in overweight men and women." *New Engl J Med* 319: 461–466 (1991)

Yamanouchi, K., T. Shinozaki, K. Chidada, T. Nishidawa, K. Ito, S. Shimizu, N. Ozawa, Y. Suzuki, H. Maeno, and K. Kato. "Daily walking combined with diet therapy is useful means for obese NIDDM patients not only to reduce body weight but also to improve insulin sensitivity." *Diabetes Care* 18: 775–778 (1995)

Zawadzki, K. M., B. B. Yaspelkis, and J. L. Ivy. "Carbohydrate-protein complex increases the rate of muscle glycogen storage after exercise." *J. Appl Physiol* 72: 1854–1859 (1992)

Chapter 10—THE BRAIN: IT'S A TERRIBLE THING TO WASTE

Benson, H. *The Relaxation Response.* William Morrow, New York, NY (1975)
———. *Timeless Healing.* Scribners, New York, NY (1996)

Blaylock, R. L. *Excitotoxins.* Health Press, Santa Fe, NM (1995)

Carrington, P. *The Book of Meditation.* Element Books, Boston, MA (1998)

DeKosy, S., S. Scheef, and C. Cotman. "Elevated corticosterone levels. A possible cause of reduced axon sprouting in aged animals." *Neuroendocrinology* 38: 33–38 (1984)

Goya, L., R. Rivero, and A. M. Pascual-Leone. "Glucocorticoids, stress, and aging," in *Hormones and Aging,* P. S. Timiras, W. B. Quay, and A. Vernadakis, eds. CRC Press, Boca Raton, FL. pp. 249–266 (1995)

Homer, H., D. Packan, and R. M. Sapolsky. "Glucocorticoids inhibit glucose transport in cultured hippocampal neurons and glia." *Neuroendocrinology* 52: 57–63 (1990)

Jacobson, L., and R. M. Sapolsky. "The role of the hippocampus in feedback regulation of the hypthalamic-pituitary-adrenocortical axis." *Endocrine Rev* 12: 118–134 (1991)

Katzman, R., and J. E. Jackson. "Alzheimer disease: Basic and clinical advances." *J Am Geriatrics Soc* 39: 516–525 (1991)

Kerr D., L. Campbell, M. Applegate, A. Brodish, and P. W. Landfield. "Chronic stress-induced acceleration of electrophysiologic and morphometric biomarkers of hippocampal aging." *J Neurosci* 11: 1316–1324 (1991)

Khalsa, D. S. *Brain Longevity*. Warner Books, New York, NY (1997)

Landfield, P. W., J. C. Waymire, and G. Lynch. "Hippocampal aging and adrenocorticoids: A quantitative correlation." *Science* 202: 1098–1102 (1978)

Newcomer, J. W., S. Craft, T. Hershey, K. Askins, and M. E. Bardgett. "Glucocorticoid-induced impairment in declarative memory performance in adult humans." *J Neurosci* 14: 2047–2053 (1994)

Roses, A. D., W. J. Strittmatter, M. A. Pericak-Vance, E. H. Corden, A. M. Saunders, and D. E. Schmechel. "Clinical application of apoplipoprotein E genotyping to Alzheimer's disease." *Lancet* 343: 1564–1565 (1994)

Sapolsky, R. M., L. Krey, and B. S. McEwen. "Stress down regulates corticosterone receptors in a site-specific manner in the brain." *Endocrinology* 114: 287–192 (1984)

Sapolsky, R. M., L. Krey, and B. S. McEwen. "Glucocorticoid-sensitive hippocampal neurons are involved in terminating the adrenocortical stress response." *Proc Natl Acad Sci USA* 81: 6174–6177 (1984)

Sapolsky, R. M., L. Krey, and B. S. McEwen. "Prolonged glucocorticoid exposure reduces hippocampal neuron number: Implications for aging." *J Neurosci* 5: 1222–1227 (1985)

Sapolsky, R. M., D. R. Packan, and W. W. Vale. "Glucocorticoid toxicity in the hippocampus: In vitro demonstration." *Brain Res* 453: 367–371 (1988)

Sapolsky, R. M., H. Uno, C. S. Rebert, and C. E. Finch. "Hippocampal damage associated with prolonged glucocorticoid exposure in primates." *J Neurosci* 10: 2897–2902 (1990)

Sapolsky, R. M. *Stress, the Aging Brain and the Mechanisms of Neuron Death*. MIT Press, Cambridge, MA (1992)

Saudners, A. M., W. J. Strittmatter, D. Schmechel, P. H. George-Hyslop, M. A. Pericak-Vance, S. H. Joo, B. L. Rosi, J. F. Gusella, D. R. Carpper-MacLachlan, and M. J. Alberts. "Association of apolipoprotein E allele ε4 with late-onset familial and sporadic Alzheimer's disease." *Neurology* 43: 1467–1472 (1993)

Stein-Behrens, B. A., E. M. Elliott, C. A. Miller, J. W. Schlling, R. Newcombe, and R. M. Sapolsky. "Glucocorticoids exacerbate kainic acid-induced extracellular accummulation of excitatory amino acids in the rat hippocampus." *J Neurochem* 58: 1730–1735 (1992)

Sheline, Y., P. W. Wang, M. H. Godo, J. B. Csernansky, and M. W. Vannier.

"Hippocampal atrophy in recurrent major depression." *Proc Natl Acad Sci USA* 93: 3908–3913 (1996)

Terry, R. D., R. DeTeresa, and L. A. Hansen. "Neocortical cell counts in the normal aging adult." *Ann Neurology* 21: 530–539 (1987)

van Eekelen, J. A., and E. R. De Kloet. "Co-localization of brain corticosteroid receptors in the rat hippocampus." *Prog Histochem Cytochem* 26: 250–258 (1992)

Vernadakis, A. "Effects of hormones on neural tissue: In vivo and in vitro studies," in *Hormones and Aging*, P. S. Tim, W. B. Quay, and A. Vernadakis, eds. CRC Press, Boca Raton, FL., pp. 291–314 (1995)

Virgin, C. E., T. P. Hu, D. R. Packan, G. C. Tombaugh, S. H. Yang, H. C. Horner, and R. M. Sapolsky. "Glucocortoids inhibit glucose transport and glutamate uptake in hippocampal astrocytes: Implications for glucocorticoid toxicity." *J Neurochem* 57: 1422–1428 (1991)

Wooley, C., E. Gould, B. S. McEwen. "Exposure to excess glucocorticoids alters dendritic morphology of adult hippocampal pyramidal neurons," *Brain Res* 531: 225–231 (1990)

Chapter 11—ANTI-AGING ZONE LIFESTYLE: THE SELF-CARE PYRAMID

Benson, H. *The Relaxation Response.* William Morrow, New York, NY (1975)

————. *Timeless Healing.* Scribners, New York, NY (1996)

Sears, B. *The Zone.* ReganBooks, New York, NY (1995)

————. *Mastering the Zone.* ReganBooks, New York, NY (1997)

————. *Zone Perfect Meals in Minutes.* ReganBooks, New York, NY (1997)

————. *Zone Food Blocks.* ReganBooks, New York, NY (1998)

Scholsberg, S., and L. Neporent. *Fitness for Dummies.* IDG Books, Foster City, CA (1996)

Chapter 12—YOUR ANTI-AGING ZONE REPORT CARE: THE TESTS YOU WANT TO PASS

Allred, J. B. "Too much of a good thing? An over-emphasis on eating low-fat food may be contributing to the alarming increase in overweight amounts of US adults." *J Am Dietetic Assoc* 95: 417–418 (1995)

Colditz, G. A. "Economic costs of obesity." *Am J Clin Nutr* 55: 503S–507S (1992)

Corti, M-C., J. M. Guraink, M. E. Saliva, T. Harris, T. S. Field, R. B. Wallace, L. F. Berkman, T. E. Seeman, R. J. Glynn, C. H. Hennekens, and R. J. Havlik. "HDL cholesterol predicts coronary heart disease mortality in older persons." *JAMA* 274: 539–544 (1995)

Drexel, H. F. W. Amann, J. Beran, K. Rentsch, R. Candinas, J. Muntwyler, A. Leuthy, T. Gasser, and F. Follath. "Plasma triglycerides and three lipoprotein cholesterol fractions are independent predictors of the extent of coronary atherosclerosis." *Circulation* 90: 2230–2235 (1992)

Gaziano, J. M., C. H. Hennekens, C. H. O'Donnell, J. L. Breslow, and J. E. Buring. "Fasting triglycerides, high-density lipoprotein, and risk of myocardinal infarction." *Circulation* 96: 2520–2525 (1997)

Golay, A., A. F. Allaz, Y. Mored, N. de Tonnac, S. Tankova, and G. Reaven. "Similar weight loss with low- or high-carbohydrate diets." *Am J Clin Nutr* 63: 174–178 (1996)

Gould, K. L. "Very low-fat diets for coronary heart disease: Perhaps, but which one?" *JAMA* 275: 1402–1403 (1996)

Gould, K. L., D. Ornish, L. Scherwitz, S. Brown, R. P. Edens, M. J. Hess, Z. Mullani, L. Bolomey, F. Dobbs, W. T. Armstrong, T. Merritt, T. Potts, S. Sparler, and J. Billings. "Changes in myocardial perfusion abnormalities by positron emission tomography after long-term, intense risk factor modification." *JAMA* 274: 894–901 (1995)

Knopp, R. H., C. E. Walden, B. M. Retzlaff, B. S. McCann, A. A. Dowdy, J. J. Albers, G. O. Gey, and M. N. Copper. "Long-term cholesterol-lowering effects of 4 fat-restricted diets in hypercholesterolemic and combined hyperlipidemic men." *JAMA* 278: 1509–1515 (1997)

Knopp, R. H. "Serum lipids after a low-fat diet." *JAMA* 279: 1345–1346 (1998)

Kaczmarski, R. J., K. M. Flegal, S. M. Campbell, and C. L. Joshnson. "Increasing prevalence of overweight among U.S. adults." *JAMA* 272: 205–211 (1994)

Hamm, P., R. B. Shekelle, and J. Stamler. "Large fluctuations in body weight during young adulthood and 25-year risk of coronary death in men." *Am J Epidemiology* 129: 312–318 (1989)

Heini, A. F., and R. L. Weinsier. "Divergent trends in obesity and fat intake patterns: An American paradox." *Am J Med* 102: 259–264 (1997)

Laws, A., A. C. King, W. L. Haskell, and G. M. Reaven. "Relation of fasting plasma insulin concentrations to high density lipoprotein cholesterol and trigylceride concentrations in man." *Arterioscler & Thromb* 11: 1636–1642 (1991)

Lee, I. M., and R. S. Paffenbarger. "Change in body weight and longevity." *JAMA* 268: 2045–2049 (1992)

Lichenstein, A. H., and L. van Horn. "Very low fat diets." *Circulation* 98: 935–939 (1998)

Markovic, T. P., A. C. Fleury, L. V. Campbell, L. A. Simons, S. Balasubramanian, D. J. Chisholm, and A. B. Jenkins. "Beneficial effect on average lipid levels from energy restriction and fat loss in obese individuals with or without Type 2 diabetes." *Diabetes Care* 21: 695–700 (1998)

Markovic, T. P., S. M. Furler, A. B. Jenkins, E. W. Kraegen, L. V. Campbell, and D. J. Chisholm. "The determinants of glycemic responses to diet restriction and weight loss in obesity and NIDDM." *Diabetes Care* 21: 687–694 (1988)

Ornish, D., S. E. Brown, L. W. Scherwitz, J. H. Billings, W. T. Armstrong, T. A. Ports, S. M. McLanahan, R. L. Kirkeeide, R. J. Brand, and K. L. Gould. "Can lifestyle changes reverse coronary heart disease?" *Lancet* 336: 129–133 (1990)

Patch, J. R., G. Miesenbock, T. Hopferwieser, V. Muhlberger, E. Knapp, J. K. Dunn, A. M. Gotto, and W. Patsch. "Relation of triglyceride metabolism and coronary artery disease." *Arteriosclerosis and Thrombosis* 12: 1336–1345 (1992)

Thompson, P. D. "More on low-fat diets." *New Engl J Med* 338: 1623–1624 (1998)

Willett, W. C., J. E. Manson, M. J. Stampfer, G. A. Colditz, B. Rosner, F. E. Speizer, and C. H. Hennekens. "Weight, weight change, and coronary heart disease in women." *JAMA* 273: 461–465 (1995)

Chapter 13—HORMONES: THE LONG COURSE

De Groot, L. J., M. Besser, H. G. Burger, J. L. Jameson, D. L. Loriaux, J. C. Marshall, W. D. Odell, J. T. Potts, and A. H. Rubenstein, eds. *Endocrinology*, 3rd ed. W. B. Saunders Co., Philadelphia, PA (1995)

Felig, P., J. D. Baxter, and L. A. Frohman. *Endocrinology and Metabolism*, 3rd ed. McGraw-Hill, New York, NY (1995)

Timiras, P. S., W. B. Quay, and A. Vernakdakis, eds. *Hormones and Aging*. CRC Press, Boca Raton, FL (1995)

Timiras, P. S., ed. *Physiological Basis of Aging and Geriatrics*, 2nd ed. CRC Press, Boca Raton, FL (1994)

Pinkey, J. A., C. D. Stenhower, S. W. Coppack, and J. S. Yudkin. "Endothelial cell dysfunction: Cause of insulin resistance syndrome." *Diabetes* 46: S9–S13 (1997)

Norman, A. W., and G. Litwack. *Hormones*, 2nd ed. Academic Press, New York, NY (1997)

Wilson, J. D., and D. W. Foster, eds. *Williams Textbook of Endocrinology*, 8th ed. W. B. Saunders Co., Philadelphia, PA (1992)

Chapter 14—INSULIN: YOUR PASSPORT TO ACCELERATED AGING

Austin, M. A., J. L. Breslow, C. H. Hennekens, J. E. Buring, W. C. Willett, and R. M. Krauss. "Low density lipoprotein subclass patterns and risk of myocardinal infarction." *JAMA* 260: 1917–1920 (1988)

Austin, M. A. "Plasma triglyceride and coronary heart disease." *Arterioscler Thromb Vasc Biol* 11: 2–14 (1991)

Baba, T., and S. Neugebauer. "The link between insulin resistance and hypertension: Effects of antihypertensive and antihyperlipidaemic drugs on insulin sensitivity." *Drugs* 47: 383–404 (1994)

Bao, W., S. R. Srinivasan, and G. S. Berenson. "Persistent elevation of plasma insulin levels is associated with increased cardiovascular risk in children and young adults." *Circulation* 93: 54–59 (1996)

Black, H. R. "The coronary artery disease paradox. The role of hyperinsulinemia and insulin resistance and implications for therapy." *J Cardiovascular Pharmacol* 15: 26S–38S (1990)

Bonora, E., J. Willeit, S. Kiechl, F. Oberhollenzer, G. Egger, R. Bonadonna, and M. Meggeo. "U-shaped and J-shaped relationships between serum insulin and coronary heart disease in the general population." *Diabetes Care* 21: 221–230 (1998)

Brandes, J. "Insulin induced overeating in the rat." *Physiol Rev* 18: 1095–1102 (1977)

Brenner, R. R. "Nutrition and hormonal factors influencing desaturation of essential fatty acids." *Prog Lipid Res* 20: 41–48 (1982)

Bruning, P. F., J. M. G. Bonfrer, P. A. H. van Noord, A. A. M. Hart, M. de Jong-Bakker, and W. J. Nooijen. "Insulin resistance and breast cancer risk." *Int J Cancer* 52: 511–516 (1992)

Busse, R., and I. Flemining. "Endothelial dysfunction in atherosclerosis." *J Vas Res* 33: 181–194 (1996)

Campbell, L. V., P. E. Marmot, J. A. Dyer, M. Borkman, and L. H. Storlien. "The high-monounsaturated fat diet as a practical alternative for non-insulin dependent diabetes mellitus." *Diabetes Care* 17: 177–182 (1994)

Cincott, A. H., E. Tozzo, and P. W. D. Scislowski. "Bromocriptine/SKF 38393 treatment ameliorates obesity and associated metabolic dysfunction in obese (ob/ob) mice." *Life Sci* 61: 951–956 (1997)

Coresh, J., P. O. Kwiterovich, and H. H. Smith. "Association of plasma triglyceride concentration and LDL particle diameter, density, and chemico-composition with premature coronary artery disease." *J Lipid Res* 34: 1687–1697 (1993)

Corti, M-C., J. M. Guraink, M. E. Saliva, T. Harris, T. S. Field, R. B. Wallace,

L. F. Berkman, T. E. Seeman, R. J. Glynn, C. H. Hennekens, and R. J. Havlik. "HDL cholesterol predicts coronary heart disease mortality in older persons." *JAMA* 274: 539–544 (1995)

Coulston, A. M., G. C. Liu, and G. M. Reaven. "Plasma glucose, insulin and lipid responses to high-carbohydrate, low-fat diets in normal humans." *Metabolism* 32: 52–56 (1983)

Davignon, J., and J. S. Cohn. "Triglycerides: A risk factor for coronary heart disease." *Atherosclerosis* 124: S57–S64 (1996)

Dek, S. B., and M. F. Walsh. "Leukotrienes stimulate insulin release from rat pancreas." *Proc Nat Acad Sci USA* 81: 2199–2202 (1985)

Depres, J-P., B. Lamarche, P. Mauriege, B. Cantin, G. R. Dagenais, S. Moorjani, and P-J. Lupien. "Hyperinsulinemia as an independent risk factor for ischemic heart disease." *New Engl J Med* 334: 952–957 (1996)

Dreon, D., H. A. Fernstrom, B. Miller, and R. M. Krauss. "Low-density lipoprotein subclass patterns and lipoprotein response to a reduced-fat diet in men." *FASEB J* 8: 121–126 (1994)

Drexel, H., F. W. Amann, J. Beran, K. Rentsch, R. Candinas, J. Muntwyler, A. Leuthy, T. Gasser, and F. Follath. "Plasma triglycerides and three lipoprotein cholesterol fractions are independent predictors of the extent of coronary atherosclerosis." *Circulation* 90: 2230–2235 (1992)

Duimetiere, P., E. Eschwege, G. Papoz, J. L. Richard, J. R. Claude, and G. Rosselin. "Relationship of plasma insulin to the incidence of myocardial infarction and coronary heart disease mortality in a middle-aged population." *Diabetologia* 19: 205–210 (1980)

Ducimetiere, P., J. L. Richard, and I. Cambrien. "The pattern of subcutaneous fat distribution in middle-aged men and risk of coronary heart disease." *Int J Obesity* 10: 229–240 (1986)

Eschwege, E., J. L. Richard, N. Thibult, P. Ducimetiere, J. M. Warsnot, J. R. Claude, and G. E. Rosselin. "Coronary heart disease mortality in relation with diabetes, blood glucose, and plasma insulin levels." *Horm Metab Res Suppl* 15: 41–46 (1985)

Fanaian, M., J. Szilasi, L. Storlien, and G. D. Calvert. "The effect of modified fat diet on insulin resistance and metabolic parameters in type II diabetes." *Diabetologia* 39: A7 (1996)

Farquhar, J. W., A. Frank, R. C. Gross, and G. M. Reven. "Glucose, insulin, and triglyceride responses to high and low carbohydrate diets in man." *J Clin Invest* 45: 1648–1656 (1966)

Fontbonne, A., E. Eschwege, F. Cambien, P. Ducimetiere, N. Thibult, J. M. Warnet, J. R. Claude, and G. E. Rosselin. "Hypertriglyceridemia as a risk factor of coronary heart disease in subjects with impaired glucose tolerance or diabetes: Results from the 11-year follow-up of the Paris Prospective Study." *Diabetologia* 32: 300–304 (1989)

Fontbonne, A. "Why can high insulin levels indicate a risk for coronary heart disease." *Diabetologia* 37: 953–955 (1994)

Foster, D. "Insulin resistance—a secret killer?" *N Engl J Med* 320: 733–734 (1989)

Gaziano, J. M., C. H. Hennekens, C. J. O'Donnell, J. L. Breslow, and J. E. Buring. "Fasting triglycerides, high-density lipoproteins and risk of mycardial infarction." *Circulation* 96: 2520–2525 (1997)

Gertler, M., H. E. Leetma, E. Saluste, J. L. Rosenberger, and R. G. Guthrie. "Ischemic heart disease, insulin, carbohydrate and lipid inter-relationship." *Circulation* 46: 103–111 (1972)

Giovannucci, E. "Insulin and colon cancer." *Cancer Causes and Control* 6: 164–179 (1995)

Gillman, M. W., A. Cupples, B. E. Millen, C. Ellison, and P. A. Wolf. "Inverse association of dietary fat with development of ischemic stroke in men." *JAMA* 278: 2145–2150 (1997)

Ginsburg, G. S., C. Safran, and R. C. Pasternak. "Frequency of low serum high-density lipoprotein cholesterol levels in hospitalized patients with desireable total cholesterol levels." *Am J Cardiol* 68: 187–192 (1991)

Gould, K. L., D. Ornish, L. Scherwitz, R. P. Edens, M. J. Hess, L. Bolomey, F. Dobbs, W. T. Armstrong, T. Merrit, T. Ports, S. Sparier, and J. Billings. "Changes in myocardial perfusion abnormalities by positron emission tomography after long-term, intense risk factor modification." *JAMA* 274: 894–901 (1995)

Gould, K. L. "Very low-fat diets for coronary heart disease: Perhaps but which one." *JAMA* 275: 1402–1403 (1996)

Haffner, S. M., L. Mykkanen, M. P. Stern, and R. Valdez, J. A. Heisserman, and R. R. Bowsher. "Relationship of proinsulin and insulin to cardiovascular risk factors in nondiabetic subjects." *Diabetes* 42: 1297–1302 (1993)

Hollenbeck, C., and G. M. Reaven. "Variations in insulin-stimulated glucose uptake in healthy individuals with normal glucose tolerance." *J Clin Endocrinol Metab* 64: 1169–1173 (1987)

Hudgins, L. C., M. Hellerstein, C. Seidman, and J. Hirsch. "Human fatty acid synthesis is stimulated by a eucaloric low fat, high carbohydrate diet." *J Clin Invest* 97: 2081–2091 (1996)

Jeppesen, J., P. Schaaf, C. Jones, M-Y. Zhou, Y. D. Chen, and G. M. Reaven.

"Effects of low-fat, high-carbohydrate diets on risk factors for ischemic heart disease in postmenopausal women." *Am J Clin Nutr* 65: 1027–1033 (1997)

Jones, P. M., and S. J. Persaud. "Arachidonic acid as a second messenger in glucose-induced insulin secretion from pancreatic beta cells." *J Endocrinol* 137: 7–14 (1993)

Job, F. P., J. Wolfertz, R. Meyer, A. Hubinger, F. A. Gries, and H. Kuhn. "Hyperinsulinism in patients with coronary artery disease." *Coronary Artery Disease* 5: 487–492 (1994)

Juhan-Vague, I., M. C. Alessi, and P. Vague. "Increased plasma plasminogen activator inhibitor 1 levels: A possible link between insulin resistance and atherothrombosis." *Diabetoglogia* 34: 457–462 (1991)

Kaplan, N. "The deadly quartet: Upper body obesity, glucose intolerance, hyper-triglyceridemia, and hypertension." *Arch Int Med* 149: 1514–1520 (1989)

Karhapaa, P., M. Malkki, and M. Laakso. "Isolated low HDL cholesterol: An insulin-resistant state." *Diabetes* 43: 411–417 (1994)

Katan, M. B., S. M. Grundy, and W. C. Willett. "Beyond low-fat diets." *N Engl J Med* 337: 563–566 (1997)

Kern, P. A., J. M. Ong, B. Soffan, and J. Carty. "The effects of weight loss on the activity and expression of adipose-tissue lipoprotein lipase in very obese individuals." *N Engl J Med* 322: 1053–1059 (1990)

Knopp, R. H., C. E. Walden, B. M. Retzlaff, B. S. McCann, A. A. Dowdy, J. J. Albers, G. O. Gey, and M. N. Cooper. "Long-term cholesterol-lowering effects of 4 fat-restricted diets in hypercholesterolemic and combined hyper-lipidemic men: the dietary alternative study." *JAMA* 278: 1509–1515 (1997)

Knopp, R. H. "Serum lipids after a low-fat diet." *JAMA* 279: 1345–1346 (1998)

Lakshmanan, M. R., C. M. Nepokroeff, G. C. Ness, R. E. Dugan, and J. W. Porter. "Stimulation by insulin of rat liver beta hydroxy methyl HMGCoA and cholesterol synthesizing activities." *Biochem Biophys Res Comm* 50: 704–710 (1973)

Lamarche, B., J. P. Espres, S. Moorjani, B. Cantin, G. R. Dagenais, and R. J. Lupien. "Triglycerides and HDL-cholesterol as risk factors for ischemic heart disease: Results from the Quebec Cardiovascular Study." *Atherosclerosis* 119: 235–245 (1996)

Lamarche, B., A. Tchernof, G. R. Dagenais, B. Cantin, P. J. Lupien, and J. P. Despres. "Small, dense LDL particles and the risk of ischemic heart disease: Prospective results from the Quebec Cardiovascular Study." *Circulation* 95: 69–75 (1997)

Lamarche, B., A. Tchernot, P. Mauriege, B. Cantin, G. R. Gagenais, P. J. Lu-pien, and J-P. Despres. "Fasting insulin and apolipoprotein B levels and low-density particle size as risk factors for ischemic heart disease." *JAMA* 279: 1955–1961 (1998)

Larsson, B., K. Svarsudd, L. Welin, L. Wilhelmssen, P. Bjorntorp, and G. Tilbin. "Abdominal adipose tissue distribution, obesity and risk of cardiovascular disease and death." *Br Med J* 288: 1401–1404 (1984)

Laws, A., A. C. King, W. L. Haskell, and G. M. Reaven. "Relation of fasting plasma insulin concentration to high density lipoprotein cholesterol and triglyceride concentration in men." *Arterioscler Thromb* 11: 1636–1642 (1991)

Laws, A., and G. M. Reaven. "Evidence for an independent relationship between insulin resistance and fasting HDL-cholesterol, triglyceride and insulin concentrations." *J Int Med* 231: 25–30 (1992)

———. "Insulin resistance and risk factors for coronary heart disease." *Clin Endocrinol Metab* 7: 1063–1078 (1993)

Lichtenstein, A. H., and L. van Horn. "Very low fat diets." *Circulation* 98: 935–939 (1998)

McKeown-Eyssen, G. "Epidemiology of colorectal cancer revisited: Are serum triglycerides and/or plasma glucose associated with risk?" *Cancer Epidemiology, Biomarkers and Prevention* 3: 687–695 (1994)

McNamara, J. R., J. L. Jenner, Z. Li, P. W. Wilson, and E. J. Schaefer. "Change in LDL particle size is associated with change in plasma triglyceride concentration." *Arterioscler Thromb Vasc Biol* 12: 1284–1290 (1992)

Metz, S., M. van Rollins, R. Strife, W. Fujimoto, and R. P. Robertson. "Lipoxygenase pathway in islet endrocrine cells—oxidative metabolism of arachidonic acid promotes insulin release." *J Clin Invest* 71: 1191–1205 (1983)

Metz, S., W. Fujimoto, and R. O. Robertson. "Modulation of insulin secretion by cyclic AMP and prostagladin E." *Metabolism* 31: 1014–1033 (1982)

Mobbs, C. V. "Genetic influences on glucose neurotoxicity, aging and diabetes: A possible role for glucose hysteresis." *Genetica* 91: 239–253 (1993)

Modan, M., J. Or, A. Karasik, Y. Drory, Z. Fuchs, A. Lusky, and A. Cherit. "Hyperinsulinemia, sex, and risk of atherosclerotic cardiovascular disease." *Circulation* 84: 1165–1175 (1991)

Nestler, J. E., N. A. Beer, D. J. Jakubowicz, C. Colombo, and R. M. Beer. "Effects of insulin reduction with benfluorex on serum dehydroepiandrosterone (DHEA), DHEA sulfate, and blood pressure in hypertensive middle-aged and elderly men." *J Clin Endocrinol Metab* 80: 700–706 (1995)

Orchard, T. J., D. J. Becker, M. Bates, L. H. Kuller, and A. L. Drash. "Plasma insulin and lipoprotein concentrations: An atherogenic association?" *Am J Epidem* 118: 326–337 (1983)

Ornish, D., S. E. Brown, L. W. Scherwitz, J. H. Billings, W. T. Armstrong,

T. A. Ports, S. M. McLanahan, R. L. Kirkeeide, R. J. Brand, and K. L. Gould. "Can lifestyle changes reverse coronary heart disease?" *Lancet* 336: 129–133 (1990)

Pek, S. B., and M. F. Walsh. "Leukotrienes stimulate insulin release from rat pancreas." *Pro Nat Acad Sci USA* 82: 2199–2202 (1984)

Perry, I. J., S. G. Wannamethee, P. H. Whincup, A. G. Shaper, M. K. Walker, and K. G. Alberti. "Serum insulin and incident coronary heart disease in middle aged British men." *Am J Epidemiol* 144: 224–234 (1996)

Pinkey, J. A., C. D. Stenhower, S. W. Coppack, and J. S. Yudkin. "Endothelial cell dysfunction: Cause of insulin resistance syndrome." *Diabetes* 46: S9–S13 (1997)

Pyorala, K. "Relationship of glucose tolerance and plasma insulin in the incidence of coronary heart disease: Results from two population studies in Finland." *Diabetes Care* 21: 131–141 (1979)

Pyorala, K., E. Savolainen, S. Kaukula, and J. Haapakowski. "Plasma insulin as a coronary heart disease risk factor." *Acad Med Scand* 701: 38–52 (1985)

Reaven, G. M. "Role of insulin resistance in human disease." *Diabetes* 37: 1595–1607 (1989)

Reaven, G. M., and B. Hoffman. "Abnormalities of carbohydrate metabolism may play a role in the etiology and clinical course of hypertension." *Trends in Pharm Sci* 9: 78–79 (1988)

———. "The role of insulin resistance and hyperinsulinemia in coronary heart disease." *Metab* 41: 16–19 (1992)

———. "Syndrome X: 6 years later." J Intern Med Suppl 736: 13–22 (1994)

Robertson, R. P., D. J. Gavarenski, D. J. Porte, and E. L. Bierman. "Inhibition of in vivo insulin secretion by prostaglandin E1." *J Clin Invest* 54: 310–315 (1974)

Robertson, R. P. "Prostaglandins, glucose homeostasis and diabetes mellitus." *Ann Rev Med* 34: 1–12 (1983)

Rodwell, V. W., J. L. Nordstrom, and Mitschelen. "Regulation of HMG-CoA reductase." *Adv Lipid Res* 14: 1–76 (1976)

Rouse, L. R., K. D. Hammel, and M. D. Jensen. "Effects of isoenergetic, low-fat diets on energy metabolism in lean and obese women." *Am J Clin Nutr* 60: 470–475 (1994)

Ruderman, N., and C. Haudenschild. "Diabetes as an atherogenic factor." *Prog in Cardiovasc Diseases* 26: 373–412 (1984)

Sacca, L., G. Perez, F. Pengo, I. Pascucci, and M. Conorelli. "Reduction of circulating insulin levels during the infusion of different prostaglandins in the rat." *Acta Endocrinol* 79: 266–274 (1975)

Salmeron, J., J. E. Manson, and W. C. Wilett. "Dietary fiber, glycemic load, and risk of non-insulin dependent diabetes mellitus in women." *JAMA* 277: 472–477 (1997)

Salmeron, J., A. Ascherio, E. Rimm, G. A. Colditz, D. Spiegelman, D. J. Jenkins, M. J. Stampfer, A. L. Wing, and W. C. Willett. "Dietary fiber, glycemic load, and risk of NIDDM in men." *Diabetes Care* 20: 545–550 (1997)

Sadur, C. N., and R. H. Eckel. "Insulin stimulation of adipose tissue lipoprotein lipase." *J Clin Invest* 69: 1119–1123 (1982)

Schapira, D. V., N. B. Kumar, G. H. Lyman, and C. E. Cox. "Abdominal obesity and breast cancer risk." *Ann Int Med* 112: 182–186 (1990)

Schwartz, M. W., D. P. Figlewicz, D. G. Baskin, S. C. Woods, and D. Porte. "Insulin in the brain: A hormonal regulation of energy balance." *Endocrine Rev* 43: 387–414 (1992)

Stern, M. P., and S. M. Haffner. "Bodyfat distribution and hyperinsulinemia as risk factors for diabetes and cardiovascular disease." *Arteriosclerosis* 6: 123–130 (1986)

Stolar, M. "Atherosclerosis in diabetes: The role of hyperinsulinemia." *Metabol* 37: 1–9 (1988)

Stout, R. "The relationship of abnormal circulating insulin levels to atherosclerosis." *Atherosclerosis* 27: 1–13 (1977)

———. "Insulin and atheroma-an update." *Lancet* i: 1077–1079 (1987)

Tchernof, A., B. Lamarche, D. Prud'Homme, A. Nadeau, S. Moorjani, F. Labrie, P. J. Lupien, and J. D. Depres. "The dense LDL phenotype: Association with plasma lipoprotein levels, visceral obesity and hyperinsulinemia in men." *Diabetes Care* 19: 629–637 (1996)

Thompson, P. D. "More on low-fat diets." *New Engl J Med* 338: 1623–1624 (1998)

Torjesen, P. A., K. J. Kirkeland, S. A. Andersson, I. Hjermann, I. Holme, and P. Urdal. "Lifestyle changes may reverse development of the insulin resistance syndrome." *Diabetes Care* 30: 26–31 (1997)

Unger, R. H. "Glucagon and the insulin glucagon ratio in diabetes and other catabolic illnesses." *Diabetes* 20: 834–838 (1971)

Unger, R. H., and P. J. Lefebvre. *Glucagon: Molecular Physiology, Clinical and Therapeutic Implication's*. Pergamon Press, Oxford (1972)

Wellborn, T. A., and K. Wearne. "Coronary heart disease incidence and cardiovascular mortality in Busselton with reference to glucose and insulin concentrations." *Diabetes Care* 2: 154–160 (1979)

Westphal, S. A., M. C. Gannon, and F. Q. Nutrall. "Metabolic response to glucose ingested with various amounts of protein." *Am J Clin Nutr* 62: 267–272 (1990)

Yam, D. "Insulin-cancer relationships: Possible dietary implication." *Med Hypothesis* 38: 111–117 (1992)

Yarnell, J. W. G., P. M. Sweetnam, V. Marks, and J. D. Teale. "Insulin in ischaemic heart disease: Are associations explained by triglyceride concentrations? The Caerphilly Prospective Study." *Br Heart J* 171: 293–296 (1994)

Yost, T. J., and R. H. Eckel. "Fat calories may be preferentially stored in reduced-obese women: A permissive pathway for resumption of the obese state." *J Clin Endocrin* 67: 259–264 (1988)

Zavaroni, I., E. Bonora, M. Pagliara, E. Dall'Aglio, L. Luchetti, G. Buonnanno, P. A. Bonati, M. Bergonzani, L. Gnudi, M. Passeri, and G. Reaven. "Risk factors for coronary artery disease in healthy persons with hyperinsulinemia and normal glucose tolerance." *N Engl J Med* 320: 702–706 (1989)

Zavaroni, I., L. Bonini, M. Fantuzzi, E. Dall'Aglio, M. Passeri, and G. M. Reaven. "Hyperinsulinemia, obesity, and syndrome X." *J Intern Med* 235: 51–56 (1994)

Zavaroni, I., E. Dall'Aglio, O. Alpi, F. Brunschi, E. Bonora, A. Pezzarossa, and U. Butturini. "Evidence for an independent relationship between plasma insulin and concentrations of high density lipoproteins cholesterol and triglycerides." *Atherosclerosis* 55: 259–266 (1985)

Zimmet, P., and S. Baba. "Central obesity, glucose intolerance and other cardiovascular risk factors." *Diabetes Res Clin Proc* 16: S167–S171 (1990)

Chapter 15—CORTISOL: WONDER DRUG OF THE 50S, MESSENGER OF AGING IN THE 90S

Cupps, T. R. and A. S. Fauci. "Corticosteroid-mediated immunoregulation in man." *Immunol Rev* 65: 133–155 (1982)

Fauci, A. S., and D. C. Dale. "The effect of in vivo hydrocortisone on subpopulation of human lymphocytes." *J Clin Invest* 53: 240–246 (1974)

Jefferies, W. *Safe Uses of Cortisone.* Charles C. Thomas, Springfield, IL (1981)

Haynes, B. F. and A. S. Fauci. "The differential effects of in vivo hydrocortisone on kinetics of subpopulations of human peripheral blood thymus-derived lymphocytes." *J Clin Invest* 61: 703–707 (1978)

Munch, A., and G. R. Crabtree. "Glucocorticoid-induced lymphocyte death," in *Cell Death in Biology and Pathology.* I. D. Bower, and R. A. Lockskin, eds. Chapman and Hall, New York, NY, pp 329–357 (1981)

Norman, A. W., and G. Litwack. *Hormones,* 2nd ed. Academic Press, New York, NY (1997)

Orth, D. N. "Cushing's syndrome." *N Engl J Med* 332: 791–803 (1995)

Romero, L. M., K. M. Raley-Susman, D. M. Redish, S. M. Brooke, and R. Sapolsky. "Possible mechanism by which stress accelerates growth of virally derived tumors." *Proc Natl Acad Sci USA* 89: 11,084–11,087 (1992)

Sapolsky, R. M., L. Krey, and B. S. McEwen. "Glucocorticoid-sensitive hippo-campal neurons are involved in terminating the adrenocorticol stress response." *Proc Natl Acad Sci USA* 81: 6174–6177 (1984)

Sapolsky, R. M., L. Krey, and B. S. McEwen. "Stress down regulates corticosterone receptors in a site-specific manner in the brain." *Endocrinology* 114: 287–292 (1984)

Sapolsky, R. M., L. Krey, and B. S. McEwen. "Prolonged glucocorticoid exposure reduces hippocampal neuron number: Implications for aging." *J Neurosci* 5: 1222–1227 (1985)

Sapolsky, R. M., D. R. Packan, and W. W. Vale. "Glucocorticoid toxicity in the hippocampus: In vitro demonstration." *Brain Res* 453: 367–371 (1988)

Sapolsky, R. M., H. Uno, C. S. Rebert, and C. E. Finch. "Hippocampal damage associated with prolonged glucocorticoid exposure in primates." *J Neurosci* 10: 2897–2902 (1990)

Selye, H. "Studies on adaptation." *Endocrinology* 21: 169–188 (1937)

Chapter 16—EICOSANOIDS: YOUR INTEL COMPUTER CHIP

Adam, O. "Polyenoic fatty acid metabolism and effects on prostaglandin biosynthesis in adults and aged persons," in *Polyunsaturated Fatty Acids and Eicosanoids*. American Oil Chemical Society Press. Champaign, IL, pp 213–219 (1987)

Aiello, L. C. and P. Wheeler. "The expensive-tissue hypothesis." *Current Anthropology* 36: 199–221 (1995)

Ascherio, A., C. H. Hennekens, and W. C. Willett. "Trans-fatty acid intake and risk of myocardial infarction." *Circulation* 89: 94–101 (1994)

Ayala, S., G. Gasper, R. R. Brenner, R. Peluffo, and W. J. Kunau. "Fate of linoleic, arachidonic and docosatetraenoic acids in rat testicles." *J Lipid Res* 14: 296–305 (1973)

Bergstrom, S., R. Rhyhage, B. Samuelsson, and J. Sorval. "The structure of prostaglandins E_1, $E_{1\alpha}$ and F_{1B}." *J Biol Chem* 238: 3555–3565 (1963)

Blond, J. P., and P. Lemarchel. "A study on the effect of alpha linolenic acid on the desaturation of dihomo gamma linolenic acid using rat liver homogenates." *Repro Nutr Dev* 24: 1–10 (1984)

Bourre, J. M., M. Piciotti, and O. Dumont. "Delta 6 desaturase in brain and liver during development and aging." Lipids 25: 354–356 (1990)

Brenner, R. R. "Nutrition and hormonal factors influencing desaturation of essential fatty acids." *Prog Lipid Res* 20: 41–48 (1982)

Burr, G. O. and M. R. Burr. "A new deficiency disease produced by rigid exclusion of fat from the diet." *J Biol Chem* 82: 345–367 (1929)

Burr, G. O. and M. R. Burr. "On the nature and role of the fatty acids essential in nutrition." *J Biol Chem* 86: 587–621 (1930)

Burr, M. L., J. F. Gilbert, and N. M. Deadman. "Effects of changes in fat, fish, and fibre intakes on death and myocardial reinfarction: Diet and Reinfarction Trial (DART)." *Lancet* ii: 757–761 (1989)

Herman, A. G., P. M. Vashmouth, W. Denolin, and A. Goursong, eds., *Cardiovascular Pharmacology of Prostglandins.* Raven Press, New York, NY (1982)

Chapkin, R. S., S. D. Somer, and K. L. Erickson. "Dietary manipulation of macrophage phospholipid classes: Selective increase of dihomogamma linolenic acid." *Lipids* 23: 776–770 (1988)

Chatzipanteli, K., S. Rudolph, and L. Axelrod. "Coordinate control of lipolysis by prostaglandin E2 and prostacyclin in rat adipose tissue." *Diabetes* 41: 927–935 (1992)

Claria, J., M. H. Lee, and C. N. Serhan. "Aspirin-triggered lipoxins are generated by human lung adrenocarcinoma cell (A549)-neutrophil interactions and are potent inhibitors of cell proliferation." *Mol Med* 2: 583–596 (1996)

Cleland, L. G., M. J. Jones, M. A. Neuman, M. D'Angel, and R. A. Gibson. "Linolenate inhibits EPA incorporation from dietary fish oil supplements in human subjects." *Am J Clin Nutr* 55: 395–399 (1992)

Coleman, R. A. and P. P. A. Humphrey. "Prostanoid receptors," in J. R. Vane and J. O'Grady, eds. *Therapeutic Applications of Prostaglandins,* Edward Arnold, London, pp 15–25 (1993)

Crawford, M. A. "Fatty acid ratios in free-living and domestic animals." *Lancet* i: 1329–1333 (1968)

Crawford, M. A. and D. Marsh. *The Driving Force: Food, Evolution, and the Future.* Harper & Row, New York (1989)

Daviglus, M. L., M. Stamler, A. J. Orencia, A. R. Dyer, K. Liu, P. Greenland, M. K. Walsh, D. Morris, and R. B. Shekelle. "Fish consumption and the 30-year risk of myocardial infarction." *N Engl J Med* 336: 1046–1053 (1997)

Dehmer, G. J., J. J. Popma, E. K. van den Ber, E. J. Eichorn, J. B. Prewitt, W. B. Campbell, L. Jennings, J. T. Willerson, and J. M. Schmitz. "Reduction in the rate of early restenosis after coronary angioplasty by a diet supplemented with n-3 fatty acids." *N Engl J Med* 319: 733–740 (1988)

Dek, S. B. and M. F. Walsh. "Leukotrienes stimulate insulin release from rat pancreas." *Proc Nat Acad Sci USA* 81: 2199–2202 (1985)

Dolecek, T. A. and G. Grandits. "Dietary polyunsaturated fatty acids and mortality in the multiple risk factor intervention trial (MRFIT)." *World Rev Nutr Diet* 66: 205–216 (1991)

Earle, C. M., E. J. Kenough, Z. S. Wisniewski, A. G. S. Tulloch, D. J. Lord, G. R. Walters, and C. Glatthear. "Prostaglandin E1 therapy for impotence, comparison with papaverine." *J Urology* 143: 57–59 (1990)

Eaton, S. B. "Humans, lipids and evolution." *Lipids* 27: 814–820 (1992)

Eaton, S. B. and M. J. Konner. "Paleolithic nutrition." *N Engl J Med* 312: 283–289 (1985)

Eaton, S. B., M. Shostalle, and M. Konner. *The Paleolithic Prescription.* Harper and Row, New York, NY (1988)

Eaton, S. B. "Stoneagers in the fast lane: Chronic degenerative diseases and evolutionary implications." *Am J Med* 84: 739–749 (1988)

Eaton, B. S. "An evolutionary perspective enhances understanding of human nutritional requirements." *J Nutr* 126: 1732–1740 (1996)

Enders, S., R. Ghorbani, V. E. Kelly, K. Georgilis, G. Lonnerman, J. W. M. van der Meer, J. G. Cannon, T. S. Rogers, M. S. Klempner, P. C. Weber, E. J. Schaefer, S. M. Wolff, and C. A. Dinarello. "The effect of dietary supplementation with n-3 polyunsaturated fatty acids on the synthesis of interleukin-1 and tumor necrosis factor by mononuclear cells." *N Engl J Med* 320: 265–271 (1989)

Ferreria, S. H., S. Moncada, and J. R. Vane. "Indomethacin and aspirin abolish prostaglandin release from the spleen." *Nature* (London) *New Biol* 231: 237–239 (1971)

Gibson, R. A. and G. M. Kneebone. "Fatty acid composition of human colostrum and mature human milk." *Am J Clin Nutr* 34: 252–256 (1981)

Giron, D. J. "Inhibition of viral replication in cell cultures treated with prostaglandin E1." *Proc Soc Exp Bio Med* 170: 25–28 (1982)

Gordon, D., M. A. Bray, and J. Morley. "Control of hymphokine secretion by prostaglandins." *Nature* 262: 401–402 (1976)

Hamberg, M. and B. Samuelsson. "Detection and isolation of an endoperoxide intermediate in prostaglandin biosyntheses." *Proc Natl Acad Sci USA* 70: 899–903 (1973)

Hamberg, M., J. Svensson, and B. Samuelsson. "Thromboxanes: A new group of biologically active compounds derived from prostaglandin endoperoxides." *Proc Nat Acad Sci USA* 72: 2994-2998 (1975)

Hamberg, M., J. Swensson, T. Wakabayashi, and B. Samuelsson. "Isolation and structure of two prostaglandin endoperoxides that cause platelet aggregation." *Proc Nat Acad Sci USA* 71: 345–349 (1974)

Hawthorne, A. B., Y. R. Mahida, A. T. Cole, and C. J. Hawkey. "Aspirin-induced gastric mucosal damage." *Br J Clin Pharmacology* 32: 77–83 (1991)

Hill, E. G., S. B. Johnson, L. D. Lawson, M. M. Mahfouz, and R. T. Holman. "Perturbation of the metabolism of essential fatty acids by dietary partially hydrogenated vegetable oil." *Proc Nat Acad Sci USA* 79: 953–957 (1982)

Honn, K. V., K. K. Nelson, C. Renaud, R. Bazaz, C. A. Diglio, and J. Timar. "Fatty acid modulation of tumor cell adhesion to microvessel endothelium and experimental metasis." *Prostaglandins* 44: 413–429 (1992)

Horrobin, D. F. "Loss of delta 6 desatures activity as a key factor in aging." *Med. Hypothesis* 7: 1211–1220 (1981)

Horrobin, D. F. (ed). *"Omega 6 Essential Fatty Acids."* Wiley-Liss. New York, NY (1990)

Huang, Y. C., J. M. Jessup, and G. L. Blackburn. "N-3 fatty acids decrease colonic epithelial cell proliferation in high-risk bowel mucosa." *Lipids* 31: S313–S316 (1996)

Jensen, R. G. *The Lipids of Human Milk.* CRC Press, Boca Raton, FL (1989)

Johnson, R. A., D. R. Morton, J. A. Kinver, R. R. Gorman, J. C. McGuire, F. F. Sun, N. Whither, S. Bunting, J. Salmon, S. Moncada, and J. R. Vane. "The chemical structure of prostaglandin X (prostacyclin)." *Prostaglandins* 12: 915–928 (1976)

Karmali, R. A. "N-3 fatty acids and cancer." *J Intern Med* 225: 197–200 (1989)

Kirtland, S. J. "Prostaglandin E1. A review." *Prostaglandins, Leukotrienes and Essential Fatty Acids* 32: 165–174 (1988)

Knapp, H. R., I. A. G. Reilly, P. Alessandrini, and G. A. FitzGerald. "In vivo indexes of platelet and vascular function during fish-oil administration in patients with atherosclerosis." *N Engl J Med* 314: 937–942 (1986)

Kromhout, D., E. B. Bosscheter, and C. L. Coulander. "The inverse relationship between fish consumption and 20-year mortality from coronary heart disease." *N Engl J Med* 312: 1205–1209 (1985)

Kunkel, S. L., J. C. Fantone, P. A. Ward, and R. B. Zurier. "Modulation of inflammatory reaction by prostaglandins." *Prog Lipid Res* 20: 633–640 (1982)

Kunkel, S. L., S. B. Thrall, R. G. Kunkel, J. R. McCormick, P. A. Ward, and R. B. Zurier. "Suppression of immune complex vasculitis in rats by prostaglandin." *J Clin Invest* 64: 1525–1529 (1979)

Kuno, S., R. Ueno, O. Hayaishi, H. Nakashima, S. Harada, and N. Yamamoto. "Prostaglandin E2, a seminal constituent, facilitates the replication of acquired immune deficiency syndrome virus in vitro." *Proc Nat Acad Sci USA* 83: 3487–3490 (1986)

Laino, C. "Trans fatty acids in margarine can increase MI risk." *Circulation* 89: 94–101 (1994)

Lands, W. E. M. *Fish and Human Health*. Academic Press. New York, NY (1986)

Leaf, A., G. E. Billman, and H. Hallaq. "Prevention of ischemia-induced ventricular fibrillation by omega-3 fatty acids." *Proc Nat Acad Sci USA* 91: 4427–4430 (1994)

Lee, T. H., R. L. Hoover, J. D. Williams, R. I. Sperling, J. Ravalese, B. W. Spur, D. R. Robinson, E. J. Corey, R. A. Lewis, and K. F. Austen. "Effect of dietary enrichment with eicosapentaenoic acid and docasahexaenoic acid in vitro neutrophil and monocyte leukotriene generation and neurophil function." *N Engl J Med* 312: 1217–1224 (1985)

Chakrin, L. W., and D. M. Bailey, eds. *The Leukotrienes*. Academic Press. New York, NY (1984)

de Lorgeril, M., P. Salen, and J. Delaye. "Effect of a Mediterranean type of diet on the rate of cardiovascular complications in patients with coronary artery disease." *J Amer Coll Cardiology* 28: 1103–1108 (1996)

Leung, K. H. and H. S. Koren. "Regulation of human natural killing: Protective effect of interferon on NK cells and suppression by PGE2." *J Immunol* 129: 1742–1747 (1982)

Liu, B., L. J. Marnett, A. Chaudhary, C. Ji, I. A. Blair, C. R. Johnson, C. A. Diglio, and K. V. Honn. "Biosynthesis of 12-hydroxy eicosatetraenoic acid by B16 amelanotic melanoma cells is a determinant of their metastatic potential." *Lab Invest* 70: 314–323 (1994)

Martin, D. D., M. E. C. Robbins, and D. H. Hussey. "The fatty acid composition of human gliomas differs from that found in non-malignant brain tissue." *Lipids* 31: 1263–1288 (1996)

Mensink, R. P., and M. B. Katan. "Effect of dietary trans fatty acids on high-density and low-density lipoprotein levels in healthy subjects." *N Engl J Med* 323: 439–445 (1990)

Metz, S., M. van Rollins, R. Strife, W. Fujimoto, and R. P. Robertson. "Lipoxygenase pathway in islet endocrine cells—oxidative metabolism of arachidonic acid promotes insulin release." *J Clin Invest* 71: 1191–1205 (1983)

Metz, S., W. Fujimoto, and R. O. Robertson, "Modulation of insulin secretion by cyclic AMP and prostagladin E." *Metabolism* 31: 1014–1033 (1982)

Meydani, S. N. "Modulation of cytokine production by dietary polyunsaturated fatty acids." *Proc Soc Exp Biol Med* 200: 189–193 (1992)

Moncada, S., R. Gryglewsk, S. Bunting, and R. Vane. "An enzyme isolated from arteries transforms prostaglandin endoperoxides to an unstable substance that inhibits platelet aggregation." *Nature* (London) 263: 663–665 (1976)

Murota S., T. Kanayasu, J. Nakano-Hayashi, and I. Morita. "Involvement of eicosanoids in angiogenesis." *Adv Prostaglandins, Thromboxanes and Leukotriene Res* 21: 623–625 (1990)

Nassar, B. A., Y. S. Huang, M. S. Manku, U. M. Das, N. Morse, and D. F. Horrobin. "The influence of dietary manipulation with n-3 and n-6 fatty acids on liver and plasma phospholipids fatty acids in rats." *Lipids* 21: 652–656 (1986)

Ninnemam, J. L. *Prostaglandins, Leukotrienes, and the Immune Response.* Cambridge University Press, New York, NY (1988)

Noguchi, M., D. P. Rose, and Miyazaki. "The role of fatty acids and eicosanoid synthesis inhibitors in breast carcinoma." *Oncology* 52: 265–271 (1995)

Oates, J. A., G. A. FitzGerald, R. A. Branch, E. K. Jackson, H. P. Knapp, and L. J. Roberts. "Clinical implications of prostaglandin and thromboxane A2 formation." *N Engl J Med* 319: 689–698 (1988)

———. "Clinical implications of prostaglandin and thromboxane A2 formation." *N Engl J Med* 319: 761–767 (1988)

Olszewski, A. J. "Fish oil decreases homocysteine in hyperlipidemic men." *Coronary Artery Dis* 4: 53–60 (1993)

Pek, S. B. and M. F. Walsh. "Leukotrienes stimulate insulin release from rat pancreas." *Proc Nat Acad Sci USA* 82: 2199–2202 (1984)

Pelikonova, T., M. Kohout, J. Base, Z. Stefka, J. Kovar, L. Kerdova, and J. Valek. "Effect of acute hyperinsulinemia on fatty acid composition of serum lipids in non-insulin dependent diabetics and healthy men." *Clin Chim Acta* 203: 329–337 (1991)

Phinney, S. "Potential risk of prolonged gamma-linolenic acid use." *Ann Int Med* 120: 692 (1994)

Prickett, J. D., D. R. Robinson, and A. D. Steinberg. "Dietary enrichment with polyunsaturated acid eicosapentaenoic acid prevents proteinuria and prolongs survival in NZB × NZW F1 mice." *J Clin Invest* 68: 556–559 (1981)

Radack, K., C. Deck, and G. Huster. "Dietary supplementation with low-dose fish oils lowers fibrinogen levels." *Ann Int Med* 11: 757–758 (1989)

Raheja, B. S., S. M. Sakidot, R. B. Phatak, and M. B. Rao. "Significance of the N-6/N-3 ratio for insulin action in diabetics." *Annals New York Acad Sci* 983: 258–271 (1993)

Reich, R. and G. R. Martin. "Identification of arachiondic acid pathways required for the invasive and metastic activity of malignant tumor cells." *Prostaglandins* 51: 10–17 (1996)

Renaud, S. and T. Paul. "Cretan Mediterranean diet for prevention of coronary heart disease." *Am J Clin Nutr* 61: 1360S–1367S (1995)

Ridker, P. M., M. Cushman, M. J. Stampfer, R. P. Tracy, and C. H. Hennekens. "Inflammation, aspirin, and the risk of cardiovascular disease in apparently healthy men." *N Engl J Med* 336: 973–979 (1996)

Ridker, P. M., R. J. Glynn, and C. H. Hennekens. "C-reactive protein adds to the predictive value of total and HDL cholesterol in determining risk of first myocardial infarction." *Circulation* 97: 2007–2011 (1997)

Robertson, R. P., D. J. Gavarenski, D. Porte, and E. L. Bierman. "Inhibition of in vivo insulin secretion by prostaglandin E_1." *J Clin Invest* 54: 310–315 (1974)

Robertson, R. P. "Prostaglandins, glucose homeostasis and diabetes mellitus." *Ann Rev Med* 34: 1–12 (1983)

Rolland, P. H., M. Martin, and M. Toga. "Prostaglandin in human breast cancer: Evidence suggesting the elevated prostaglandin production is a marker of high metastatic potential." *J Nat Cancer Inst* 64: 1061–1070 (1980)

Rose, D. P., J. M. Conolly, and M. Coleman. "Effect of omega-3 fatty acids on the progression of metastases after the surgical excision of human breast cancer cell solid tumors growing in nude mice." *Clin Cancer Res* 2: 1751–1756 (1996)

Rose, D. P. "Dietary fatty acids and cancer." *Am J Clin Nutr* 66: 998S–1003S (1997)

Roth, G. J. and P. W. Majerus. "The mechanism of the effect of aspirin on human platelets." *J Clin Invest* 50: 624–632 (1975)

Roth, G. J. and C. J. Siok. "Acetylation of the NH2-terminal series of prostaglandin synthesase by aspirin." *J Biol Chem* 253: 3782–3784 (1975)

Sacca, L., G. Perez, F. Pengo, I. Pascucci, and M. Conorelli. "Reduction of circulating insulin levels during the infusion of different prostaglandins in the rat." *Acta Endocrinol* 79: 266–274 (1975)

Samuelsson, B. "On incorporation of oxygen in the conversion of 8, 11, 14 eicoatrienoic acid into prostaglandin E." *J Am Chem Soc* 89: 3011–3013 (1965)

Schofield, J. G. "Prostaglandin E_1 and the release of growth hormone in vitro." *Nature* 228: 179 (1970)

Schror, K. and H. Sinziner, eds. *Prostaglandins in Clinical Research.* Alan R. Liss, New York, NY (1989)

See, J., W. Shell, O. Matthews, C. Canizales, M. Vargos, J. Giddings, and J. Cerrone. "Prostaglandin E_1 infusion after angioplasty in humans inhibits abrupt occlusion and early restenosis." *Adv Prost Thromboxane and Leukotriene Res* 17: 266–270 (1987)

Serhan, C. N. "Lipoxin biosynthesis and its impact in inflammatory and vascular events." *Biochim Biophys Acta* 1212: 1–25 (1994)

Serhan, C. N. "Lipoxins and novel aspirin-triggered 15-epilipoxins."*Prostaglandins* 53: 107–137 (1997)

Simopoulos, A. P., and J. Robinson. *The Omega Plan.* Harper Collins, New York, NY (1998)

Sinclair, A., and R. Gibson. *Essential Fatty Acids and Eicosanoids."* American Oil Chemical Society, Champaign, IL (1992)

Sinzinger, H., and W. Rogatti, eds. *Prostaglandin E1 in Atherosclerosis.* Springer-Verlag. New York, NY (1986)

Smith, D. L., A. L. Willis, N. Nguyen, D. Conner, S. Zahedi, and J. Fulks. "Eskimo plasma constituents, dihomo gamma linolenic acid, eicosapentaenoic acid and docosahexaenoic acid inhibit the release of atherogenic mitogens." *Lipids* 24: 70–75 (1989)

Stone, K. J., A. L. Willis, M. Hurt, S. J. Kirtland, P. B. A. Kernoff, and G. F. McNichol. "The metabolism of dihomo gamma linolenic acid in man." *Lipids* 14: 174–180 (1979)

Thaler-Dao, H., A. Crastes de Paulet, and R. Paoletti. "Icosanoids and Cancer." Raven Press, New York, NY (1984)

Vane, J. R., and J. O'Grady, eds., *Therapeutic Applications of Prostaglandins.* Edward Arnold, London. (1993)

Vane, J. R. "Inhibition of prostaglandin synthesis as a mechanism of action of aspirin-like drugs." *Nature* (London) *New Biol* 231: 232–235 (1971)

von Euler, U. S. "On the specific vasodilating and plain muscle stimulating substances from accessory genital glands in men and certain animals (prostaglandins and vesiglandin)." *J Physiol* (London) 88: 213–234 (1936)

Watkins, W. D., M. B. Petersen, and J. R. Fletcher, eds., *Prostaglandins in Clinical Practice.* Raven Press. New York, NY (1989)

Westphal, S. A., M. C. Gannon, and F. Q. Nutrall. "Metabolic response to glucose ingested with various amounts of protein." *Am J Clin Nutr* 62: 267–272 (1990)

Willett, W. C., M. J. Stampfer, G. A. Colditz, F. E. Speizer, B. A. Rosner, L. A. Sampson, and C. H. Hennekens. "Intake of trans fatty acids and risk of coronary heart disease among women." *Lancet* 341: 581–585 (1993)

Willis, A. *Handbook of Eicosanoids, Prostglandins and Related Lipids.* CRC Press, Boca Raton, FL (1987)

Williams, L. L., D. M. Doody, and L. A. Horrocks. "Serum fatty acid proportions are altered during the year following acute Epstein-Barr virus infection." *Lipids* 23: 981–988 (1988)

Yam, D., A. Eliraz, B. Eliraz, and M. Elliot. "Diet and disease-the Israeli paradox: Possible dangers of a high omega-6 polyunsaturated fatty acid diet." *Isr J Med Sci* 32: 1134–1143 (1996)

Zurier, R. B. "Prostaglandins, immune responses and murine lupus." *Arth Rheum* 25: 804–809 (1982)

Zurier, R. B. "Eicosanoids and inflammation," in W. D. Watkins, M. B. Peterson, and J. R. Flectcher, eds., *Prostaglandins in Clinical Practice*, Raven Press, New York, NY, pp. 79–96 (1989)

Chapter 17—SEX AND THE ZONE FOR MEN: THE SECRETS OF VIAGRA

Andersson, K-E., and G. Wagner. "Physiology of penile erection." *Physiol Rev* 75: 191–236 (1995)

Burnett, A. L. "The role of nitric oxide in the physiology of erection." *Bio Reprod* 52: 485–489 (1995)

Earle, C. M., E. J. Kenough, Z. S. Wisniewski, A. G. S. Tulloch, D. J. Lord, G. R. Walters, and C. Glatthear. "Prostaglandin E1 therapy for impotence, comparison with papaverine." *J Urology* 143: 57–59 (1990)

Godschalk, M., J. Chen, P. G. Katz, and T. Mulligan. "Prostaglandin E1 as treatment for erectile failure in elderly men." *J Am Geriatr Soc* 42: 1263–1265 (1994)

Goldstein, I., T. F. Lue, H. Padma-Nathan, R. C. Rosen, W. D. Steers, and P. A. Wicker. "Oral sildenafil in the treatment of erectile dysfunction." *N Engl J Med* 338:1397–1404 (1998)

Heller, C. G., and G. B. Meyers. "The male climacteric: Its symptomatology, diagnosis and treatment." *JAMA* 126: 472–479 (1944)

Lamm, S. *The Virility Solution.* Simon & Shuster, New York, NY (1998)

Linet, O. I., and F. G. Orginc. "Efficacy and safety of intracavernosal alprostadil in men with erectile dysfunction." *N Engl J Med* 334: 1–7 (1996)

Lochmann, A., and I. Gallmetzer. "Erectile dysfunction of arterial origin as possible primary manifestation of atherosclerosis." *Minerva Cardioangiol* 44: 243–246 (1996)

Murdock, M. I. "Prostaglandin E-1: A problem-free medication." *Impotence Worldwide* 9: 2–3 (1993)

Rajfer, J., W. J. Aronson, P. A. Bush, F. J. Doresey, and L. J. Ignarro. "Nitric oxide as a mediator of relaxation of the corpus cavernosum in response to nonadrenergic, noncholinergic neurotransmission." *N Engl J Med* 326: 90–94 (1992)

Werner, A. A. "The male climacteric." *JAMA* 112: 1441–1443 (1939)

Chapter 18—SEX AND THE ZONE FOR FEMALES: WHERE HAS THE FERTILITY GONE?

Bruning, P. F., J. M. G. Bonfrer, P. A. H. van Noodr, A. A. M. Hart, M. de Jong-Bakker, and W. J. Nooijen. "Insulin resistance and breast cancer." *Int J Cancer* 52: 511–516 (1992)

Brush, M. G., Watson, D. F. Horrobin, and M. S. Manku. "Abnormal essential fatty acid levels in plasma of women with premenstrual syndrome." *Am J Obstet Gynecol* 150: 363–366 (1984)

Carlson, S., and A. Werkman. "A randomized trial of visual attention of preterm infants fed docosahexaenoic acid until two months." *Lipids* 31: 85–90 (1996)

Cerin, A., A. Collins, B. M. Landgren, and P. Eneroth. "Hormonal and biochemical profiles of premenstrual syndrome: Treatment with essential fatty acids." *Acta Obstet Gynecol Scand* 72: 337–343 (1993)

Gibson, R. A., and G. M. Kneebone. "Fatty acid composition of human colostrum and mature human milk." *Am J Clin Nutr* 34: 252–256 (1981)

Gibson, R. A., M. A. Neuman, and M. Makrides. "Effect of dietary docosahexenoic acid on brain composition and neural function in term infants." *J Lipid Res* 34: S177–S181 (1996)

Holman, R. T., S. B. Johnson, and P. L. Ogburn. "Deficiency of essential fatty acids and membrane fluidity during pregnancy and lactation." *Proc Natl Acad Sci USA* 88: 4835–4839 (1991)

Horwood, L. J. and D. M. Fergusson. "Breast feeding and later cognitive and accademic outcomes." *Pediatrics* 101: E9 (1998)

Johnson, D. L., P. R. Swank, V. M. Howie, C. D. Baldwin, and M. Owen. "Breast feeding and children's intelligence." *Psychol Reports* 79: 1179–1185 (1996)

Kiddy, D. S., D. Hamilton-Fairley, M. Seppala, R. Koistinem, V. H. Jones, M. J. Reed, and S. Franks. "Diet-induced changes in sex hormone binding globulin and free testosterone in women with normal or polycystic ovaries: Correlation with serum insulin and insulin-like growth factor." *Clin Endocrinol* 31: 757–763 (1989)

Kiddy, D. S., D. Hamilton-Fairley, A. Bush, F. Short, V. Anyaoku, M. J. Reed, and S. Franks. "Improvement in endocrine and ovarian function during dietary treatment of obese women with polycystic ovary syndrome." *Clin Endocrinol* 36: 105–111 (1992)

Lanting, C. I., V. Fidler, M. Huisman, B. C. L. Touwen, and E. R. Boersma. "Neurological differences between 9-year-old children fed breast-milk or formula-milk as babies" *Lancet* 344: 1319–1322 (1994)

Lindheim, S. R., S. C. Presser, E. C. Ditkoff, M. A. Vijod, F. Z. Stanczyk, and

R. A. Lobo. "A possible bimodal effect of estrogen on insulin sensitivity in postmenopausal women and the attenuating effect of added progestin." *Fertil Steril* 60: 664–667 (1993)

Lucas, A., R. Morley, T. J. Cole, G. Lister, and C. Leeson-Payne. "Breast milk and subsequent intelligence quotient in children born perterm." *Lancet* 339: 261–264 (1992)

Nestler, J. E., and D. J. Jakubowicz. "Decreases in ovarian cyctochrone P450c17α activity and serum free testosterone after reduction of insulin secretion in polycystic ovary syndrome." *N Engl J Med* 335: 617–623 (1996)

Puolakka, J., L. Makarainen, L. Viinikka, and O. Ylikorkala. "Biochemical and clinical effects of treating the premenstrual syndrome with prostaglandin synthesis precursors." *J Reprod Med* 30: 149–153 (1985)

Schapira, D. V., N. B. Kumar, G. H. Lyman, and C. E. Cox. "Abdominal obesity and breast cancer risk." *Ann Int Med* 112: 182–186 (1990)

Uauy, R., P. Peirano, D. Hoffman, P. Mena, D. Birch, and E. Birch. "Role of essential fatty acids in the function of the developing nervous system." *Lipids* 31: S167–S176 (1996)

Velazquez, E. M., S. Mendoza, T. Hamer, E. Sosa, and C. J. Glueck. "Metformin therapy in polycystic ovary syndrome reduces hyperinsulinemia, insulin resistance, hyperandrogenemia, and systolic blood pressure while facilitating normal menses and pregnancy." *Metabolism* 43: 647–654 (1994)

Watkins, B. A., M. F. Seifert, and K. G. Allen. "Importance of dietary fat in modulating PGE_2 responses and influence of vitamin E on bone morphometry." *World Rev Nutr Diet* 82: 250–259 (1997)

Chapter 19—ESTROGEN: DOES EVERY WOMAN NEED IT?

Asbell, B. *The Pill.* Random House, New York, NY (1995)

Best, J. M., P. B. Berger, V. M. Miller, and A. Lerman. "The effect of estrogen replacement therapy on plasma nitric oxide and endothelin-1 levels in postmenopausal women." *Ann Int Med* 128: 285–268 (1998)

Bruning, P. F., J. M. G. Bonfrer, P. A. H. van Noord, A. Am. Hart, M. de Jong-Bakker, and W. J. Nooijen. "Insulin resistance and breast cancer." *Int J Cancer* 52: 511–516 (1992)

Colditz, G., W. C. Willett, M. J. Stampfer, B. Rosner, F. E. Speizer, and C. H. Hennekens. "Menopause and the risk of coronoary heart disease in women." *N Engl J Med* 316: 1105–1109 (1987)

Colditz, G. A., S. E. Hankinson, D. J. Hunter, W. C. Willet, M. J. Stampfer, C. Hennekens, B. Rosner, and F. E. Speizer. "The use of estrogen and progestins and the risk of breast cancer in postmenopausal women." *N Engl J Med* 332: 1589–1593 (1995)

Collaborative Group on Hormonal Factors in Breast Cancer. "Breast cancer and hormonal contraceptives: Collaborative reanalysis of individual data on 53,297 women with breast cancer and 100,239 women without breast cancer from 54 epidemiological studies." *Lancet* 347: 1713–1727 (1996)

Coney, S. *The Menopause Industry.* Hunter House, Alameda, CA (1994)

Follingstad, A. H. "Estriol, the forgotten estrogen?" *JAMA* 239: 29–30 (1978)

Haffner, S. M., M. S. Katz, and J. F. Dunn. "Increased upper body and overall adiposity is associated with decreased sex hormone binding globulin in post-menopausal women." *Int J Obes* 15: 471–478 (1991)

Henderson, V. W., A. Paganini-Hill, C. K. Emanuel, M. E. Dunn, and J. G. Buckwalter. "Estrogen replacement therapy in older women. Comparisions between Alzeheimer's disease cases and nondemented control subjects." *Arch Neurol* 51: 896–900 (1994)

Hollenbeck, C., and G. M. Reavan. "Variations in insulin-stimulated glucose uptake in healthy individuals with normal glucose tolerance." *J Clin Endocrinol Metab* 64: 1169–1173 (1987)

Hulley, S., D. Grady, T. Bush, C. Furberg, D. Derrington, B. Riggs, and E. Vittinghoff. "Randomized trial of estrogen plus progestin for secondary prevention of coronary heart disease in postmenopausal women." *JAMA* 280: 605–613 (1998)

Kaye, S. A., A. R. Folsom, J. T. Soler, R. J. Prineas, and J. D. Potter. "Associations of body mass index and fat distribution with sex hormone concentration in postmenopausal women." *Int J Epidemiol* 20: 151–156 (1991)

Laux, M., and C. Conrad. *Natural Women. Natural Menopause.* HarperCollins, New York, NY (1998)

Lee, J. R. "Osteoporosis reversal: The role of progesterone." *Int Clin Nutr Rev* 10: 384–391 (1990)

————. *What Your Doctor May Not Tell You About Menopause.* Warner Books, New York, NY (1996)

Lemon, H. M., H. H. Wotiz, L. Parsons, and P. J. Mozden. "Reduced estriol excretion in patients with breast cancer prior to endocrine therapy." *JAMA* 196: 112–120 (1996)

Lindheim, S. R., S. C. Presser, E. C. Ditkoff, M. A. Vijod, F. Z. Stanczyk, and R. A. Lobo. "A possible biomodal effect of estrogen on insulin sensitivity in postmenopausal women and the attenuating effect of added progestin." *Fertil Steril* 60: 664–667 (1993)

Manson, J. E. "Postmenopausal hormone therapy and atherosclerotic disease." *Am Heart J* 128: 1137–1343 (1994)

Nabulsi, A. A., A. R. Folsom, A. White, W. Patsch, G. Heiss, K. K. Wu, and

M. Szko. "Association of hormone-replacement therapy with various cardio-vascular risk factors in postmenopausal women." *New Engl J Med* 328: 1069–1075 (1993)

PEPI Trial. "Effects of estrogen or estrogen/progestin regimens on heart disease risk factors in postmenopausal women." *JAMA* 273: 199–208 (1995)

Phillips, S. M. and B. B. Sherwin. "Effects on estrogen on memory function in surgically menopausal women." *Pscyhoneuroendocrinology* 17: 485–495 (1992)

Prior, J. C. "Progesterone as a bone-trophic hormone." *Endocrine Revs* 11: 386–398 (1990)

Schapira, D. V., N. B. Kumar, G. H. Lyman, C. E. Cox. "Abdominal obesity and breast cancer risk." *Ann Int Med* 112: 182–186 (1990)

Sherwin, B. B. "Sex hormones and psychological functioning in postmenopausal women." *Exp Gerontology* 29: 423–430 (1994)

Simpkin, J. W., M. Singh, and J. Bishop. "The potential role for estrogen replacement therapy in the treatment of cognitive decline and neurodegeneration associated with Alzheimer's disease." *Neurobiol Aging* 15: S195–S197 (1994)

Stanford, J. L., N. S. Weiss, L. F. Voigt, J. R. Daling, L. A. Habel, and M. A. Rossing. "Combined estrogen and progestin hormone replacement therapy in relation to breast cancer in middle-aged women." *JAMA* 274: 178–179 (1995)

Stephanson, J. "More evidence links NSAID's, estrogen use with reduced Alzheimer's risk." *JAMA* 275: 1389–1390 (1996)

Tang, M. X., D. Jacobs, Y. Stern, K. Marder, P. Schofield, B. Gurland, H. Andrews, and R. Mayeux. "Effect of estrogen during menopause on risk and age at onset of Alzheimer's disease." *Lancet* 348: 429–432 (1996)

Wilson, R. *Feminine Forever*. M. Evans & Co., New York, NY (1966)

Ziel, H. K., and W. D. Finkle. "Increased risk of endometrial carcinoma among users of conjugated estrogens." *N Engl J Med* 293: 1167–1170 (1975)

Chapter 20—TESTOSTERONE: HORMONE OF STRENGTH, HORMONE OF DESIRE

Adams, M. R., J. K. Williams, and J. R. Kaplan. "Effects of androgens on coronary artery atherosclerosis and atherosclerosis-related impairment of vascular responsiveness." *Aterioscler Thromb Vasc Biol* 15: 562–570 (1995)

Ajayi, A. A. "Testosterone increases human platelet thromboxane A_2 receptor density and aggregation responses." *Circulation* 91: 2742–2747 (1995)

Bahr, R. *The Virility Factor*. GP Putnam's Sons. New York, NY (1992)

Bancroft, J., and F. C. W. Wu. "Changes in erectile responsiveness during androgen replacement therapy." *Arch Sex Behav* 12: 59–66 (1983)

Barrett-Connor, E. "Lower endogenous androgen levels and dyslipidemia in men with non-insulin-dependent diabetes millitus." *Ann Int Med* 117: 807–811 (1992)

Barrett-Connor E. "Testosterone and risk factors for cardiovascular disease in men." *Diabetes and Metabolism* 21: 156–161 (1995)

Bhasin, S., W. T. Storer, N. Berman, C. Callegari, B. R. Clevenger, J. Phillips, T. J. Bunnell, R. Tricker, A. Shirazi, and R. Casaburi. "The effect of supraphysiologic doses of testosterone on muscle size and strength in normal men." *N Engl J Med* 335: 1–7 (1996)

Carruthers, M. *Maximizing Manhood.* HarperCollins, London, (1997)

Chamness, S. L., D. D. Richer, J. K. Crone, C. L. Dembeck, M. P. Maguire, A. L. Burnett, and T. S. Chang. "The effect of androgen on nitric oxide synthase in the male reproductive tract of the rat." *Fert Stertil* 63: 1101–1107 (1995)

Claustres, M., and C. Sultan. "Androgen and erythropoiesis: Evidence for an androgen receptor in the erythroblasts from human bone marrow cultures." *Hormone Res* 29: 17–22 (1988)

Davis, S. R., P. McCloud, B. J. Strauss, and H. Burger. "Testosterone enhances estradiol's effect on postmenopausal bone density and sexuality." *Maturitas* 21: 227–236 (1995)

Deyssig, R., and M. Weissel. "Ingestion of androgenic-anabolic steroids induces mild thyroid impairment in the male body builders." *Int J Sports Med* 12: 408–412 (1993)

Diamond, J. *Male Menopause.* Sourcebooks, Inc., Naperville, IL (1997)

Ekblom, B., and B. Bergland. "Effect of erythropoietin administration of maximal aerobic power." *Scand J Med Sci Sports* 1: 88–93 (1991)

Erfurth, E. M., and L. E. Hagman. "Decreased serum testosterone and free triiodothyronine levels in healthy middle-aged men indicate an age effect at the pituitary level." *Eur J Endcrinol* 132: 663–667 (1995)

Fiatarone, M. A., E. C. Marks, N. D. Ryan, C. N. Meredith, L. A. Lipsitz, and W. J. Evans. "High-intensity strength training in nonagenarians: Effects on sketletal muscle." *JAMA* 263: 3029–3034 (1990)

Frankle, M. A., R. Eichberg, and S. B. Zachariah. "Anabolic-endrogenic steroids and a stroke in an athlete: Case report." *Arch Phys Med Rehab* 69: 682–683 (1988)

Glueck, C. J., H. I. Glueck, D. Stroop, J. Spiers, T. Hamer, and T. Tracy. "Endogenous testosterone, fibrinolysis, and coronary heart disease risk in hyperlipidemic men." *J Lab Clin Med* 122: 412–420 (1993)

Goh, H.H., D. F. Loke, and S. S. Ratnam. "The impact of long-term testosterone replacement therapy on lipids and lipoprotein profiles in women." *Maturitas* 21: 65–70 (1995)

Haffner, S. M., R. A. Valdez. L. Mykkanen, M. P. Stern, and M. S. Katz. "Decreased testosterone and dehydroepiandrosterone sulfate concentrations are associated with increased insulin and glucose concentration in nondiabetic men." *Metab* 43: 599–603 (1994)

Heller, C. G., and G. B. Myers. "The male climacteric: Its symptomatology, diagnosis and treatment." *JAMA* 126: 472–479 (1994)

Hill, A. *The Testosterone Solution.* Prima Publishing, Rocklin, CA (1997)

Jeppesen, L. L., H. S. Jorgensen, H. Nakayama, H. O. Raaschou, T. S. Olsen, and K. Winther. "Decreased serum testosterone in men with acute ischemic stroke." *Arterioscler Thromb Vas Biol* 16: 749–754 (1996)

Jackson, J. A., M. W. Riggs, and A. M. Spiekerman. "Testosterone dificiency as a risk factor for hip fractures in men: A case-control study." *Am J Med Sci* 304: 4–8 (1992)

Khaw, T-K., and E. Barrett-Conor. "Lower endogenous androgens predict central adiposity in men." *Ann of Epidemiol* 2: 675–682 (1992)

Kirschner, M. A. "Hirsutism and virilism in women." *Endocrin Metab* 6: 55–93 (1984)

Kraemer, W. J. "Influence of the endocrine system on resistance training adaptations." *National Strength and Conditioning Assoc J* 14: 47–53 (1992)

Kreuz, L. E. "Suppression of plasma testosterone levels and psychological stress." *Arch Gen Psychiatry* 26: 479–482 (1972)

Lamb, D. R. "Anabolic steroids in athletes: How well do they work and how dangerous are they?" *An J Sports Med* 12: 31–38 (1994)

Lichtenstein, M. J., J. M. Yarnell, P. C. Elwood, A. D. Beswick, P. M. Sweetnam, V. Marks, D. Teale, and D. Riad-Fahmy. "Sex hormones, insulin, lipids and prevalent ischemic heart disease." *Amer J Epidemiol* 126: 647–657 (1987)

Lochmann, A., and J. Gallmetzer. "Erectile dysfunction of arterial origin as possible primary manifestation of atherosclerosis." *Minerva Cardioangiol* 44: 243–246 (1996)

Marin, P., S. Holmang, L. Jonsson, L. Sjostrom, H. Kvist, G. Holm, G. Lindstedt, and P. Bjorntorp. "The effects of testosterone on body composition and metabolism in middle-aged obese men." *Int J Obes* 16: 991–997 (1992)

Marin, P., M. Krotkiewski, and P. Bjorntrop. "Androgen treatment of middle-aged, obese men: Effects on metabolism, muscle and adipose tissue." *Eur J Med* 1: 329–336 (1992)

Marin, P. "Testosterone and regional fat distribution." *Obesity Res* 3: 609S–612S (1995)

Marques-Vidal, P., P. Sie, J. P. Cambou, H. Chap, and B. Perret. "Relationships of plasminogen activator inhibitor activity and lipoprotein (a) with insulin, testosterone, 17 beta-estradiol, and testosterone binding globulin in myocardial infarction patients and healthy controls." *J Clin Endocrinol Metab* 80: 1794–1798 (1995)

Mazur, A. "Aging and endocrinology." *Science* 279: 305–306 (1998)

Moller, J., and H. Einfeldt. *Testosterone Treatment of Cardiovascular Diseases.* Springer-Verlag, Berlin. (1984)

Nicklas, B. J., A. J. Ryan, M. M. Treuth, S. M. Harman, M. R. Blackman, B. F. Hurley, and M. A. Rogers. "Testosterone, growth hormone and IGF-1 responses to acute and chronic resistive exercise in men aged 55–70 years." *Int J Sports Med* 16: 445–450 (1994)

Parrott, A. C., P. Y. Choi, and M. Davies. "Anabolic steroid use by amateur athletes: Effects upon psychological mood states." *J Sport Med Phy Fitness* 34: 292–298 (1994)

Phillips, G. B., T. Y. Jung, L. M. Resnick, M. Barbagallo, J. A. Laragh, and J. E. Sealey. "Sex hormones and hemostatic risk factors for coronary heart disease in men with hypertension." *J Hypertension* 11: 699–702 (1993)

Phillips, G. B., T. Y. Jung, L. M. Resnick, M. Barbagallo, J. A. Laragh, and J. E. Sealey. "Sex hormones and hemostatic risk factors for coronary heart disease in men with hypertension." *J Hypertension* 11: 699–702 (1993)

Poggi, U. L., A. E. Arquelles, J. Rosner, N. P. de Lalorde, M. H. Cassini, and M. C. Volmer. "Plasma testosterone and serum lipid in male survivors of myocardial infarction." *J Steroid Biochem* 7: 229–237 (1976)

Polderman, K. H., C. D. A. Stehouwer, G. J. Van de Damp, G. A. Kedder, F. W. A. Verheugt, and L. J. G. Gooren. "Influence of sex hormones on plasma endothelin levels." *Ann Int Med* 118: 429–432 (1993)

Pope, H. J., and D. I. Katz. "Psychiatric and medical effects of anabolic-androgen steroid use: A controlled study of 160 athletes." *Arch Gen Psychiatry* 51: 375–382 (1994)

Rako, S. *The Hormone of Desire.* Harmony Books, New York, NY (1996)

Rogozkin, V. A. *Metabolism of Anabolic Androgenic Steroids.* CRC Press, Boca Raton, FL (1991)

Sand, R., and J. Studd. "Exogenous androgens in postmenopausal women." *Am J Med* 98: 76S–79S (1995)

Savvas, M., J. W. Studl, S. Norman, A. T. Leather, T. J. Garnett, and J. Fogellman. "Increase in bone mass after one year of percutaneous oestradiol and testosterone implants in post-menopausal women who have previously received long-term oral osetrogens." *Brit J Obstet Gynaecol* 99: 767–760 (1992)

Schofield, J. G. "Prostglandin E₁ and the release of growth hormone in vitro." *Nature* 228: 179 (1970)

Shahidi, N. T. "Androgens and erythropoiesis." *New Engl J Med* 289: 72–80 (1973)

Shippen, E., and W. Fryer. *The Testosterone Syndrome*. M. Evans & Co., New York, NY (1998)

Simon, D., M. A. Charles, K. Nahoul, G. Ossaud, J. Kremski, V. Hully, E. Joubert, L. Papoz, and E. Esehwege. "Association between plasma total testosterone and cardiovascular risk factors in healthy adult men: The Telecom study." *J Clin Endocrinol Metab* 82: 682–685 (1997)

Simon, D., P. Preziosi, E. Barret-Connor, M. Roger, M. Saint-Paul, K. Nahral, and L. Papoz. "Interrelationship between plasma testosterone and plasma insulin in healthy adult men: The Telecom study." *Diabetologia* 35: 173–177 (1992)

Tenover, J. S., "Effects of testosterone supplementation in the aging male." *J Clin Endocrinol Metab* 75: 1092–1098 (1992)

Tenover, J. S. "Androgen administration to aging men." *Endocrinol Metab clin North Am* 23: 877–892 (1994)

Tibblin, G., A. Adlerberth, G. Lindstedt, and P. Bjorntrop. "The pituitary-gonadal axis and health in elderly men." *Diabetes* 45: 1605–1609 (1996)

Urban, R. J., Y. H. Bodenbury, C. Gilikson, J. Foxworth, A. L. Coggan, R. R. Wolfe, and A. Ferando. "Testosterone administration to elderly men increases muscle strength and protein synthesis." *Am J Physiol* 269: E820–E826 (1995)

Van Goozen, S. H., P. T. Cohen-Kettenis, L. J. Looren, N. H. Frijda, and E. Van de Poll. "Activating effects of androgens on cognitive performance: Causal evidence in a group of female-to-male transsexuals." *Neuropsychologia* 32: 1153–1154 (1994)

Wang, C., G. Alexander, N. Berman, B. Salehian, T. Davidson, V. McDonald, B. Steiner, L. Hull, C. Callegari, and R. T. Swerdloff. "Testosterone replacement therapy improves mood in hypogondal men." *J Clin Endocrinol Metabl* 81: 578–583 (1996)

Werner, A. A. "The male climacteric." *JAMA* 112: 1441–1443 (1939)

Zgliczynski, S., M. Ossowski, J. Slowinska-Srzedricka, A. Brzezinsha, W. Zgliczynski, P. Soszynski, E. Chotkowski, M. Srzednicki, and Z. Sadowski. "Effect of testosterone replacement therapy on lipids and lipoproteins in hypogonadic and elderly men." *Atherosclerosis* 121: 35–43 (1996)

Zumoff, B., G. W. Strain, D. L. K. Miller, and W. Rosner. "Twenty-four hour mean plasma testosterone concentration declines with age in normal pre-menopausal women." *J Endocrin Metab* 80: 1429–1430 (1995)

Zvara, P., R. Sioufi, H. M. Schipper, L. R. Begin, and G. B. Brach. "Nitric oxide mediated erectile activity in the testosterone dependent event: A rat erection model." *Int J Impotence Res* 7: 209–219 (1995)

Chapter 21—GROWTH HORMONE: TURNING BACK THE HANDS OF TIME?

Benbassat, C. A., K. C. Maki, and T. G. Unterman. "Circulating levels of insulin-like growth factor (IGF) binding protein-1 and -3 in aging men: Relationships to insulin glucose, IGF, and dehydroepiandrosterone sulfate levels and anthropometric measures." *J Clin Endocrinol Metab* 82: 1484–1491 (1997)

Crist, D. M., G. T. Peake, P. A. Egan, and D. L. Waters. "Body composition response to exogenenous GH during training in highly conditioned adults." *J Appl Physiol* 65: 579–584 (1988)

Fazio, S., D. Sabatini, C. Capaldo, C. Vigorito, A. Giordano, R. Guida, F. Pardo, B. Biondi, and L. Sacca. "A preliminary study of growth hormone in the treatment of dilated cardiomyopathy." *N Engl J Med* 334: 809–814 (1996)

Fiatarone, M. A., E. C. Marks, N. D. Ryan, C. N. Meredith, L. A. Lipsitz, and W. J. Evans. "High-intensity strength training in nonagenarians: Effect of skeletal muscle." *JAMA* 263: 3029–3034 (1990)

Gama, R., J. D. Teale, and V. Marks. "The effect of synthetic very low calorie diets on the GH-IGF-1 axis in obese subjects." *Clin Chim Acta* 188: 31–38 (1990)

Hartman, M. L., P. E. Clayton, M. L. Johnson, et al. "A low-dose euglycemic infusion of recombinant human insulin-like growth factor-1 rapidly suppresses fasting-enhanced pulsatile growth hormone secretion in humans." *J Clin Invest* 91: 2453–2462 (1993)

Jorgensen, J., N. Vahl, T. Tansen, S. Fisker, C. Hagen, and J. S. Christiansen. "Influence of growth hormone and adrogens on body composition in adults." *Hormone Res* 45: 94–98 (1996)

Klatz, R. *Grow Young with HGH*. Harper Collins, New York, NY (1997)

Kraemer, W. J. "Influence of the endocrine system on resistance training adaptations." *National Strength and Conditioning Association Journal* 14: 47–53 (1992)

Lee, P. D. K., C. A. Conover, and D. R. Powell. "Regulation and function of insulin-like growth factor-binding protein-1." *Proc Soc Exp Biol Med* 204: 4–29 (1993)

McCarty, M. "Up-regulation of IGF binding protein as an anticarcinogenic strategy." *Med Hypothesis* 48: 297–308 (1997)

Miller, E. E., S. G. Cella, M. Parenti, Deghenghi, V. Loctelli, V. deGennaro Colonna, A. Torsell, and D. Cocchi. "Somatrotropic dysregulation in old mammals." *Horm Res* 43: 39–45 (1995)

Morley, J. E., F. Kaiser, W. J. Raum, H. M. Perry, J. F. Flood, J. Jensen, A. J. Silver, and E. Roberts. "Potentially predicative and manipulatable blood serum correlates of aging in the healthy male; progressive decreases in bioavailable testosterone, dehydroepiandrosterone sulfate, and the ratio of insulin-like growth factor 1 to growth hormone." *Proc Natl Acad Sci USA* 94: 7537–7542 (1997)

Papadakis, M. A., D. Grady, D. Black, M. J. Tierney, G. A. W. Gooding, M. Schambelan, and C. Grunfeld. "Growth hormone replacement in healthy older men improves body composition, but not functional ability." *Ann Intern Med* 124: 708–716 (1996)

Regelson, W., and C. Colman. *The Super-Hormone Promise.* Simon & Schuster, New York, NY (1996)

Rogozkin, V. A. *Metabolism of Anabolic Androgenic Steroids.* CRC Press, Boca Raton, FL (1991)

Roth, J. S. M. Gluck, R. S. Yalow, and S. A. Berson. "The influence of blood glucose on the plasma concentration of growth hormone." *Diabetes* 13: 335–361 (1964)

Rudman, D. A. Feller, H. S. Nagrag, G. A. Gergans, P. Y. Lalitha, A. F. Goldberg, R. A. Schlenker, L. Cohn, I. Rudman, and D. E. Mattson. "Effects of human growth hormone in men over 60 years of age." *New Engl J Med* 323: 1–6 (1990)

Schofield, J. G. "Prostglandin E_1 and the release of growth hormone in vitro." *Nature* 228: 179 (1970)

Sonntag, W. E., X. Xu, R. L. Ingram, and A. D'Costa. "Moderate calorie restriction alters the subcellular distribution of somatostatin mRNA and increases growth hormone pulse amptitude in aged animals." *Neuroendocrinology* 61: 601–608 (1995)

Takahoski, Y., D. M. Kipmis, and W. H. Daughaday. "Growth hormone secretion during sleep." *J Clin Invest* 47: 2079–2090 (1968)

Tannenbaum, G. S., and J. B. Martin. "Evidence for an endogenous ultradian rhythm governing growth hormone secretion in the rat." *Endocrinology* 115: 1952–1957 (1986)

Thissen, J-P., J-M. Ketelslegers, and L. E. Underwood. "Nutritional regulation of the insulin-like growth factors." *Endocrine Rev* 15 80–101 (1994)

Uberti, E. C., M. R. Ambrosio, S. B. Cella, A. R. Margutti, G. Trasforini, A. E. Rigamonti, E. Pertrone, and E. E. Muller. "Defective hypothalamic growth hormone (GH)-releasing hormone activity may contribute to declining GH secretion with age in man." *J Clin Endocrinol Metab* 82: 2885–2888 (1997)

Weltman, A., J. Y. Weltman, R. Schurrer, W. S. Evans, J. D. Veldhuis, and A. D. Rogal. "Endurance training amplifies the pulsatile release of growth hormone: Effects of training intensity." *J Appl Physiol* 72: 2188–2196 (1992)

Yamshita, S., S. Melmed. "Effects of insulin on rat anterior pituitary cells: Inhibition of growth hormone secretion and mRNA levels." *Diabetes* 35: 440–447 (1986)

Chapter 22—SEROTONIN: YOUR MORALITY HORMONE

Abdulla, Y. H., and K. Hamadah. "Effect of ADP on PGE formation in blood platelets from patients with depression, mania, and schizophrenia." *Br J Psychiatry* 127: 591–595 (1975)

Adams, P. B., S. Lawson, A. Sanigorski, and A. J. Sinclair. "Arachidonic acid to eicosapentaenoic acid ratio in blood correlates positively with clinical symptoms of depression." *Lipids* 31: S157–S161 (1996)

Brus, R., Z. S. Herman, R. Szhilnik, and J. Zabawska. "Mediation of central prostaglandin effects by serotonergic neurons." *Psychopharmacology* 64: 113–120 (1979)

Calabrese, J. R., R. G. Shwerer, B. Barma, A. D. Gulledge, R. Valenzula, A. Butkus, S. Subichin, and N. E. Drupp. "Depression, immumocompetence, and prostaglandins of the E series." *Psychiatry Research* 17: 41–47 (1986)

Cincott, A. H., E. Tozzo, and P. W. D. Scislowski. "Bromocriptine/SKF 38393 treatment ameliorates obesity and associated metabolic dysfunction in obese (ob/ob) mice." *Life Sci* 61: 951–956 (1997)

Debnath, P. K., S. K. Bhattacharya, A. K. Sanyal, M. K. Poddar, and J. J. Ghosh. "Prostaglandins: Effect of prostaglandin E_1 on brain, stomach and intestinal serotonin in rat." *Biochemical Pharmacology* 27: 130–132 (1978)

Klerman, G. L., and M. M. Weissman. "Increasing rates of depression." *JAMA* 261: 2229–2235 (1989)

Hamazaki, T., S. Sawazaki, and M. Kobayashi. "The effects of docosahexaenoic acid on agression in young adults." *J Clin Invest* 97: 1129–1134 (1996)

Nishino, S., R. Ueno, K. Ohishi, T. Sakai, and O. Hayaishi. "Salivary prostaglandin concentrations: Possible state indicators for major depression." *Amer J Psychiatry* 146: 365–368 (1989)

Norden, M. J. *Beyond Prozac*. ReganBooks, New York, NY (1996)

Ohishi, K., R. Eno, S. Mishimo, T. Sakai, and O. Hyaishi. "Increased level of salivary prostaglandins in patients with major depression." *Biological Psychiatry* 23: 326–334 (1988)

Roy, A., and M. S. Kafka. "Platelet adrenoceptors and prostaglandin responses in depressed patients." *Psychiatry Research* 30: 181–189 (1989)

Sanyal, A. K., K. Srivastava, and S. K. Bhattacharya. "The antinociceptive effect of intracerebroventricularly administered prostagladin E₁ in the rat." *Psychpharmacology* 60: 159–163 (1979)

Sharpe, M., K. Hawton, A. Clements, and P. J. Cowen. "Increased brain serotonin function in men with chronic fatigue syndrome." *Brit Med J* 315: 164–165 (1997)

Stevens, L. J., S. S. Zentall, and J. R. Burgess. "Essential fatty acid metabolism in boys with attention-deficit hyperactivity disorder." *Am J Clin Nutr* 62: 761–768 (1995)

Stevens, L. J., S. S. Aentall, M. L. Abate, T. Kuczek, and J. R. Burgress. "Omega-3 fatty acids in boys with behavior, learning, and health problems." *Physiology and Behavior* 59: 915–920 (1996)

Vikkunen, M. E., D. F. Horrobin, and M. S. Manku. "Plasma phospholipid essential fatty acids and prostaglandins in alcoholic, habitually violent, and impulsive offenders." *Biological Psychiatry* 22: 1087–1096 (1987)

Winokur, A., G. Maislin, J. L. Phillips, and J. D. Amsterdam. "Insulin resistance after oral glucose tolerance testing in patients with major depression." *Amer J Psychiatry* 145: 325–330 (1988)

Wurtman, J. J. *The Serotonin Solution.* Ballantine Books, New York, NY (1996)

Chapter 23—THYROID: THE MYSTERY OF METABOLISM

Anitschkkow, N. "On variations in the rabbit aorta in experimental cholesterol feeding." *Beitr Path Ana v Allegern Path* 56: 379–386 (1913)

Barnes, B. O., and C. W. Barnes. *Solved: The Riddle of Heart Attacks.* Robinson Press, Fort Collins, CO (1976)

Barnes, B. O., and L. Galton. *Hypothyroidism: The Unsuspected Illness.* Harper & Row, New York, NY (1976)

Brent, G. A. "The molecular basis of thyroid action." *N Engl J Med* 331: 847–853 (1994)

Giustna, A., and W. B. Wehrenberg. "Influence of thyroid hormones on the regulation of growth hormone secretion." *J Endocrin* 133: 646–653 (1995)

Fishberg, A. M. "Arteriosclerois in thyroid deficiency." *JAMA* 82: 463–471 (1924)

Friedland, I. B. "Investigations on the influence of thyroid preparations on experimental hypercholesterolemia and atherosclerosis." *Z Ges Exp Med* 87: 683–695 (1933)

Greenspan, S. L., A. Klibanski, J. R. Rowe, and D. Elahi. "Age related alternations in pulsatile secretion of TSH: Role of dopaminergic regulation." *Am J Physiol* 260: E486–E491 (1991)

Greer, M. A., ed. *The Thyroid Gland.* Raven Press, New York, NY (1990)

Malysheva, L. V. "Tisue respiration rate in certain organs in experimental hypercholesterolemia and atherosclerosis." *Fed Proc* 56: T562–T568 (1964)

Murray, G. R. "Note on the treatment of myxoedema by hypodermic injections of an extract of the thyroid gland of sheep." *Brit Med J* ii: 796–799 (1891)

Pasquini, A. M., and A. M. Adamo. "Thyroid hormones and the central nervous system." *Dev Neuosci* 16: 161–168 (1994)

Rosenthal, M. S. *The Thyroid Sourcebook.* Lowell House, Los Angeles, CA (1996)

Ves-Losada, A., and R. O. Peluffo. "Effect of L-triiodthyronine on liver microsomal delta 6 and delta 5 desaturase activity of male rats." *Mol Cell Biochem* 121: 149–153 (1993)

Chapter 24—DHEA AND MELATONIN: THE HAPPAS BROTHERS?

Barlow-Walden, L. R., R. J. Reiter, M. Ale, A. Menendez-Pelaez, L. D. Chen, and B. Poeggeler. "Melatonin stimulates brain peroxidase activity." *Neurochem Int* 26: 497–502 (1995)

Barrett-Connor, E., K. T. Kaw, and S. S. C. Yen. "A prospective study of dehydroepiandrosterone sulfate mortality and cardiovascular disease." *N Engl J Med* 315: 1519–1524 (1986)

Belanger, A., B. Candas, A. Dupont, L. Cusan, P. Diamond, J. L. Gomez, and F. Labrie. "Changes in serum concentrations of conjugated and unconjugated steroids in 40–80 year-old men." *J Clin Endocrin Metab* 79: 1086–1090 (1994)

Cagnacci, A., J. A. Elliott, and S. S. Yen. "Melatonin: A major regulator of the circadian rhythm of core temperature in humans." *J Clin Endocrin Metab* 75: 447–452 (1992)

Cagnoli, C. M., C. Atabay, E. Kharlamova, and H. Marney. "Melatonin protects neurons from singlet oxygen induced apoptosis." *J Pineal Res* 18: 222–226 (1995)

Dilman, V. M., V. N. Anisimov, M. Ostroumova, V. K. Khavinson, and V. G. Morozov. "Increase in lifespan of rats following polypeptide pineal extract treatment." *Exp Pathology* 17: 539–545 (1979)

Dorgan, J. F., F. Z. Stanczyk, C. Longcope, H. E. Stephenson, L. Chang, R. Miller, C. Franz, R. T. Falk, and L. Kahle. "Relationship of serum dehydroepiandrosterone (DHEA), DHEA sulfate, and 5-androstene-3β,17βdiol to risk of breast cancer in postmenopausal women." *Cancer Epidem, Biomarkers & Prevention* 6: 177–181 (1997)

Eich, D. M., J. E. Nestler, D. E. Johnson, G. H. Dworkin, D. Ko, A. S. Wechsler, and M. L. Hess. "Inhibition of accelerated coronary atherosclerosis with dehydroepiandrosterone in the hetretrop rabbit model of cardiac transplantation." *Circulation* 87: 261–269 (1993)

Field, A. E. R., G. A. Colditz, W. C. Willett, C. Longcope, and J. B. McKinalay. "The relation of smoking, age, relative weight, and dietary intake to serum adrenal steroids, sex hormones, and sex hormone-binding globulin in middle aged men." *J Clin Endocrinol Metab* 79: 1310–1316 (1994)

Fleshner, M., C. R. Pugh, D. Tremblay, and J. W. Rudy. "DHEA-S selectively impairs contextual-fear conditioning: Support for the antiglucocorticoid hypothesis." *Behavioral Neurosci* 111: 512–517 (1997)

Gazzah, N., A. Gharib, I. Delton, P. Moliere, G. Durand, R. Christon, M. Lagarde, and N. Sarda. "Effect of an n-3 fatty acid-deficient diet on the adenosine-dependent melatonin release in cultured rat pineal." *J Neurochem* 61: 1057–1063 (1993)

Haffner, S. M., R. A. Valdez, L. Mykkanen, M. P. Stern, and M. S. Katz. "Decreased testosterone and DHEA sulfate concentrations are associated with increased insulin and glucose concentration in nondiabetic men." *Metab* 43: 599–603 (1994)

Hardeland, R., R. J. Reiter, R. Poeggler, and D. X. Tan. "The significance of the metabolism of the neurohormone melatonin: anti-oxidative protection and formation of bioactive substances." *Neuroscience and Behavioral Rev* 17: 347–357 (1993)

Kalimi, M., and W. Regelson. "Physicochemical characterization of (^{3}H) DHEA binding in rat liver." *Biochem Biophys Res Comm* 156: 22–29 (1988)

Kalimi, M., Y. Shafagoj, R. Loria, D. Radgett, and W. Regelson. "Anti-glucocorticoid effects of dehydroepiandrosterone (DHEA)." *Mol Cell Biochem* 131: 99–104 (1994)

Kunkel, S. L., J. C. Fantone, P. A. Ward, and R. B. Zurier. "Modulation of inflammatory reaction by prostaglandins." *Prog Lipid Res* 20: 633–640 (1982)

Labrie, F., A. Belanger, L. Cusan, and B. Candas. "Physiological changes in dehydroepiandrosterone are not reflected by serum levels of active androgens and estrogens, but of their metabolites: Intracrinology." *J Clin Endocrinol Metab* 82: 2403–2409 (1997)

Lane, M. A., D. J. Baer, W. V. Rumpler, R. Weindruch, D. K. Ingram, E. M. Tilmont, R. G. Cutler, and G. S. Roth. "Calorie restriction lowers body temperature in rhesus monkeys, consistent with a postulalted anti-aging mechanism in rodents." *Proc Natl Acad Sci USA* 93: 4159–4164 (1996)

Lane, M. A., D. K. Ingram, S. S. Ball, and G. S. Roth. "Dehydroepiandrosterone sulfate: A biomarker of primate aging slowed by calorie restriction. *J Clin Endocrinol Metab* 82: 2093–2096 (1997)

Lavallee, B., P. R. Provost, Z. Kahwash, J. E. Nestler, and A. Belanger. "Effect of insulin on serum levels of dehydroepiandrosterone metabolites in men." *Clinical Endrocinology* 46: 93–100 (1997)

Leblhuber, F. E., E. Windhager, C. Neubauer, J. Weber, F. Reisecker, and E. Dienstl. "Antiglucocorticoid effects of DHEAS in Alzheimer's disease." *Am J Psychiatry* 149: 1125–1126 (1992)

Martinuzzo, M., M. M. Del Zar, D. P. Cardinali, L. O. Carreras, and M. I. Vacas. "Melatonin effect on arachidonic acid metabolism to cyclooxygenase derivatives in human platelets." *J Pineal Res* 11: 111–115 (1991)

May, M., E. Hollmes, W. Rogers, and M. Poth. "Protection from glucocorticoid induced thymic involution by dehydroepiandrosterone." *Life Sci* 46: 1627–1631 (1990)

Morales, A. J., J. J. Nolan, J. C. Nelson, and S. S. Yen. "Effects of replacement dose of dehydroepiandrosterone in men and women of advancing age." *J Clin Endocrinol Metab* 78: 1360–1367 (1994)

Nair, N. P., N. Hariharasubmenian, C. Pilapil, I. Issue, and J. X. Thavundayil. "Plasma melatonin–an index of brain aging in humans?" *Biological Psychiatry* 21: 141–150 (1986)

Nestler, J. E., K. S. Usiskin, C. O. Barascine, D. F. Welty, J. N. Clore, and W. G. Blackard. "Suppression of serum dehydroepiandrosterone sulfate levels by insulin: An evaluation of possible mechanisms." *J Clin Endocrinology and Metabolism* 69: 1040–1046 (1989)

Nestler, J. E., J. N. Clore, and W. G. Blackard. "Dehydroepiandrosterone: The 'missing link' between hyperinsulinemia and atherosclerosis." *FASEB J* 6: 3073–3075 (1992)

Nestler, J. E., and Z. Kahwash. "Sex-specific action of insulin to actuely increase the metabolic clearance rate of dehydroepiandrosterone in humans." *J Clin Invest* 94: 1483–1489 (1992)

Nestler, J. E., M. A. McClaanahan, J. N. Clore, and W. G. Blackard. "Insulin inhibits adrenal 17,20 lyase activity in man." *J Clin Endrocrinology and Metabolism* 74: 362–367 (1992)

Nestler, J. E. "Insulin and adrenal androgens." *Seminar in Reproductive Endocrinol* 12: 1–5 (1994)

Nestler, J. E., N. A. Beer, D. J. Jakubowicz, C. Colombo, and R. M. Beer.

"Effects of insulin reduction with benfluorex on serum dehydroepiandrosterone (DHEA), DHEA sulfate, and blood pressure in hypertensive middle-aged and elderly men." *J Clin Endocrinol Metab* 80: 700–706 (1995)

Oaknin-Bendahan, S., Y. Anis, and N. Zisapel. "Effects of long-term administration of melatonin and putative antagonist on the aging rat." *Neuro Report* 6: 785–788 (1995)

Orlock, C. *Know Your Body Clock.* Citadel Press, New York, NY (1993)

Orentreich, N., J. L. Brind, R. L. Rizer, and J. H. Vogelman. "Age changes and sex differences in serum dehydroepiandrosterone sulfate concentration throughout adulthood." *J Clin Endocrin and Metab* 59: 551–555 (1984)

Ozasa, H., M. Kitz, T. Inove, and T. Mori. "Plasma dehydroepiandrosterone to cortisol ratios as an indicator of stress to gynecologic patients." *Gynecol Oncol* 37: 178–182 (1990)

Pierpaoli, W., A. Dall'Ara, E. Pedrinis, and W. Regelson. "The pineal control of aging: The effects of melatonin and pineal grafting on the survival of older mice." *Ann NY Acad Sci* 621: 291–313 (1991)

Pierpaoli, W., and W. Regelson. "Pineal control of aging: Effect of melatonin and pineal grafting on aging mice." *Proc Natl Acad Sci USA* 94: 787–791 (1994)

Pierpaoli, W., and W. Regelson. *The Melatonin Miracle.* Simon & Schuster, New York, NY (1995)

Poeggeler, B., R. J. Reiter, D. X. Tan, L. D. Chen, and L. C. Manchester. "Melatonin, hydroxyl radical-mediated oxidative damage and aging: A hypothesis." *J Pineal Res* 14: 151–168 (1993)

Prickett, J. D., D. R. Robinson, and A. D. Steinberg. "Dietary enrichment with polyunsaturated acid eicosapentaenoic acid prevents proteinuria and prolongs survival in NZBxNZW F1 mice." *J Clin Invest* 68: 556–559 (1981)

Regelson, W., and M. Kalimi. "Dehydroepiandrosterone—the multifunctional steroid." *Ann NY Acad Sci* 719: 564–575 (1994)

Regelson, W., and C. Colman. *The Super-Hormone Promise.* Simon & Schuster, New York, NY (1996)

Reiter, R. J., D. X. Tan, B. Poeggler, A. Menendez-Pelaez, L. D. Chen, and S. Saarela. "Melatonin as a free radical scavenger: Implications for aging and age-related diseases." *Ann NY Acad Sci* 719: 1–12 (1994)

Reiter, R. J., D. Melchoiorrie, F. Sewerynak, B. Poeggeler, L. Barlow-Walden, J. Chuang, G. G. Ortiz, and D. Acuna-Castroviejo. "A review of the evidence supporting melatonin's role as an anti-oxidant." *J Pineal Res* 18: 1–11 (1995)

Reiter, R. J., and J. Robinson. *Melatonin.* Bantam Books, New York, NY (1995)

Sewerynek, E., D. Melchiorri, G. G. Ortiz, B. Poeggeler, and R. J. Reiter. "Melatonin reduces H_2O_2-induced lipid peroxidation in honogenates of different rat brain regions." *J Pineal Res* 19: 51–56 (1995)

Stokkan, K-A., R. J. Reiter, and M. K. Vaughan. "Food restriction retards aging of the pineal gland." *Brain Res* 545: 66–72 (1991)

Touitou, Y., A. Bogdan, and A. Auzeby. "Activity of melatonin and other pineal indoles on the in vitro synthesis of cortisol, cortisone, and adrenal androgens." *J Pineal Res* 6: 341–350 (1989)

Vacas, M. I., M. M. Del Zar, M. Martinuzzo, C. Falcon, L. O. Carreras, and D. P. Cardinali. "Inhibition of human platelet aggregation and thromboxane B_2 production by melatonin." *J Pineal Res* 11: 135–139 (1991)

Walker, R. F., K. M. McMahon, and E. B. Pivorun. "Pineal gland structure and respiration as affected by age and hypocaloric diet." *Exp Gerontology* 13: 91–99 (1978)

Wolf, O. T., O. Neumann, D. H. Hellhammer, A. C.. Geiben, C. J. Strasburger, R. A. Dressendorder, K-M. Pirke, and C. Kirschbaum. "Effects of two-week physiological dehydroepiandrosterone substitution on cognitive performance and well-being in healthy elderly women and men." *J Clin Endocrinology and Metabolism* 82: 2363–2367 (1997)

Chapter 25—NITRIC OXIDE: THE NEW KID ON THE BLOCK

Best, J. M., P. B. Berger, V. M. Miller, and A. Lerman. "The effect of estrogen replacement therapy on plasma nitric oxide and endothelin-1 levels in post-menopausal women." *Ann Int Med* 128: 285–268 (1998)

Dawon, T. M., and V. L. Dawson. "Nitric oxide: Actions and pathological roles." *The Neuroscientist* 1: 920 (1994)

Drexler, H., A. M. Zeller, K. Meinzer, and H. Just. "Correction of endothelial dysfunction in coronary microcirculation of hypercholesterolaemic patients by L-arginine." *Lancet* 338: 1546–1550 (1991)

Furchgott, R. F. and J. V. Zawadzi. "The obligatory role of endothelial cells in the relaxation of arterial smooth muscle by aceylcholine." *Nature* 288: 373–376 (1980)

Ignarro, L. J., G. M. Buga, K. S. Wood, R. E. Byrns, and G. Chaudhuri. "Endo-thelium-derived relaxing factor produced and released from artery and vein is nitric oxide." *Proc Nat Acad Sci USA* 84: 9265–9269 (1987)

Landino, L. M., B. C. Crews, M. D. Timmons, J. D. Morrow, and L. J. Marnett. "Peroxynitrite: The coupling product of nitric oxide and superoxide, activates prostaglandin synthesis." *Proc Natl Acad Sci USA* 93: 15069–15074 (1996)

Moncada, S., R. M. J. Palmer, and E. A. Higgs. "Nitric oxide: Physiology, pathophysiology, and pharmacology." *Pharmacological Reviews* 43: 109–142 (1991)

Murad, F., C. K. Mittal, W. P. Arnold, S. Katsuki, and H. Kimura. "Guanylate cyclase: Activation by azide, nitro compounds, nitric oxide, and hydroxyl radical are inhibited by hemoglobin and myoglobin." *Adv Cyclic Nucleotide Res* 9: 145–158 (1978)

Lancaster, J., ed., *Nitric Oxide.* Academic Press, New York, NY (1996)

Palmer, R. M. J., D. S. Ashton, and S. Moncada. "Vascular endothelial cells synthesize nitric oxide from L-arginine." *Nature* 333: 664–666 (1988)

Polderman, K. H., C. D. A. Stehouwer, G. J. van Kamp, and L. J. G. Gooren. "Effects of insulin infusion on endothelium-derived vasoactive substances." *Diabetologia* 39: 1284–1292 (1996)

Salvermini, D., T. P. Misko, J. L. Masferret, K. Siebert, M. G. Currie, and P. Needleman. "Nitric oxide activates cyclooxygenase enzymes." *Proc Natl Acad Sci USA* 90: 7240–7244 (1993)

Swierkosz, T. A., J. A. Mitchell, T. D. Warner, R. M. Botting, and J. R. Vane. "Co-induction of nitric oxide synthase and cyclooxygenase interactions between nitric oxide and prostanoids." *Br J Pharmacol* 114: 1335–1342 (1995)

Tousoulis, D., G. Davies, C. Tentolouria, T. Crake, and P. Poutouzas. "Coronary stenosis dilation induced by L-arginine." *Lancet* 349: 1812–1813 (1997)

Chapter 26—ANTI-AGING SUPPLEMENTS: BEYOND THE ANTI-AGING ZONE LIFESTYLE PYRAMID

Alpha Tocopherol, Beta Carotene, Cancer Prevention Study Group. "The effect of vitamin E and beta carotene on incidences of lung cancer and other cancers in male smokers." *N Eng J Med* 330: 1029–1035 (1994)

Arsenian, M. A. "Magnesium and cardiovascular disease." *Prog in Cardiovascular Diseases* 35: 271–310 (1993)

Ascherio, A., C. H. Hennekens, and W. C. Willett. "Trans-fatty acid intake and risk of myocardial infarction." *Circulation* 89: 94–101 (1994)

Baggio, E., R. Gandini, A. C. Plancher, M. Passeri, and G. Camosino. "Italian multicenter study on the safety and efficacy of coenzyme Q10 as adjunctive therapy in heart failure." *Molec Aspects Med* 15: S287–S294 (1994)

Block, G., B. Patterson, and A. Safar. "Fruit, vegetables and cancer prevention." *Nutr Cancer* 18: 1–29 (1992)

Blaylock, R. L., *Excitotoxins.* Health Press, Santa Fe, NM (1994)

Blot, W. J., J. Y. Li, P. R. Taylor, W. Gauo, S. M. Damsey, G. Q. Wang, C. S. Yang, S. F. Zheng, M. Gail, and G. Y. Li. "Nutritional intervention trials in Linxion, China." *J Nat Cancer Res* 85: 1483–1492 (1993)

Colditz, G. A., L. G. Branch, R. J. Lipnick, W. C. Willett, B. Rosener, B. M. Posner, and C. H. Hennekens. "Increased green and leafy vegetable intake and lowered cancer deaths in an elderly population." *Am J Clin Nutr* 41: 32–36 (1985)

Hill, E. G., S. B. Johnson, L. D. Lawson, M. M. Mahfouz, and R. T. Holman. "Perturbation of the metabolism of essential fatty acids by dietary partially hydrogenated vegetable oil." *Proc Nat Acad Sci USA* 79: 953–957 (1982)

Lindheim, S. R., S. C. Presser, E. C. Ditkoff, M. A. Vijod, F. Z. Stanczyk, and R. A. Lobo. "A possible bimodal effect of estrogen on insulin sensitivity in postmenopausal women and the attenuating effect of added progestin." *Fertil Steril* 60: 664–667 (1993)

Maurer, K., R. Ihl, T. Dierks, and L. Frolich. "Clinical efficacy of gingko biloba special extract EGb 761 in dementia of Alzheimer type." *J Psychiatric Res* 31: 645–655 (1997)

Mohr, A., V. W. Bowry, and R. Stocker. "Dietary supplementation with coenzyme Q10 results in increased levels of ubiquininol-10 within circulating lipoproteins and increased resistance of human low-density lipoproteins to the initiation of lipd peroxidation." *Biochem Biophys Acta* 1126: 247–254 (1992)

Murray, M. T. *Encyclopedia of Nutritional Supplements.* Prima Publishing, Rocklin, CA (1996)

PEPI Trial. "Effects of estrogen or estrogen/progestin regimens on heart disease risk factors in postmenopausal women." *JAMA* 273: 199–208 (1995)

Polyp Prevention Group. "A clinical trial of antioxidant vitamins to prevent colorectal ademona." *N Engl J Med* 331: 141–147 (1994)

Rimm, E. B., M. J. Stampfer, A. Acherio, E. Giovannucci, G. A. Colditz, and W. C. Willett. "Vitamin E consumption and risk of coronary heart disease in men." *N Eng J Med* 328: 1450–1456 (1993)

Roberts, H. J. *Aspartame: Is it Safe?* Charles Press, Philadelphia, PA (1990)

Stampfer, M. J., C. H. Hennekens, J. E. Mason, G. A. Colditz, B. Rosner, and W. C. Willett. "Vitamin E consumption and risk of coronary disease in women." *N Eng J Med* 32: 1444–1449 (1993)

Sears, B. *Zone Perfect Meals in Minutes.* ReganBooks, New York, NY (1997)

Shekelle, R. B., M. Lepper, and S. Liu. "Dietary vitamin A and risk of cancer in the Western Electric Study." *Lancet* ii: 1185–1190 (1981)

Steinmetz, K. A., and J. C. Potter. "Vegetables, fruit and cancer." *Cancer Causes Control* 325: 325–357 (1991)

Willett, W. C., M. J. Stampfer, G. A. Colditz, F. E. Speizer, B. A. Rosner, L. A. Sampson, and C. H. Hennekens. "Intake of trans fatty acids and risk of coronary heart disease among women." *Lancet* 341: 581–585 (1993)

Yamshita, S., and S. Melmed. "Effects of insulin on rat anterior pituitary cells: Inhibition of growth hormone secretion and mRNA levels." *Diabets* 35: 440–447 (1986)

Ziegler, R. G., A. F. Subar, D. E. Craft, G. Ursin, B. H. Patterson, and B. T. Graubard. "Does beta carotene explain why reduced cancer risk is associated with vegetable and fruit intake?" *Cancer Res* 52: 2060s–2066s (1992)

Chapter 27—THE SKIN ZONE: BEAUTY IS SKIN DEEP

Abraham, W., and D. T. Downing. "Preparation of model membranes for skin permeability studies using stratum corneum lipids." *J Invest Dermatol* 93: 809–813 (1989)

Bittiner, B. S., I. Cartwright, W. F. G. Tucker, and S. S. Bleehen. "A double-blind, randomized, placebo-controlled trial of fish oil in psoriasis." *Lancet* i: 378–380 (1988)

Blumenkrantz, N., and J. Sondergaard. "Effect of prostaglandin E_1 and $F_{1\alpha}$ on biosynthesis of collagen." *Nature* 239: 246–247 (1972)

Burr, G. O., and Burr, M. M. "A new deficiency disease produced by the rigid exclusion of fat from the diet." *J Biol Chem* 82: 345–367 (1929)

———. "On the nature of fatty acids essential in nutrition." *J Biol Chem* 85: 587–621 (1930)

Fauler, J., C. Neumann, D. Tsikas, and J. Frolich. "Enhanced synthesis of cysteinyl leukotrienes in psoriasis." *J INvest Dermatol* 99: 8–11 (1992)

Furstenberger, G., H. Richter, N. E. Fusenia, and F. Marks. "Arachidonic acid and prostaglandin E2 release and enhanced cell proliferation induced by phrobel ester TPA in a murine epidermal cell line." *Cancer Lett* 11: 191–198 (1981)

Furstenberger, G., M. H. Gross, and F. Marks. "Involvement of prostaglandins in the process of skin tumor promotion," in H. Thaler-Dao, A. Crastes de Paulet, and R. Paoletti, eds., *Icosanoids and Cancer,* Raven Press, Boca Raton, FL (1984)

Koosis, V., and J. Sondergaard. "PGE_1 in normal skin: Methodological evaluation, topographical distribution and data related to sex and age." *Arch Dermatol Res* 275: 9–13 (1983)

Ruzicka, T., ed. *Eicosanoids and the Skin.* CRC Press, Boca Raton, FL (1990)

Wertz, P. W., W. Abraham, L. Landmann, and D. T. Downing. "Preparation of liposomes from stratum corneum lipids." *J Invest Dermatol* 87: 582–584 (1986)

Ziboh, V. A., K. A. Cohen, C. M. Ellis, C. Miller, R. A. Hamilton, K. Kragballe, C. R. Hydrich, and J. J. Voorhees. "Effects of dietary supplemenation of fish oil on neutrophil and epidermal fatty acids." *Arch Dermatol* 122: 1277–1282 (1986)

Ziboh, V. A., and C. A. Miller. "Essential fatty acids and polyunsaturated fatty acids: Significance in ceutaneous biology." *Ann Rev Nutr* 10: 433–450 (1990)

Chapter 28—EMOTIONS: THE MIND-BODY-DIET CONNECTION

Benson, H. *The Relaxation Response.* William Morrow, New York, NY (1975)

———. *Timeless Healing.* Schribners, New York, NY (1996)

Carrington, P. *The Book of Meditation.* Element Books, Boston, MA (1998)

Cousins, N. *Anatomy of an Illness.* Bantam Books, New York, NY (1983)

Khalsa, D. S. *Brain Longevity.* Warner Books, New York, NY (1997)

Norman, A. W., and G. Litwack. *Hormones,* 2nd ed., Academic Press, New York, NY (1997)

Pert, C. *Molecules of Emotion.* Schribners, New York, NY (1997)

Pert, C., S. H. Snyder, "Opiate receptor: demonstration in nervous tissue." *Science* 179: 1011–1014 (1973)

INDEX